1991
YEAR BOOK OF
NEONATAL AND
PERINATAL
MEDICINE

The 1991 Year Book® Series

Year Book of Anesthesia®: Drs. Miller, Kirby, Ostheimer, Roizen, and Stoelting

Year Book of Cardiology®: Drs. Schlant, Collins, Engle, Frye, Kaplan, and O'Rourke

Year Book of Critical Care Medicine®: Drs. Rogers and Parrillo

Year Book of Dentistry®: Drs. Meskin, Currier, Kennedy, Leinfelder, Matukas, and Rovin

Year Book of Dermatology®: Drs. Sober and Fitzpatrick

Year Book of Diagnostic Radiology®: Drs. Hendee, Keats, Kirkpatrick, Miller, Osborn, Reed, and Thompson

Year Book of Digestive Diseases®: Drs. Greenberger and Moody

Year Book of Drug Therapy®: Drs. Lasagna and Weintraub

Year Book of Emergency Medicine®: Drs. Wagner, Burdick, Davidson, Roberts, and Spivey

Year Book of Endocrinology®: Drs. Bagdade, Braverman, Halter, Horton, Kannan, Molitch, Morley, Odell, Rogol, Ryan, and Sherwin

Year Book of Family Practice®: Drs. Berg, Bowman, Dietrich, Green, and Scherger

Year Book of Geriatrics and Gerontology®: Drs. Beck, Abrass, Burton, Cummings, Makinodan, and Small

Year Book of Hand Surgery®: Drs. Dobyns, Chase, and Amadio

Year Book of Health Care Management: Drs. Heyssel, King, and Steinberg, Ms. Avakian, and Messrs. Berman, Brock, Kues, and Rosenberg

Year Book of Hematology®: Drs. Spivak, Bell, Ness, Quesenberry, and Wiernik

Year Book of Infectious Diseases®: Drs. Wolff, Barza, Keusch, Klempner, and Snydman

Year Book of Infertility: Drs. Mishell, Paulsen, and Lobo

Year Book of Medicine®: Drs. Rogers, Des Prez, Cline, Braunwald, Greenberger, Utiger, Epstein, and Malawista

Year Book of Neonatal and Perinatal Medicine: Drs. Klaus and Fanaroff

Year Book of Neurology and Neurosurgery®: Drs. Currier and Crowell

Year Book of Nuclear Medicine®: Drs. Hoffer, Gore, Gottschalk, Sostman, Zaret, and Zubal

Year Book of Obstetrics and Gynecology®: Drs. Mishell, Kirschbaum, and Morrow

Year Book of Occupational and Environmental Medicine: Drs. Emmett, Brooks, Harris, and Schenker

Year Book of Oncology: Drs. Young, Longo, Ozols, Simone, Steele, and Weichselbaum

Year Book of Ophthalmology®: Drs. Laibson, Adams, Augsburger, Benson, Cohen, Eagle, Flanagan, Nelson, Reinecke, Sergott, and Wilson

Year Book of Orthopedics®: Drs. Sledge, Poss, Cofield, Frymoyer, Griffin, Hansen, Johnson, Springfield, and Weiland

Year Book of Otolaryngology–Head and Neck Surgery®: Drs. Bailey and Paparella

Year Book of Pathology and Clinical Pathology®: Drs. Brinkhous, Dalldorf, Langdell, and McLendon

Year Book of Pediatrics®: Drs. Oski and Stockman

Year Book of Plastic, Reconstructive, and Aesthetic Surgery: Drs. Miller, Cohen, McKinney, Robson, Ruberg, and Whitaker

Year Book of Podiatric Medicine and Surgery®: Dr. Kominsky

Year Book of Psychiatry and Applied Mental Health®: Drs. Talbott, Frances, Freedman, Meltzer, Perry, Schowalter, and Yudofsky

Year Book of Pulmonary Disease®: Drs. Green, Loughlin, Michael, Mulshine, Peters, Terry, Tockman, and Wise

Year Book of Speech, Language, and Hearing: Drs. Bernthal, Hall, and Tomblin

Year Book of Sports Medicine®: Drs. Shephard, Eichner, Sutton, and Torg, Col. Anderson, and Mr. George

Year Book of Surgery®: Drs. Schwartz, Jonasson, Robson, Shires, Spencer, and Thompson

Year Book of Ultrasound: Drs. Merritt, Mittelstaedt, Carroll, and Nyberg

Year Book of Urology®: Drs. Gillenwater and Howards

Year Book of Vascular Surgery®: Drs. Bergan and Yao

Roundsmanship '91–'92: A Year Book® Guide to Clinical Medicine: Drs. Dan, Feigin, Quilligan, Schrock, Stein, and Talbott

1991
The Year Book of
NEONATAL AND
PERINATAL
MEDICINE

Editors
Marshall H. Klaus, M.D.
Director of Academic Affairs, Children's Hospital Oakland, California;
Adjunct Professor of Pediatrics, University of California, San Francisco
Avroy A. Fanaroff, M.B.B.Ch. (Rand), F.R.C.P.E.
Professor and Vice Chairman, Department of Pediatrics, Case Western
Reserve University; Director, Division of Neonatology, Rainbow Babies
and Childrens Hospital, Cleveland, Ohio

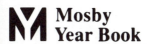

Mosby
Year Book

St. Louis   Baltimore   Boston   Chicago   London   Philadelphia   Sydney   Toronto

Editor-in-Chief, Year Book Publishing: Nancy Gorham
Sponsoring Editor: Nancy G. Puckett
Manager, Medical Information Services: Edith M. Podrazik
Senior Medical Information Specialist: Terri Strorigl
Senior Medical Writer: David A. Cramer, M.D.
Assistant Director, Manuscript Services: Frances M. Perveiler
Associate Managing Editor, Year Book Editing Services: Elizabeth Fitch
Production Coordinator: Max F. Perez
Proofroom Manager: Barbara M. Kelly

Mosby–Year Book, Inc.
11830 Westline Industrial Drive
St. Louis, MO 63146

Editorial Office:
Mosby-Year Book, Inc.
200 North LaSalle St.
Chicago, IL 60601

International Standard Serial Number: 8756-5005
International Standard Book Number: 0-8151-5138-1

Table of Contents

The material in this volume represents literature reviewed up to November 1990.

Journals Represented

Mosby–Year Book subscribes to and surveys nearly 850 U.S. and foreign medical and allied health journals. From these journals, the Editors select the articles to be abstracted. Journals represented in this YEAR BOOK are listed below.

American Heart Journal
American Journal of Cardiology
American Journal of Diseases of Children
American Journal of Epidemiology
American Journal of Human Genetics
American Journal of Obstetrics and Gynecology
American Journal of Perinatology
American Journal of Physiology
American Journal of Public Health
American Journal of Roentgenology
Anesthesiology
Annals of Neurology
Archives of Disease in Childhood
Biology of the Neonate
British Journal of Obstetrics and Gynaecology
British Journal of Plastic Surgery
British Journal of Psychiatry
British Journal of Urology
British Medical Journal
Chest
Child Development
Developmental Medicine and Child Neurology
Diagnostic Microbiology and Infectious Disease
Early Human Development
International Journal of Epidemiology
Israel Journal of Medical Sciences
Journal of Applied Physiology
Journal of Child Neurology
Journal of Clinical Endocrinology and Metabolism
Journal of Clinical Ultrasound
Journal of Developmental and Behavioral Pediatrics
Journal of Family Practice
Journal of Infectious Diseases
Journal of Neurology
Journal of Obstetrics and Gynaecology
Journal of Pediatric Surgery
Journal of Pediatrics
Journal of Perinatology
Journal of Thoracic and Cardiovascular Surgery
Journal of Ultrasound in Medicine
Journal of the American College of Cardiology
Journal of the American Medical Association
Lancet
Laryngoscope
Nature
Neurology
Neuropediatrics
New England Journal of Medicine

Obstetrics and Gynecology
Paediatric and Perinatal Epidemiology
Pain
Pediatric Infectious Disease Journal
Pediatric Research
Pediatrics
Plastic and Reconstructive Surgery
Prenatal Diagnosis
Psychoneuroendocrinology
Radiology
S.A.M.J./S.A.M.T.–South African Medical Journal
Science
Surgical Neurology
Thrombosis and Haemostatis

STANDARD ABBREVIATIONS

The following terms are abbreviated in this edition: acquired immunodeficiency syndrome (AIDS), central nervous system (CNS), cerebrospinal fluid (CSF), computed tomography (CT), electrocardiography (ECG), and human immunodeficiency virus (HIV).

Introduction

Penning this introduction heralds the completion of the fifth edition of the YEARBOOK OF NEONATAL AND PERINATAL MEDICINE. It signifies that the exhaustive review of the perinatal literature has been concluded, the articles selected, and the commentaries written. It remains for you, the reader, to render the verdict on the completed product.

As always the material available for review has been extensive and fascinating. The frontiers of neonatal and perinatal medicine have been expanded and manipulation of the fetus has reached new heights. Major surgical procedures, such as correction of diaphragmatic hernia, have now been successfully undertaken on the fetus and are now under evaluation. Perhaps more fascinating is the concept of reconstituting the bone marrow with stem cells from cord blood and the emerging role of cytokines in the pathogenesis of disease. The ability to control these cytokines will prevent many disorders and even open new avenues for therapy.

Old disorders such as congenital syphilis have reemerged and, together with the cocaine epidemic and HIV infections, tax the public health systems to their limits and even beyond. It was inspiring and at the same time very nostalgic to include the long-term follow-up by Northway of his original cohorts of infants with bronchopulmonary dysplasia (BPD). We are a little wiser concerning this disorder but, despite surfactant, steroids, and all forms of ventilators, BPD is still very prevalent.

We are grateful to Dr. Henry Halliday for writing the opening commentary and review on surfactant therapy, still very much a topic of interest in neonatal-perinatal medicine. We have once again called on many of our colleagues and friends to offer their opinions and words of wisdom regarding some of the articles selected. They have graciously given of their time and their thoughtful contributions add considerably to the quality of the book. The staff at Mosby–Year Book has once again provided superb assistance facilitating timely completion of the project. We acknowledge not only Carla White and Nancy Gorham from the Editorial staff also the great folks, literally behind the scenes, who find all the interesting articles from even the most obscure journals. We continue to have fun working on the YEAR BOOK, and hope that the readers will continue to enjoy our efforts.

Avroy A. Fanaroff, M.B.B.Ch.
Marshall H. Klaus, M.D.

Surfacant Replacement

HENRY L. HALLIDAY, M.D., F.R.C.P.
Consultant Neonatologist and Honorary Lecturer,
Neonatal Intensive Care Unit, Royal Maternity Hospital;
Dept. of Child Health, The Queen's University of Belfast, Northern Ireland

I take it as a great compliment to be asked to write on this topic, and to follow such a great researcher and clinician as Dr. Don Shapiro who so tragically died on October 15th, 1989.

In 1990 four further randomized controlled trials (RCTs) of surfactant replacement were reported (1–4). There are now at least 32 RCTs that can be used in a meta-analysis to assess the effects of surfactants in prevention and treatment of respiratory distress syndrome (RDS) (5) (Table 1). An odds ratio (OR) of less than 1 suggests that treatment is superior to control and vice versa. If the 95% confidence intervals (CI) are also less than 1 then the difference between treated and control babies is statistically significant.

TABLE 1.—Typical Odds Ratios and 95% Confidence Invervals (CI) for the Effects of Surfactants in Prophylaxis and Treatment Trials

	N	Odds Ratio	95% CI	N	Odds Ratio	95% CI
Prophylaxis		Natural Surfactant			Synthetic Surfactant	
Neonatal death	9	0.55	0.38–0.80	7	0.65	0.50–0.86
PTX	9	0.31	0.22–0.44	3	0.62	0.40–0.96
IVH	7	0.90	0.62–1.30	2	0.87	0.60–1.27
PDA	8	1.17	0.88–1.57	4	1.33	1.01–1.75
BPD	6	0.59	0.40–0.86	6	0.99	0.75–1.31
Death or BPD	6	0.43	0.30–0.63	3	0.84	0.64–1.09
Treatment		Natural Surfactant			Synthetic Surfactant	
Neonatal Death	13	0.60	0.47–0.76	5	0.61	0.46–0.80
PTX	12	0.34	0.26–0.43	4	0.52	0.42–0.65
IVH	9	0.93	0.68–1.27	2	0.83	0.65–1.05
PDA	10	1.14	0.85–1.53	3	0.72	0.60–0.87
BPD	8	0.94	0.64–1.39	4	0.71	0.50–1.00
Death or BPD	9	0.61	0.45–0.84	3	0.56	0.45–0.72

N = number of trials; *PTX* = pneumothorax; *IVH* = intraventricular hemorrhage; *PDA* = patent ductus arteriosus; BPD = bronchopulmonary dysplasia.
Data obtained from the Perinatal Clinical Trials Database, Oxford (5).

For neonatal death the ORs for both prophylaxis and treatment with both natural and synthetic surfactants are about 0.60 with 95% CI all less than 1. This means that surfactant replacement reduces the odds of death by about 40%. Similar or greater significant reductions are also found for pneumothorax and other pulmonary air leaks, but for intraventricular hemorrhage and bronchopulmonary dysplasia (BPD), although the ORs are less than 1, the 95% CI generally cross unity, showing that these reductions are not significant. For patent ductus arteriosus (PDA) the ORs are generally greater than 1, suggesting an increase in this complication that is significant for prophylaxis with synthetic surfactants (see Table 1). A number of questions remain to be resolved.

Synthetic or Natural Surfactants?

Although a number of surfactants have now been licensed for use in Japan, the United States, and Europe (Table 2) there have been no comparative trials of synthetic or natural preparations. In April 1991 a multicenter trial comparing Survanta and Exosurf is scheduled to begin in the United States (Lucey JF, personal communication) and other comparative trials are being planned in Europe.

Prophylaxis or Treatment?

At the recent Ross Laboratories Special Conference on "Hot Topics in Neonatology 1990" in Washington four trials comparing very early or prophylactic administration of natural surfactants with late administration (or rescue) were reported (6–9). These trials showed conflicting results that the moderator, Dr. Mary Ellen Avery, scored at 2 for prophylaxis and 2 for treatment. The trials of Konishi et al. (6) and Merritt et al. (7) enrolled only babies with immature lung profiles, the former favoring prophylaxis and the latter treatment. In the larger study there was an increase in moderate or severe developmental delay in the babies treated prophylactically (7). In two trials of calf lung surfactant extract (CLSE), both with considerable numbers of babies, one showed improved survival with prophylaxis (8) and the other showed an increased incidence of BPD and longer hospital stay in the babies treated at birth (9). I think it is fair to say that the jury is still out on this one.

Without lung maturity tests about half of babies less than 31 weeks given surfactant prophylactically will be treated unnecessarily. The United Kingdom trial of Exosurf (OSIRIS) is recruiting 6,000 babies and will compare early and late treatment. We eagerly await the results of this trial, which should be completed by April 1991.

Single or Multiple Doses?

In 1990 two studies of natural surfactants that attempted to answer this question were completed (10, 11). In the study by Dunn et al. (10) using CLSE only relatively mature (30–36 weeks) preterm babies with RDS were enrolled. Improved oxygenation in the babies given multiple doses of surfactant was demonstrated but duration of ventilation was not

TABLE 2.—Surfactant Preparations in Clinical Use

Brand Name (Common Name) Company	Composition	Dose of Phospholipids (mg/kg)	No of Doses	P or T	Approved
Synthetic					
Pumactant (ALEC) Britannica	DPPC: PG 7:3 w/w Phospholipid 50 mg/ml	100	4	P	UK (NPB)
Exosurf (Colfosceril Palmitate Wellcome Foundation	DPPC 13.5 mg/ml Hexadecanol 1.5 mg/ml Tyloxapol 1.0 mg/ml	67.5	2–4	P,T T	USA UK
Natural					
Survanta (Beractant) Abbott	Bovine Mince with Tripalmitin, Palmitic acid	100	3	P,T	USA (TIND) Germany
Surfactant TA	"	100	3	P,T	Japan
Alveofact (SF-RI 1) Boehringer–Thomae	Bovine Lavage Phospholipid 41.7 mg/ml	50	4	T	Germany Holland
Curosurf Chiesi	Porcine Mince Phospholipid 80 mg/ml	200	3	T	Trials
Human Surfactant	Amniotic Fluid 5% protein Phospholipid 20 mg/ml	60	3–4	P,T	Trials
CLSE e.g. Infasurf	Calf lung lavage	100	3	P,T	Trials

P = prophylaxis; T = treatment; CLSE = calf lung surfactant extract; ALEC = artificial lung expanding compound; NPB = named patient basis; TIND = treatment investigational new drug (special FDA protocol); DPPC = dipalmitoylphosphatidylcholine; PG = phosphatidylglycerol.

decreased. Speer et al. (11) studied 357 babies who were both immature (700–2000 g) and had severe RDS (needing at least 60% oxygen) and found that babies given multiple doses of Curosurf had a significantly lower rate of pneumothorax and mortality.

These studies support the recommendations of multiple doses for treatment with human surfactant, Survanta, Exosurf, and ALEC (Pumactant).

What Dose Is Needed?

The dosage of surfactant used in clinical trials over the past 10 years has varied from 25 to 200 mg of phospholipids per kilogram body weight (5). Two recent trials have compared different doses of surfactant (12, 13). Konishi et al. (12) showed that treatment of established RDS with 120 mg/kg of Surfactant TA improved oxygenation and reduced the incidence of BPD compared to 60 mg/kg. Gortner et al. in an interim analysis (13) of their trial comparing 100 mg/kg and 50 mg/kg of a bovine surfactant (SF-RI 1) showed improved oxygenation with the higher dose. Using Curosurf in a pilot trial of 32 babies we have also found improved oxygenation but no difference in 28-day outcome for babies treated with 200 mg/kg compared to 100 mg/kg (Halliday and Speer, unpublished results). A large European multicenter trial is under way to compare high and low initial doses with repeated doses if needed (Curosurf 4). This trial will recruit 2,000 babies and be completed by the end of 1991.

Larger doses are probably better than smaller ones but how much is optimal? Certainly more than the 5 mg/kg estimated to form the air/liquid interface in the lung and perhaps as much as the 100 to 250 mg/kg estimated to form the total pulmonary surfactant pool (14).

How Should It Be Administered?

All surfactants are administered intratracheally through an endotracheal tube in one or more boluses. With most natural surfactants two bolus doses are used with the infant positioned so that each dependent lung receives surfactant. After instillation the baby is either manually ventilated for a short time or reconnected to the ventilator. A feeding tube is used to deliver the surfactant into the lower trachea. With Exosurf an endotracheal adaptor that has a side port is used. The surfactant is administered slowly so that it does not accumulate in the endotracheal tube, with a minimum recommended time for administration of the full dose of 4 minutes.

In one small study, Curosurf was administered by a slow infusion over 5 to 10 minutes through a fine polyethylene catheter positioned in the lower trachea (Nars and Rudin, unpublished results). The acute improvement in oxygenation was less marked and sustained for only 5 to 6 hours in these 11 babies, compared to those treated by a divided bolus dose.

In a study in Kuwait, in a neonatal unit with no facilities for assisted ventilation, 14 babies weighing more than 1,500 g with severe RDS were intubated only for the administration of the bovine form of Curosurf (15). Twelve babies showed the expected acute responses and 1 of the 2 nonresponding babies was subsequently found to have streptococcal pneumonia. Thirteen babies survived without sequelae.

More studies of methods of adminstration are obviously needed, particularly since acute responses seem to vary with the duration of instillation. Studies comparing the incidence of potentially adverse hemodynamic effects in rapid and slow instillation procedures should be performed.

What About Adverse Effects?

Adverse effects have been reported relatively infrequently. The incidence of PDA is higher with both natural and synthetic surfactants (see Table 1). It has been suggested by Fujiwara (3) that the development of PDA accounts for most relapses after surfactant treatment. The judicious use of Doppler ultrasound and intravenous indomethacin means that in most cases this complication has minimal effects. However, it has been reported that, in babies of less than 27 weeks gestation who develop PDA, pulmonary hemorrhage can occur. This complication has been reported with Exosurf and also with some of the natural surfactants.

Patent ductus arteriosus has also been suggested as a cause of hemodynamic instability, particularly after instillation of natural surfactants in treatment studies. These hemodynamic effects are variable, with some reports suggesting no change in blood pressure and cerebral blood flow velocities (16, 17) and some suggesting reduction of these measurements (18, 19). The babies showing altered cerebral blood flow velocities generally have suffered from severe asphyxia (18) and may not be typical of those usually treated with surfactant. Asphyxia has been shown to lessen the acute response to surfactant (20).

Using near infrared spectroscopy (NIRS) it has been shown that cerebral oxygenation improves after surfactant treatment (19, 21), but this may be associated with transient depression of cerebral electrical activity (19). This also occurs if babies on ventilators are exposed to repeated suctioning or develop a pneumothorax, but there is no evidence that this short suppression of electroencephalogram activity has any adverse effects on the baby (19).

It has been speculated that the rapid improvement of pulmonary mechanics after giving surfactant may in some infants cause overdistension of the lungs with hyperinflation and perhaps hypocarbia (19, 21). It is also possible that circulatory changes with PDA may also have an influence. Further studies of the timing, dose, mode of administration, and ventilator management after surfactant are urgently needed.

One study has looked specifically for evidence of cerebral ischemia after surfactant administration (22). The authors serially measured creatine kinase isoenzyme (CK-BB) levels and antibodies to brain antigens and performed cerebral ultrasound and could find no evidence of any adverse effect of Curosurf on cerebral function in preterm babies (22). In addition, follow-up studies of babies treated with surfactant are now being reported that give no cause for concern despite increased survival of immature babies (23).

Follow-Up Studies?

There have been ten reported studies of long-term outcome of babies treated with surfactant (23); seven with natural surfactants and three with synthetic surfactants (Table 3). The rates of neurologic handicap are not increased by the use of surfactants despite the increased survival of immature babies. The apparent differences in long-term outcome between natural surfactant treated babies (about 70% normal) and syn-

TABLE 3.—Handicaps and Late Deaths in 10 Follow-Up Studies of Infants
Treated With Surfactants

NATURAL SURFACTANTS (N=7)

	Treated (N=156)	Control (N=118)	P Value (Chi square)
Late Deaths	4	4	–
Major Handicap	20 (12.8%)	16 (3.6%)	0.85
Minor Handicap	26 (16.7%)	21 (17.8%)	0.80
Normal Babies	110 (70.5%)	81 (68.6%)	0.75

SYNTHETIC SURFACTANTS (N=3)

	Treated (N=167)	Control (N=171)	P Value (Chi square)
Late Deaths	7	6	–
Major Handicap	14 (8.4%)	9 (5.3%)	0.25
Minor Handicap	11 (6.6%)	7 (4.1%)	0.30
Normal Babies	142 (85.0%)	155 (90.6%)	0.15

thetic surfactant treated babies (about 85% normal) can be accounted for by both the greater gestational age and the prophylaxis design of the latter studies. In prophylaxis trials about half of the babies entered as controls do not develop RDS and would be expected to have an improved outcome.

Costs of Surfactant?

Table 2 lists the surfactants currently being used, some in clinical trials and some available commercially. Exosurf is available in the United States at $450 per vial and in the United Kingdom at £314.29. Up to four doses are needed, so this form of therapy is not cheap. Three studies have looked at costs; Maniscalco et al. (24) showed a savings of $18,500 (U.S. dollars) per surviving baby and Shennan et al. (25) a saving of $10,000 (Canadian dollars) per survivor when CLSE was used prophylactically. In Belfast Tubman et al. (26) showed that the cost per extra survivor was £13,720, which is similar to the costs of caring for any very low birth weight baby. The quality adjusted life year (QALY) was £710, which is much less than that for hemodialysis or coronary artery by-pass surgery (26).

As surfactant replacement improves survival it may lead to increased costs of neonatal health care, but the real bonus is the increased numbers of surviving healthy babies and also decreased costs of producing a healthy baby.

Other Uses of Surfactants

Don Shapiro's group in Rochester has very recently reported acute responses and successful outcome in seven full-term babies with pneumonia and seven with meconium aspiration syndrome after treatment with CLSE (27). Multicenter controlled trials of surfactant-TA for these indications seem warranted.

Secondary surfactant deficiency has also been implicated in adult respiratory distress syndrome (ARDS). Some recent reports suggest that natural surfactant replacement may improve outcome (27, 28). More studies using both synthetic and natural surfactants are needed.

Surfactant deficiency has been found in the lungs of babies dying of sudden infant death syndrome (SIDS) but it is still not clear if lower concentrations of phosphatidylcholine are a primary or secondary phenomenon (30). It is difficult to envisage how replacement therapy could be used to reduce the incidence of SIDS.

The Future?

On the basic science front characterization of the surfactant apoproteins (31) has permitted relationships between structure and function to be further defined (32). Surfactant apoprotein B (SP-B) can now be expressed in *Escherichia coli* (33) so that genetically engineered surfactants will soon be available for clinical trials. These and other developments would surely have been much appreciated by Don Shapiro, and perhaps the greatest tribute that can be paid to him is that his research continues to be published posthumously (27, 34).

References

1. Horbar JD, Soll RF, Schachinger H, et al: A European multicenter randomized controlled trial of single dose surfactant therapy for idiopathic respiratory distress syndrome. *Eur J Pediatr* 149:416–423, 1990.
2. Soll RF, Hoekstra RE, Fangman JJ, et al: Multicenter trial of single-dose modified bovine surfactant extract (Survanta) for prevention of respiratory distress syndrome. *Pediatrics* 85:1092–1102, 1990.
3. Fujiwara T, Konishi M, Chida S, et al: Surfactant replacement therapy with a single postventilatory dose of a reconstituted bovine surfactant in preterm neonates with respiratory distress syndrome: Final analysis of a multicenter, double-blind, randomized trial and comparison with similar trials. *Pediatrics* 86:753–764, 1990.
4. Bose C, Corbet A, Bose G, et al: Improved outcome at 28 days of age for very low birth weight infants treated with a single dose of a synthetic surfactant. *J Pediatr* 117:947–953, 1990.
5. Soll RF: 1. Prophylactic administration of synthetic surfactant. 2. Prophylactic administration of natural surfactant. 3. Synthetic surfactant treatment of RDS. 4. Natural surfactant treatment of RDS, in Chalmers I (ed): *Oxford Database of Perinatal Trials*. Version 1.1, Disk Issue 3, February 1990.
6. Konishi M, Fujiwara J, Chida S, et al: A prospective, randomized trial of early versus late administration of a single dose of Surfactant-TA, in *Ross Laboratories Special Conference: Hot Topics 1990 in Neonatology*. Washington, DC, 1990, pp233–250.
7. Merritt TA, Hallman M, Berry C, et al: Results of the randomized, placebo controlled trial of human surfactant: Is prophylaxis better than rescue? in *Ross Lab-*

oratories Special Conference: Hot Topics 1990 in Neonatology. Washington, DC, 1990, pp255–260.

8. Kendig JW, Notter RH, Cox C, et al: Immediate prophylactic versus rescue administration of surfactant in very premature infants, in *Ross Laboratories Special Conference: Hot Topics 1990 in Neonatology.* Washington, DC, 1990, pp261–265.

9. Dunn MS, Shennan AT, Zayack D, et al: Bovine surfactant replacement therapy in neonates of less than 30 weeks gestation: A randomized controlled trial of prophylaxis versus treatment, in *Ross Laboratories Special Conference: Hot Topics 1990 in Neonatology.* Washington, DC, 1990, pp313–315.

10. Dunn MS, Shennan AT, Possmayer F: Single- versus multiple-dose surfactant replacement therapy in neonates of 30 to 36 weeks' gestation with respiratory distress syndrome. *Pediatrics* 86:564–571, 1990.

11. Speer CP, Curstedt T, Robertson B, et al: Randomized European multicenter trial of surfactant replacement in neonatal respiratory distress syndrome: Single versus multiple doses of Curosurf (abstract). *Pediatr Res* 28:281, 1990.

12. Konishi M, Fujiwara T, Naito T, et al: Surfactant replacement therapy in neonatal respiratory distress syndrome: A multicenter, randomized trial—comparison of high v low dose of surfactant-TA. *Eur J Pediatr* 147:20–25, 1988.

13. Gortner L, Bernsau U, Hellwege HH, et al: Surfactant treatment in very premature infants: A multicenter controlled sequential clinical trial of high-dose versus standard-dose of bovine surfactant, in *Ross Laboratories Special Conference: Hot Topics 1990 in Neonatology.* Washington, DC, 1990, pp266–273.

14. Hallman M: Recycling of surfactant: A review of human amniotic fluid as a source of surfactant for treatment of respiratory distress syndrome. *Rev Perinat Med* 6:197–226, 1989.

15. Victorin LH, Deverajan LV, Curstedt T, et al: Surfactant replacement in spontaneously breathing babies with hyaline membrane disease: A pilot study. *Biol Neonate* 58:121–126, 1990.

16. McCord B, Halliday HL, McClure G, et al: Changes in pulmonary and cerebral blood flow after surfactant treatment of severe respiratory distress syndrome, in Lachman B (ed): *Surfactant Replacement Therapy in Neonatal and Adult Respiratory Distress Syndrome.* Berlin, Springer-Verlag, 1988, pp195–200.

17. Jorch G, Rabe H, Michel E, et al: Acute and protracted effects of intratracheal surfactant application on internal carotid blood flow velocity, blood pressure and carbon dioxide tension in very low birthweight infants. *Eur J Pediatr* 148:770–773, 1989.

18. Cowan F, Silverman M, Wertheim D, et al: Changes in cerebral blood flow velocity, blood pressure and heart rate after administration of surfactant. Presented at the 5th Curosurf Workshop, Sestri Levante, 1990.

19. Svenningsen NW: Cerebral function and oxygenation in babies receiving surfactant. Presented at the International Symposium on Surfactant in Clinical Practice, Parma, Italy, June 1990.

20. Collaborative European Multicenter Study Group: Factors influencing the clinical response to surfactant replacement therapy in babies with severe respiratory distress syndrome. *Eur J Pediatr* 1991, in Press.

21. Edwards AD, Reynolds EOR: Cerebral oxygenation and haemodynamics investigated by near infrared spectroscopy: Preliminary results from infants receiving Curosurf. Presented at the 5th Curosurf Workshop, Sestri Levante, 1990.

22. Amato M, Hüppi P, Markus D, et al: Neurological function of immature babies after surfactant replacement therapy. *Neuropediatrics* 21:43, 1990.

23. Halliday HL: Follow-up studies of surfactant replacement. Presented at the International Symposium on Surfactant in Clinical Practice, Parma, Italy, June 1990.

24. Maniscalco WM, Kendig JG, Shapiro DL: Surfactant replacement therapy: Impact on hospital charges for premature infants with respiratory distress syndrome. *Pediatrics* 83:1–6, 1989.

25. Shennan A, Dunn M, Possmayer F: Cost-effectiveness of single dose surfactant

prophylaxis in infants of less than 30 weeks gestation (abstract). *Pediatr Res* 25:231, 1989.

26. Tubman TRJ, Halliday HL, Normand C: Cost of surfactant replacement treatment for severe neonatal respiratory distress syndrome: A randomised controlled trial. *Br Med J* 301:842–845, 1990.
27. Auten RL, Notter RH, Kendig JW, et al: Surfactant treatment of full-term newborns with respiratory failure. *Pediatrics* 87:101–107, 1991.
28. Nosaka S, Sakai T, Yonekura M, et al: Surfactant for adults with respiratory failure (letter). *Lancet* 336:947–948, 1990.
29. Richman PS, Spragg RG, Robertson B, et al: The adult respiratory distress syndrome: First trials with surfactant replacement. *Eur Respir J* 2(suppl 3):109–111, 1989.
30. James D, Berry PJ, Fleming P, et al: Surfactant abnormality and the sudden infant death syndrome: A primary or secondary phenomenon? *Arch Dis Child* 65:774–778, 1990.
31. Curstedt T, Johansson J, Persson P, et al: Hydrophobic surfactant-associated polypeptides: SP-C is a lipopeptide with two palmitoylated cysteine residues, whereas SP-B lacks covalently linked fatty acyl groups. *Proc Natl Acad Sci USA* 87:2985–2989, 1990.
32. Takahashi A, Waring AJ, Amirkhanian J, et al: Structure-function relationships of bovine pulmonary surfactant proteins: SP-B and SP-C. *Biochim Biophys Acta* 1044:43–49, 1990.
33. Yao L-J, Richardson C, Ford C, et al: Expression of mature pulmonary surfactant-associated protein B (SP-B) in *Escherichia coli* using truncated human SP-B cDNAs. *Biochem Cell Biol* 68:559–566, 1990.
34. Hennes HM, Lee MB, Rimm AA, et al: Surfactant replacement therapy in respiratory distress syndrome: Meta-analysis of clinical trials of single-dose surfactant extracts. *Am J Dis Child* 145:102–104, 1991.

1 The Fetus

Successful Repair In Utero of a Fetal Diaphragmatic Hernia After Removal of Herniated Viscera From the Left Thorax
Harrison MR, Adzick NS, Longaker MT, Goldberg JD, Rosen MA, Filly RA, Evans MI, Golbus MS (Univ of California, San Francisco; Wayne State Univ, Detroit)
N Engl J Med 322:1582–1584, 1990   1–1

Pulmonary hypoplasia in congenital diaphragmatic hernia is believed to be a developmental consequence of compression of the developing lung that can be reversed by removing the herniated viscera from the chest before birth. After a decade of studies documenting the natural history of untreated human fetal diaphragmatic hernia in 200 fetuses, assessing the pathophysiology and technical feasibility of repair in a primate model, and proving that hysterotomy did not endanger maternal safety, repair of a diaphragmatic hernia was attempted in 6 highly selected fetuses over 6 years. Four fetuses were doomed by technical problems; the other 2 fetuses had technically successful repair but died after birth.

Successful repair of a fetal diaphragmatic hernia was undertaken at 24 weeks' gestation. The fetus was continuously monitored by pulse oximetry, ECG, and sonography, while the herniated viscera (intestines, dilated stomach, and spleen) and part of the liver were removed from the left chest. The large diaphragmatic defect was closed with a Gore-Tex patch, and the air in the left chest cavity was replaced with warm Ringer's lactate. The abdominal cavity was enlarged with a second patch to accommodate the reduced viscera. Weekly sonography showed a reexpanded left lung. The male infant, born at 32 weeks' gestation, required ventilatory support for 4 weeks. At 8 months of age the infant was developing normally.

The majority of fetuses with diaphragmatic hernia will die despite optimal prenatal and postnatal care. Their condition is usually detected early in gestation, with a large volume of herniated viscera (particularly a dilated stomach), a large mediastinal shift, and subsequent hydramnios. Before 24 weeks' gestation the family has 3 choices: terminate the pregnancy, continue it, or opt for fetal repair. Because no management option is demonstrably superior, the family's choice should be respected. If repair is elected it is best performed before the 28th week of gestation to allow adequate growth of the lung before birth and lower the risk of inducing preterm labor. Although the feasibility of in utero repair of fetal diaphragmatic hernia has been established, further studies are warranted to define both efficacy and cost effectiveness.

▶ We have asked Richard J. Powers, M.D., a neonatologist from Children's Hospital Oakland, California, to comment on this article:

▶ The use of fetal surgery for congenital diaphragmatic hernia is an exciting but risky approach to a complex problem. One could possibly justify the risks to both mother and fetus if the outcome of this congenital defect were indeed as low as the authors cite. They report the survival rate for such babies to be only 25%, thus justifying an aggressive prenatal approach. Reviewing the outcome for babies with diaphragmatic hernia admitted to the intensive care nursery (ICN) at Children's Hospital Oakland and the population data from national and regional databases, this estimate is substantially low.

Of 32 babies with diaphragmatic hernia admitted to our ICN over a 30-month review period, 23 (72%) survived after conventional surgery. This overall rate includes babies with isolated diaphragmatic hernias, possibly eligible for fetal surgery, as well as those with diaphragmatic hernia and other anomalies who would not be eligible for fetal surgery. Since the introduction of extracorporeal membrane oxygenation (ECMO) in April 1987, 18 (75%) of 24 babies admitted with diaphragmatic hernia have survived, including 8 (73%) of the 11 babies requiring ECMO.

Confirming our findings, the National Neonatal ECMO Registry of infants receiving ECMO since 1975 shows that 62% of 620 babies with diaphragmatic hernia survived. Assuming that figure represents only the most serious cases, a higher overall survival rate would be expected if babies not requiring ECMO were included.

The authors sugggest that data from tertiary care institutions are skewed because some babies with diaphragmatic hernia die at their hospital of birth before their admission to a level III ICN (2,3). However, the rigorously maintained regional database of the California Birth Defects Monitoring Program (CBDMP) appears to refute this suggestion and confirms the higher survival rates.

In the CBDMP database population of 452,287 deliveries occurring throughout the area of California surveyed from 1983 to 1986, the incidence of diaphragmatic hernia was 3.36 per 10,000 or 152 babies, of whom 3 were stillborn; the data to 1985 have been published (4). Of the 149 liveborn babies, 70 (47%) had multiple congenital anomalies or recognized syndromes; 29% of the infants with multiple anomalies and 16% with recognized syndromes survived. Of the 79 babies with isolated diaphragmatic hernia, 62% survived. As these figures predate the now widespread use of ECMO for diaphragmatic hernia in this region, the survival rate at present would presumably be even higher. The data from the CBDMP also suggest a much smaller "hidden mortality" rate than Harrison et al. (2) propose, showing only 6 babies (7.5%) with isolated diaphragmatic hernia who died before surgery was attempted.

It is most important to have an accurate, current picture of the survival rates for a fetus with diaphragmatic hernia before decisions are made to expose the mother and fetus to the attendant risk of fetal surgery.—R.J. Powers, M.D.

References

1. Harrison MR, et al: *N Engl J Med* 322:1582, 1990.
2. Harrison MR, et al: *J Pediatr Surg* 13:227, 1978.
3. Adzick NS, et al: *J Pediatr Surg* 24:654, 1989.
4. Torfs CP, et al: *Teratology* 39:486, 1989.

In-Utero Transplantation of Fetal Liver Haematopoietic Stem Cells in Monkeys

Harrison MR, Slotnick RN, Crombleholme TM, Golbus MS, Tarantal AF, Zanjani ED (Univ of California, San Francisco; California Primate Research Ctr, Davis; Univ of Nevada, Reno)
Lancet 2:1425–1427, 1989

1–2

A previous study showed that injection of allogeneic fetal stem cells into preimmune fetal lambs resulted in hematopoietic chimerism. Because many genetic disorders are potentially curable by transplantation of hematopoietic stem cells (HSCs), a study in fetal rhesus monkeys was undertaken to evaluate the potential of in utero HSC transplantation for permanent engraftment as treatment of congenital hemoglobinopathies. Five pregnant rhesus monkeys, at 60 to 62 days' gestation, were given in utero intraperitoneal injection of fetal liver cells, 10^8 to 10^9 cells/kg estimated fetal recipient body weight, obtained from opposite sex donors of 59 to 68 days' gestation. Peripheral blood and bone marrow samples were taken from the transplant recipients at birth and at monthly intervals for up to 2 years for karyotype analysis.

Donor cell engraftment was evident in 4 of 5 in utero HSC transplant recipients at birth; the samples were inadequate for the other recipient. The chimerism involved the lymphoid, erythroid, and myeloid lineages with 2.9% to 8.0%, 5.3% to 12.5%, and 8.5% to 15.4% of donor cells engrafted, respectively. Furthermore, engraftment persisted for up to 2 years without evidence of graft-vs.-host disease.

Hematopoietic stem cells from preimmune incompatible fetuses easily engraft in immature fetal recipients, resulting in stable hematopoietic chimerism without rejection of graft-vs.-host disease. The fetus appears to be an ideal donor and recipient of HSCs, and fetus-to-fetus transplantation may offer the first effective therapy of a genetic disorder in utero.

▶ The table is being set. Throughout the world scientists are working furiously and jockeying for positions at the front of the pack attempting to correct specific genetic disorders. The fetus has proved to be an excellent model, as exemplified by the above report. The concept that the introduction of totipotent stem cells will ultimately populate the recipient fetus with necessary cells to rectify the underlying single gene defects is popular. As demonstrated by Harrison and associates it is also practical. Stem cells can be introduced into a fetus without apparent undesirable side effects. It remains to be demonstrated that these cells will not only be permanently engrafted but also function and remedy the underlying defects. Modified attenuated retroviruses with specific genes added is another approach under consideration. The race is on and the future is now.

Life is a wave which in no two consecutive moments of its existence is composed of the same particles.—John Tyndall

A.A. Fanaroff, M.B.B.Ch.

The Risks of Early Cordocentesis (12–21 Weeks): Analysis of 500 Procedures
Orlandi F, Damiani G, Jakil C, Lauricella S, Bertolino O, Maggio A (Ospedale V Cervello, Palermo, Italy)
Prenat Diagn 10:425–428, 1990   1–3

The intravascular route opens many possibilities for direct fetal treatment, but cordocentesis generally has been limited to relatively advanced gestational ages. The safety of early cordocentesis was examined in a series of 500 procedures done between 12 and 21 weeks' gestation, all by the same operator. Exclusion of therapeutic abortions left 370 concluded pregnancies available for follow-up.

The rate of fetal loss was 4.3% in this series, and that of preterm delivery was 5.9%. No fetal deaths preceded therapeutic abortion. Cord bleeding occurred in 13% of cases with a normal outcome and in 31% intrauterine fetal deaths. The mean duration of the procedure was 7 minutes, but 14 minutes in the cases with fetal loss.

Cord bleeding, fetal bradycardia, prolonged procedure time, and anterior insertion of the placenta are associated with an adverse outcome after early cordocentesis. After 19 weeks' gestation fetal loss dropped from 5% to 2.5%. The authors suggest that fetal blood sampling be discontinued after 10 minutes.

▶ The authors are to be congratulated for being so open in publishing their experiences with cordocentesis. The higher mortality before 21 weeks' gestation suggests that other techniques such as choriovillus sampling would be more appropriate for several of the indications described in this report. It is interesting that when cordocentesis was initially introduced it was suggested that it be limited to a small number of centers that would develop a unique expertise. Now, 5 years after its introduction, cordocentesis is not just done in a few centers in the United States as originally recommended.—M.H. Klaus, M.D.

Fetal Blood Sampling From the Intrahepatic Vein: Analysis of Safety and Clinical Experience With 214 Procedures
Nicolini U, Nicolaidis P, Fisk NM, Tannirandorn Y, Rodeck CH (Royal Postgraduate Med School, London)
Obstet Gynecol 76:47–53, 1990   1–4

To determine the efficacy and safety of using the intrahepatic vein as an alternative approach to fetal blood sampling, transabdominal fetal blood sampling was performed under ultrasonic guidance at the intrahepatic vein on 214 occasions in 177 fetuses. Intravascular transfusion was also attempted at the same site on 72 occasions in 42 fetuses. Liver enzyme levels were measured before and after transfusion in 13 nonhydropic fetuses with Rh alloimmunization and 13 consecutive nonhydropic fetuses in whom the site of sampling/transfusion was the placental cord insertion.

An adequate fetal blood sample (>1 mL) was obtained in 91.1% of the samplings. Intravascular transfusion resulted in satisfactory fetal hematocrit and platelet concentration in 89.9% of transfusions. Complica-

Median or Mean Basal Levels of Fetal Liver Enzymes

	Intrahepatic vein	P	Placental cord insertion
Gamma glutamyl transpeptidase	69	NS	100
Range	43–498		22–693
Alkaline phosphatase	159	NS	152
Confidence interval	124–194		133–173
Aspartate transaminase	14	NS	11
Range	3–64		3–51
Alanine transaminase	0	NS	1
Range	2–5		0–5

NS = not significant.
(Courtesy of Nicolini U, Nicolaidis P, Fisk NM, et al: *Obstet Gynecol* 76:47–53, 1990.)

tions included fetal bradycardia (2.3%), intraperitoneal bleeding (2.3%), and needle dislodgement (8.7%). Among fetuses at low risk, only 1 intrauterine death occurred 3 weeks after the procedure and 1 spontaneous abortion occurred in a twin pregnancy. In fetuses with Rh or Kell alloimmunization or perinatal alloimmune thrombocytopenia, the survival rate was 86%. Of the 9 (2.9%) procedure-related deaths in these fetuses, only 1 occurred after intrahepatic transfusion; the other 8 occurred after transfusion at the placental cord insertion. There were no significant differences in fetal liver enzyme levels 2 to 5 weeks after the procedure when sampling/transfusions at the intrahepatic vein were compared with placental cord insertion (table).

The intrahepatic vein is an alternate site of fetal sampling/transfusion when difficulties arise or failure occurs at the placental cord insertion. This approach minimizes the risks of fetal blood loss, fetal-maternal hemorrhage, and cord tamponade.

▶ The mental image of moving from a primary site, the placental cord attachment, to the intrahepatic vein for fetal blood sampling and not securing the needle during the infusion is a little harrowing. Nonetheless, there is some experience, strengthened by the addition of these 177 patients, suggesting that the procedure is both safe and efficacious. It is apparent that the infants subjected to direct fetal blood sampling represent a select and extremely high-risk group. The technical success rate (91%) and the apparently low morbidity make the intrahepatic vein a reasonable alternative sampling site. Indications for intrahepatic vein sampling were mainly situations in which the placental cord attachment was inaccessible (failed attempts, 14.9%), difficult to visualize or approach, or twin gestations where "attribution of the placental insertion was uncertain." These are unequivocal indications. Less clear are the cases with "concerns about fetal-maternal hemorrhage." Although there was no evidence of fetal trauma and only minimal enzymatic changes not necessarily attributable to the procedure, there is no long-term evidence of safety. Continued and close follow-up of these infants is mandatory. See also Abstract 1–5.

I am not in the giving vein today.—Shakespeare

A.A. Fanaroff, M.B.B.Ch.

Intrauterine Intravascular Transfusion for Severe Erythroblastosis Fetalis: How Much to Transfuse?
Plecas DV, Chitkara U, Berkowitz GS, Lapinski RH, Alvarez M, Berkowitz RL (Mount Sinai School of Medicine, New York; Univ of Belgrade, Yugoslavia)
Obstet Gynecol 75:965–969, 1990   1–5

Infusion volumes are still not established for intrauterine intravascular transfusion in the treatment of fetal anemia in erythroblastosis fetalis. Intrauterine intravascular infusions in 28 women with severe red cell isoimmunization were evaluated to define guidelines for estimating the blood volume required for an intravascular transfusion.

A total of 81 intrauterine intravascular transfusions were performed between 19 and 34 weeks of gestation. A total of 1 to 6 transfusions were performed for each patient, with a mean 40 mL of blood transfused; the mean interval between transfusions was 18 days (range, 5–27 days). Each transfusion was to achieve a final hematocrit of 35% to 50%. Multiple regression analysis showed that factors most predictive of total volume of blood required for transfusion were hematocrit increase and either estimated fetal weight or gestational age. Among fetuses with no signs of fetal hydrops, the rate of decline in hematocrit per day was 1.1%. Factors that affected the rate of decrease in hematocrit after transfusion in the nonhydropic fetus were hematocrit increase, gestational age, and hematocrit of the transfused blood.

Infusion volumes for intrauterine intravascular transfusions should be guided by the hematocrit increase and either estimated fetal weight or gestational age. It appears that previously established guidelines used in intraperitoneal infusions are not applicable for intravascular transfusions. Still, the adequacy of transfusion must be confirmed in each patient by a posttranfusion hematocrit.

▶ The tale of erythroblastosis fetalis remains a major triumph for medical science. The time from when the disorder was first recognized until uniform screening of pregnant women and the equally wide use of prophylaxis was about 40 years. There remains a small pool of women who, for various reasons, still give birth to affected infants or in whom the fetus may be jeopardized. This report deals with the intravascular transfusion of 28 such fetuses with hydrops or severe anemia. The purpose was to establish the volume of blood for infusion into the fetus. One is reminded of the stunning differences between the current direct intravascular transfer into the fetus compared with the rather crude methodology of intraperitoneal transfusion, the only technique available until 1984. It comes as no surprise that there are only broad guidelines for the volume to be transfused. The needs are ultimately dependent on fetal weight, gestational age, hematocrit, and status (i.e., presence of hydrops), in addition to the hematocrit of the donor blood. Although only a few subjects were studied, the rate of decline of the hematocrit was more than doubled in the hydropic infants. Although complex equations were derived, the bottom line is that the fetus needs to be transfused up to the "desired hematocrit." This can be readily measured before discontinuing the transfusion, hence obviating these equations. See also Abstract 1–4.

The more things change, the more they remain the same.—*Alphonse Karr*

A.A. Fanaroff, M.B.B.Ch.

Effects of Intravascular, Intrauterine Transfusion on Prenatal and Postnatal Hemolysis and Erythropoiesis in Severe Fetal Isoimmunization
Millard DD, Gidding SS, Socol ML, MacGregor SN, Dooley SL, Ney JA, Stockman JA III (Northwestern Univ, Chicago)
J Pediatr 117:447–454, 1990   1–6

The hematologic course of isoimmunized fetuses was studied to evaluate the effects of intravascular, intrauterine transfusion (IUT) on prenatal hemolysis and erythropoiesis and postnatal anemia in severe fetal isoimmunization. In a prospective study, serial determinations of hemoglobin, Kleihauer-Betke stains to detect fetal hemoglobin-containing erythrocytes, and plasma erythropoietin (EPO) were performed prenatally, at birth, and postnatally in 12 isoimmunized fetuses (mean gestational age, 26 weeks) treated with IUT. Sensitizing antibody titer and reticulocyte count were also measured in 5 fetuses.

Before the first and final IUT and at birth, the mean values for hemoglobin were 6.1, 9.1, and 11.3 g/dL; the reticulocyte counts were 22.7%, .5%, and .9%; fetal hemoglobin-containing erythrocytes were 100%, 1.6%, and 1.5%; and the EPO levels were 12, 56, and 756 mU/mL, respectively. All but 1 fetus who died in utero were born by cesarean section at a mean gestational age of 35 weeks. Only 1 infant required exchange transfusion. Profound anemia developed postnatally in all 10 surviving infants, and all but 1 required simple blood transfusions. Before the first postnatal blood transfusion, the mean hemoglobin concentration was 6.2 g/dL, the mean reticulocyte count was .8%, the mean EPO level was 23 mU/mL, and the sensitizing antibody titer remained markedly increased. The EPO levels increased in the fetus or neonate only when hemoglobin level decreased to less than 5 g/dL.

Intravascular transfusions in isoimmunized fetuses partially correct fetal anemia, suppress fetal erythropoiesis, and thereby decrease fetal hemolysis. Postnatally, these infants have a progressive, often prolonged anemia with an absence of reticulocytosis, relatively low EPO levels, and increased titers of sensitizing antibody that typically persist for months. These data suggest that the intrauterine and postnatal anemia in isoimmunized fetuses treated with IUT may be caused by both hemolysis of newly formed erythrocytes by circulating antibody and suppressed erythropoiesis.

▶ The few residual pregnancies complicated by isoimmunization continue to yield important physiologic data such as that presented above. It is reassuring to note the high survival rate for these compromised fetuses. Furthermore, intrauterine transfusions obviated the need for postnatal exchange transfusion with a single exception and permitted intrauterine growth and maturation, minimizing the major problems associated with very early delivery. By suppressing the bone marrow and erythropoiesis the intrauterine transfusion effectively reduces hemolysis. However, there is a profound postnatal anemia that needs to be closely monitored and corrected. There is interesting speculation regarding the ontogeny of EPO production, its shift from the liver to kidney, and the various responses to hypoxia. Further studies will no doubt transform some of this speculation to hard facts. It suffices for now to be aware that EPO levels are lower than anticipated, to closely follow the hemoglobin levels of the infants, and to patiently await the explanations thereafter. As an added wrinkle, whereas intrauterine transfusions are beneficial for the fetus it is worth noting that fetal-maternal hemorrhage occurring at the time of the transfusion may increase sensitization in subsequent pregnancies. Nicolini reported that 27 of 68 intrauterine transfusions resulted in fetal-maternal hemorrhage (1). The clinical significance of this observation is uncertain.—A.A. Fanaroff, M.B.B.Ch.

Reference

1. Nicolini U, et al: *Br Med J* 297:1379, 1988.

Intravenous Pancuronium Bromide for Fetal Neuromuscular Blockade During Intrauterine Transfusion for Red-Cell Alloimmunization

Moise KJ Jr, Deter RL, Kirshon B, Adam K, Patton DE, Carpenter RJ Jr (Baylor Univ, Houston)
Obstet Gynecol 74:905–908, 1989   1–7

Administration of neuromuscular blocking agents directly to the fetus before intrauterine procedures has become widely accepted. Intravenous injection of pancuronium bromide into the umbilical cord to achieve temporary fetal paralysis was used in 12 fetuses that underwent 34 intrauterine procedures for the treatment of severe red cell alloimmunization.

Fetal neuromuscular blockade was successful in all fetuses and occurred within 30 seconds of injection. The same initial dose, .2 mg/kg of fetal weight estimated by ultrasound, was used in all fetuses. The most important factors affecting the duration of action of intravenous pancuronium were adjusted dose and fetal hematocrit, and the relationship among these 3 was best described by this equation: duration (hours) = 5.24 + 10.30 adjusted dose (mg/kg) − .16 hematocrit (%) (R^2 = .49; $P<$ .001). There were no deleterious effects of intrauterine paralysis in the neonates.

Intravenous pancuronium bromide is a safe and effective method for suspending fetal movement during intrauterine procedures for red cell alloimmunization. Because anemia makes the fetus sensitive to the effects of pancuronium bromide, a lower dose should be used in anemic infants to avoid prolonged neuromuscular blockade.

▶ It is the right, nay the obligation, of an armchair critic to be critical. That pancuronium is effective in suspending fetal movement is indisputable. Whether it should be used at all for intrauterine procedures is debatable. My impression, and remember it has been gained from the comfort of my chair, not from the front lines attempting an infusion on a mobile target, is that is is not necessary to paralyze the fetus. Support for this stand comes from reports of other investigators who not only did not immobilize the fetus but even left the needle free. At least the data are available with regard to the onset of action, dose, and expected duration of action. On the basis of the limited experience to date with paralyzing agents it is premature to conclude that it is "safe."—A.A. Fanaroff, M.B.B.Ch.

Water and Salt Conservation in the Human Fetus and Newborn. I: Evidence for a Role of Fetal Prolactin

Pullano JG, Cohen-Addad N, Apuzzio JJ, Ganesh VL, Josimovich JB (Univ of Medicine and Dentistry of New Jersey–New Jersey Med School, Newark)
J Clin Endocrinol Metab 69:1180–1186, 1989   1–8

Prolactin (PRL) may play a role in maintaining osmotic equilibrium in the fetus. In this study, the specific role of fetal PRL in human fetal and neonatal salt and water conservation was evaluated in 94 women with uncomplicated pregnancies who delivered at 34 to 44 weeks' gestation. Ultrasonic estimation of amniotic fluid (AF) volume and sampling of maternal blood, AF, cord blood, and 2-hour neonatal blood were performed to analyze PRL, osmolality, sodium ion concentrations, hematocrit, total serum solids, and total protein concentrations.

There was a lack of correlation between gestational age and fetal PRL, hematocrit, total serum solids, and total protein concentrations. There was a significant correlation between maternal and fetal cord serum osmolality and sodium ion concentrations, as well as parallel changes in cord blood hematocrit, total serum solids, and total protein concentrations. There was reduced estimated AF volume and increased AF osmolality in the face of elevated cord serum osmolality and sodium ion concentrations. A shift toward normal cord hematocrit and total serum solids was observed over the first 2 hours of neonatal life after an initially increased or decreased cord serum osmolality, sodium ion concentrations, hematocrit, or total serum solids. A positive correlation was observed for PRL levels of 230 µg/L or less and cord serum osmolality, sodium ion concentrations, and hematocrit. The entire range of cord serum PRL levels correlated positively with changes in AF osmolality and sodium ion concentrations, and inversely with neonatal changes in hematocrit and total serum solids.

Osmotic equilibrium exists between maternal and fetal circulations, and any disturbances in this balance lead to changes in fetal and neonatal water excretion. The signal for fetal PRL secretion appears to be cord serum osmolality or sodium ion concentrations. Fetal PRL also provides sustained antidiuretic effect in the newborn period that leads to restoration of the neonate's extracellular fluid volume.

▶ The fetus, ordinarily surrounded by an abundance of water, does not need to conserve water. On the other hand, the intimate relationship between the 3 compartments renders the fetus vulnerable to water loss in the face of maternal hyperosmolar dehydration. This is an interesting multipurpose report. First, it confirms earlier studies correlating maternal and fetal cord serum osmolality with a slightly higher value in the fetal compartment. Then it adds new data concerning the importance of fetal pituitary PRL in osmoregulation of the human fetus and newborn at term. The cord serum osmolality is a signal for PRL release and PRL has an antidiuretic effect. Finally, the next logical series of experiments are defined. We recognize how finely the fluid balance of the fetus is orchestrated and how the regulatory-counterregulatory mechanisms to maintain intravascular volume are all fully tested and operational before delivery. See also Abstract 1–11.

What am I, Life? A thing of watery salt
Held in cohesion by unresting cells,
Which work they know not why, which never halt,
Myself unwitting where their master dwells.—*John Masefield*

A.A. Fanaroff, M.B.B.Ch.

Benefits of Placental Biopsies for Rapid Karyotyping in the Second and Third Trimesters (Late Chorionic Villus Sampling) in High-Risk Pregnancies

Holzgreve W, Miny P, Gerlach B, Westendorp A, Ahlert D, Horst J (Zentrum für Frauenheilkunde; Westfälische Wilhelms-Univ, Münster, Germany)
Am J Obstet Gynecol 162:1188–1192, 1990   1–9

Late chorionic villus sampling provides special benefits in high-risk pregnancies, particularly when the more established method of cordocentesis can sometimes be difficult, such as in abnormal amniotic fluid volume. Late placental biopsies were performed for rapid karyotyping in 301 women at 12 to 41 weeks of gestation, with peaks at 22 to 23 weeks and 31 to 32 weeks. The indications for placental biopsies were suspicious ultrasonographic findings in 22 patients, late booking or unsuccessful amniotic fluid cell culture in 48, and confirmation of abnormal result after chorionic villus sampling or amniocentesis in 28.

Rapid karyotyping demonstrated cytogenetic anomalies in 45 (20%) of 225 pregnancies with suspicious ultrasonographic findings. Oligohydramnios and polyhydramnios were key ultrasonographic findings in 86 (38%) of 225 pregnancies and were associated with of abnormal chromosomal findings in 10 (22%) of 45 pregnancies. All but 1 pregnancy was terminated in 28 patients in whom rapid karyotyping confirmed previous abnormal results of chorionic villus sampling or amniocentesis. For the 48 patients in whom placental biopsy confirmed normal chromosomal counts in all but 3, pregnancy resulted in live births or is still ongoing, except for the 2 pregnancies terminated by ornithine transcarbamylase deficiency and β-thalassemia and 1 pregnancy with trisomy 21. No complications were associated with placental biopsies.

Placental biopsies for rapid karyotyping in the second and third trimesters provide beneficial information that may influence obstetric and perinatal management. Suggestive findings on ultrasonography appear to justify the exclusive use of direct preparation. Compared with the pipette method, placental biopsies can be easily performed even in pregnancies with abnormal amniotic fluid volume.

▶ We have become increasingly more aggressive in establishing diagnoses in the fetus. This report summarizes the authors' experience with second and third trimester biopsies. Results are available promptly and there were apparently few mishaps with the procedure. There is always the chance of discrepant results from trophoblastic tissue but this was observed on two occasions only, both with mosaicism. The detection of abnormal karyotypes in 20% of the group with abnormal ultrasound findings, notably if amniotic fluid volume was abnormal too, is the basis for justifying the procedure. The biopsies may be used to confirm metabolic and other genetic disorders including hemophilia, β-thalassemia, ornithine transcarbamylase deficiency as well as viral infections such as rubella. As a larger experience accumulates, and a central registry is established in Europe, the role of placental biopsy will be set.

Placental bed biopsy is also used to study placentation in normal and abnormal pregnancies. Tissue is obtained at cesarean section or immediately after vaginal delivery. Morphologic and immunologic studies provide insight into hypertensive disorders of pregnancy and intrauterine growth retardation (1).

A world of made is not a world of born.—ee cummings

A.A. Fanaroff, M.B.B.Ch.

Reference

1. Robertson WB, et al: *Am J Obstet Gynecol* 155:401, 1986.

Embryoscopy: Description and Utility of a New Technique
Cullen MT, Reece EA, Whetham J, Hobbins JC (Yale Univ)
Am J Obstet Gynecol 162:82–86, 1990   1–10

Embryoscopy is a new invasive technique for direct visualization of the first-trimester conceptus. Under ultrasonographic guidance, a rigid fiberoptic endoscope is passed transcervically into the chorionic cavity without disturbing the amnion (Fig 1–1). The light source is a xenon lamp rated at 6,000 K. At present, the length of time required to insert the scope and observe the embryo is about 2 minutes.

Embryoscopy was performed in 100 patients scheduled for elective termination of pregnancy. Gestational ages ranged from 5 weeks to 13 weeks. The embryo was visualized and anatomical survey was completed in all but 4 cases. Complications included amniotic rupture in 5 cases, 1 of which occurred at 11 weeks. One fetal death occurred at 7 weeks' gestation, but pathologic examination revealed no trauma to the embryo; there was no evidence of uterine perforation or any other maternal morbidity. Further testing is necessary before embryoscopy can be applied routinely; however, when it is performed at appropriate gestational ages (7.5 to 11 menstrual weeks), the risk of amniotic rupture is minimal.

▶ James D. Goldberg, M.D., Assistant Professor of Obstetrics, Gynecology, and Reproductive Sciences at the School of Medicine, University of California, San Francisco, offers the following comment:

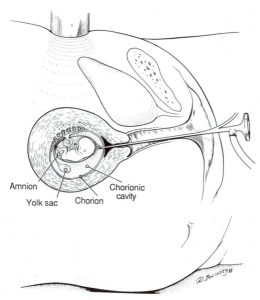

Amnion
Yolk sac   Chorion   Chorionic
cavity

Fig 1–1.—Technique of embryoscopy. The endoscope is passed under ultrasonographic guidance into the chorionic space. (Courtesy of Cullen MT, Reece EA, Whetham J, et al: *Am J Obstet Gynecol* 162:82–86, 1990.)

▶ Advances in prenatal diagnosis continue to provide new and improved options to at-risk couples. The focus in recent years has been on the development of earlier diagnostic techniques, allowing couples with an affected fetus the option of pregnancy termination with decreased medical and psychological risks. This report describes a new technique, first trimester embryoscopy. After seeing the incredibly clear pictures of the developing embryo provided by this technique, it is tempting to readily accept this as a major new fetal diagnostic tool. There are several potential problems with this approach, some of which are pointed out by the authors. First, the authors have not demonstrated the superiority of this approach for detecting structural fetal anomalies as compared with high resolution vaginal ultrasound. Also, normal developmental variants at this stage of gestation must be assessed before using this technique diagnostically. In addition, these procedures were performed on women undergoing termination of pregnancy, and thus the longer term complications of early chorion penetration or light to the developing eye have not been addressed. The potential for fetal therapy remains an intriguing one, but much work remains to be done in this area. At present this is a technique in search of an indication. I think the authors' final sentence should be strongly emphasized, "Further testing is necessary before its widespread routine clinical use."—J.D. Goldberg, M.D.

Foetal Wound Healing in a Large Animal Model: The Deposition of Collagen Is Confirmed
Burd DAR, Longaker MT, Adzick NS, Harrison MR, Ehrlich HP (Shriners Burns Inst, Boston; Univ of California, San Francisco)
Br J Plast Surg 43:571–577, 1990   1–11

Wound healing in the fetus occurs without scarring. Because collagen is a major structural protein of scar tissue, the presence and nature of collagen deposition in fetal wounds was investigated using a well-developed large animal model. A previous study showed that the cellular and matrix sequence of events in polyvinyl alcohol sponges implanted in adult incision wounds reflect the events of incisional wound healing in postnatal skin. In 8 pregnant ewes, at 75 and 100 days' gestation (term = 145 days), polyvinyl alcohol sponges were implanted in incisions made at the back of the fetus, and the incision was closed. Collagen deposition was studied histologically with trichrome staining and biochemically at 5 to 20 days after implantation. The results were compared to those of sponges implanted in nonpregnant adult animals.

Trichrome staining showed collagen deposition in all fetal and adult sponges. Likewise, amino acid analysis of acid hydrolysates of the pooled sponges showed increased levels of hydroxyproline, a biochemical marker for collagen. Type I collagen was extracted in sponges between 10 and 20 days, but decreased thereafter. There was also a progressive rise in the breaking strength of the wound tissue.

These data confirm the deposition of collagen during fetal wound healing in a large animal model. It has been suggested that macrophages are the major effector cells that mobilize fibroblasts and control the deposition of matrix of repair. The suppression of non–site-specific macrophages in combination with activation of site-specific fibroblasts may be a potential mechanism for achieving scarless healing in postnatal wounds.

Studies in Fetal Wound Healing. VI: Second and Early Third Trimester Fetal Wounds Demonstrate Rapid Collagen Deposition Without Scar Formation
Longaker MT, Whitby DJ, Adzick NS, Crombleholme TM, Langer JC, Duncan BW, Bradley SM, Stern R, Ferguson MWJ, Harrison MR (Univ of California, San Francisco; Univ of Manchester, England)
J Pediatr Surg 25:63–69, 1990   1–12

Wound healing in the fetus is rapid and without scar formation. The mechanisms that underlie the lack of scarring in fetal wounds remain unknown, but they may relate to the dynamics of collagen deposition. Several models have been used to study collagen deposition in fetal wounds, but these models create an artificial wound environment that affects the results.

Deposition of collagen types I, III, IV, and VI during wound healing

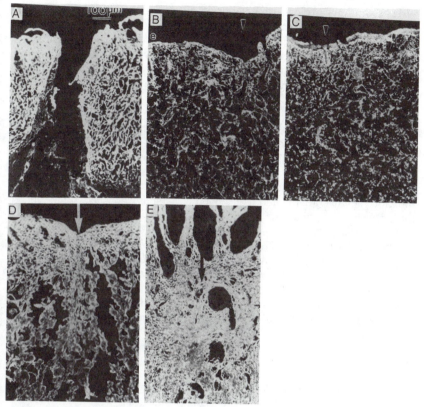

Fig 1–2.—A, 75-day fetus 24 hours post wounding (PW). Collagen type VI staining throughout dermis. No collagen deposition is seen in wound. **B,** 75-day fetus 15 days PW. Collagen type VI staining shows wound well healed and normal collagen pattern without scar formation. **C,** 75-day fetus 15 days PW. Collagen type 1 staining was similar to type VI. Again there is lack of scar formation. **D,** 120-day fetus 7 days PW. Collagen type VI staining showed wound epithelialized and collagen deposited in wound as bands parallel to original wound. **E,** adult wound 14 days PW. Collagen type VI staining showed dense scar tissue at wound site with closely packed collagen fibers. Bar = 100 μm. (Courtesy of Longaker MT, Whitby DJ, Adzick NS, et al: *J Pediatr Surg* 25:63–69, 1990.)

was studied in the fetal lamb of 75, 100, and 120 days' gestation and in the adult. To study fetal wounds without artificially altering the wound environment, a highly sensitive immunohistochemical technique that uses antibodies to collagen types I, III, IV, and VI was applied.

Epithelialization was complete by 48 hours in the 75- and 100-day fetuses and by 72 hours in the 120-day fetus, compared to 7 days in the adult wounds. Wound collagen deposition occurred in a normal dermal and mesenchymal pattern in second and early third trimester fetal lambs (Fig 1–2). The time at which collagen deposition was first seen and the final pattern varied among the 3 fetal groups. In 120-day fetus minimal mesenchymal scarring was observed at 14 days. In contrast, in adults the collagen was disorganized and formed a dense mesenchymal scar by 14 days (Fig 1,E).

These findings are consistent with previous findings that the fetus heals rapidly and without scar formation. There may be a spectrum of fetal wound healing as a function of gestational age with scar formation occurring in the last half of the third trimester. If verified, this information may be pertinent for the timing of fetal intervention for craniofacial anomalies, so that surgeons can take advantage of the unique fetal wound healing qualities.

▶ The observation by this group that fetal wounds are repaired after 2 weeks without a scar is a major discovery that will lead eventually to important surgical advances in the care of adults. Interestingly, for up to a week scar tissue is present in the wound of a fetus but by 14 days this is no longer apparent. Control of the rearranging of the repair tissue appears to be an important part of the process. This group noted that though collagen is deposited in the wound more rapidly than in the adult it is deposited in a normal dermal and mesenchymal pattern. In a further paper (1) by this group they suggest that part of the mechanism for the scarless healing is the role of hyaluronic acid, a glycosaminoglycan component of amniotic fluid. Amniotic fluid contains a factor that stimulates cells around the wound site to produce hyaluronic acid. The present evidence is that amniotic fluid plays an important role in scarless healing. Though fetal surgery may never be clinically indicated on a large scale this finding alone has been worth the intensive exploration of fetal surgery.—M.H. Klaus, M.D.

Reference

1. Longaker M, et al: *J Pediatr Surg* 25:430, 1990.

2 Genetics and Teratology

The Candidate Wilms' Tumour Gene Is Involved in Genitourinary Development

Pritchard-Jones K, Fleming S, Davidson D, Bickmore W, Porteous D, Gosden C, Bard J, Buckler A, Pelletier J, Housman D, van Heyningen V, Hastie N (Western Gen Hosp; Univ of Edinburgh, Scotland; Massachusetts Inst of Technology, Cambridge)

Nature 346:194–197, 1990

2–1

Wilms' tumor is an embryonic kidney tumor believed to arise through aberrant mesenchymal stem cell differentiation. It is thought to result from loss of function of a "tumor suppressor" gene. An increased frequency of urinary tract and genitalia abnormalities has been associated with both sporadic and syndrome-associated Wilms' tumors. A Wilms' tumor gene lies at chromosomal position 11p13. This discovery led to the isolation of a candidate Wilms' tumor gene that encoded a zinc-finger protein likely to be a transcription factor. Northern blot analysis and in situ hybridization were used to investigate the expression of the candidate Wilms' tumor gene.

In situ messenger RNA hybridization was performed on sections of human embryos and Wilms' tumors. The candidate Wilms' tumor gene was specifically expressed in the condensed mesenchyme, renal vesicle, and glomerular epithelium of the developing kidney, in the related mesonephric glomeruli, and in cells approximating these structures in tumors. The genital ridge, fetal gonad, and mesothelium are the other main sites of expression.

This candidate is indeed a Wilms' tumor gene. The associated genital abnormalities are apparently pleiotropic effects of mutation in the Wilms' tumor gene itself, in support of recent genetic analysis. This gene seems to have a specific role in kidney development and a wider role in mesenchymal-epithelial transitions.

▶ John Johnson, M.D., Associate Director of Medical Genetics at Children's Hospital Oakland, California, offers his commentary on this article:

▶ The discovery of a Wilms' tumor gene in the chromosome 11p region long suspected of containing such a gene is yet another success for the "positional cloning" technique. This is a strategy of gene cloning in the absence of functional information about the gene, but with linkage studies or chromosomal rearrangements giving clues to gene location. One of the challenges of this

17

method is to develop functional information concerning an isolated gene to prove that it is indeed the one of interest. This study provides such information to solidify the earlier discoveries of a probable Wilms' tumor gene.

In this study, RNA transcribed from the candidate Wilms' tumor gene was studied in two formats, by Northern blot analysis and by in situ hybridization. Both techniques indicate which tissues produce RNA, but the in situ method provides additional information regarding anatomical distribution on a microscopic level. These studies show that the Wilms' tumor gene is expressed in early podocyte and glomerular epithelial cells within the fetal metanephric blastema. There is no expression in the ureteric bud, the structure that interacts with the blastema in forming the kidney. Expression was also detected in other genitourinary structures, including the sex cord epithelium (but not the germ cells) and the germinal ridge.

Northern blot analysis and in situ hybridization were also performed on Wilm's tumors, showing normal-sized RNA but a 500-fold variation in expression. The expression was highest in tumors with epithelial expression and lowest in those with stromal preponderance as assessed histologically and by in situ studies. Although mutations of the Wilms' tumor gene are to be expected in such tumors, the level of resolution on a Northern blot is not sufficient to show point mutations or rearrangements. In addition, some Wilms' tumors result from alterations of a different gene not mapped to chromosome 11.

This study contributes to confirmation of the identity of the Wilms' tumor candidate gene. Future studies will most likely add to this by finding mutations in tumors and by elucidating the Wilms' tumor protein function, hypothesized to involve tumor suppression. The extrarenal expression of the gene may explain involvement of other genitourinary tissues in the WAGR complex (Wilms' tumor, aniridia, genitourinary malformation, retardation), the DRASH syndrome (pseudohermaphroditism with Wilms' tumor), and occasional associations of Wilms' tumor with other genitourinary malformations. However, it is also possible that these conditions result from contiguous gene syndromes (multiple adjacent genetic defects) or involvement of other genes, such as the postulated second Wilms' tumor gene. The aniridia gene has recently been physically separated from the Wilms' tumor gene.—J. Johnson, M.D.

Type 1 Neurofibromatosis Gene: Identification of a Large Transcript Disrupted in Three NF1 Patients
Wallace MR, Marchuk DA, Andersen LB, Letcher R, Odeh HM, Saulino AM, Fountain JW, Brereton A, Nicholson J, Mitchell AL, Brownstein BH, Collins FS (Univ of Michigan; Washington Univ, St Louis)
Science 249:181–186, 1990   2–2

The lack of a reliable cellular phenotypic marker for von Recklinghausen neurofibromatosis (NF1), a common autosomal disorder, had impeded direct attempts to identify the gene. The gene has been mapped genetically to 17q11.2. Information from 2 patients having balanced translocations in this region have narrowed the possible interval.

Chromosome jumping studies and artificial yeast chromosome technology now have identified a 13-kilobase transcript from this region, *NF1LT*, which is definitely interrupted by 1 of the translocations and probably is interrupted by both. Studies with the RNA polymerase chain reaction using primers from the translated region showing that *NF1LT* is expressed in many human tissues, including B lymphoblasts, skin fibroblasts, spleen, lung, and muscle. The transcript also is expressed in colon and breast cancer lines and in an NF1 neurofibrosarcoma cell line.

These findings, as well as the high mutation rate of NF1 that is consistent with a large locus, suggest that *NF1LT* is the NF1 gene. Other genes in the region may have a role in NF1. Homozygous loss of *NF1LT* expression could lead to increased expression of *EV12* and *NF1-c2*, which may be ultimately responsible for some of the phenotypic features of NF1.

▶ John Johnson, M.D., Associate Director of Medical Genetics at Children's Hospital Oakland, California, has offered his insights on this article as well:

▶ The gene accounting for the common form of von Recklinghausen disease, NF1, is the second major gene to be isolated by Dr. Francis Collins within the last year (the gene for cystic fibrosis being the other). The work preceding this achievement included linkage studies locating the gene on chromosome 17, and the discovery of 2 NF1 patients with chromosome 17 translocations within 60,000 base pairs of each other, suggesting that they had suffered a gene disruption and providing a "pinpoint" location for the gene.

Initial efforts to locate the gene within the region bounded by the 2 translocations resulted in the unusual discovery of 3 genes, 1 a mouse oncogene homologue and another a brain protein, none of which proved to be abnormal in any NF1 patients. At this point, Collins' group decided to move outside the region and to find DNA segments conserved in other species, an approach that has been helpful in identifying genes. With such a clone in hand they found a homologue in a peripheral nerve cDNA library, or a collection of functional gene fragments from this relevant tissue. They used this cDNA probe to demonstrate that 1 of the translocations deleted some of the apparently functional material, suggesting that a gene might have indeed been disrupted in this patient and that this caused the patient to develop NF1.

The next step was a study of RNA to look for an active gene. The cDNA probe revealed that many neural tissues contained a huge transcript (RNA) about 13,000 bases in length, the second largest RNA in humans. Further studies showed that the transcript is present in humerous nonneural tissue types. These properties are consistent with a gene expected to cause NF1, a large gene with a high mutation rate and activity in many tissues, as reflected in diverse malignancies.

The convincing evidence indicating that a given gene causes a clinical disorder is the demonstration of alterations in patients with the disease that are never observed in normal individuals. Collins' group decided to evaluate patients with "new mutation" NF1, meaning that their parents have no evidence of the disorder. In 1 such patient, a small DNA insertion in the probable NF1 gene was found in the patient and was not observed in the parents or in any other normal (or affected) individual. Since this report, other rearrangements and point mutations have been found in this gene, confirming its role as the cause of NF1.

The cDNAs isolated in this study include about 2,000 of the 13,000 functional base pairs and predict 6 exons (expressed gene regions), which are spread out over a 33,000 basepair chromosomal region. The authors could not make any functional predictions based on the cDNA sequences, but a Utah group (Ray White), which simultaneously isolated the gene using a similar approach, sequenced other parts of it and found significant homology with a group of proteins that are GTPase activators. The prototype is called GAP (*GTPase Activating Protein*), and is involved in regulating the *ras* (oncogene) protein product by stimulating conversion of GTP (guanosine triphosphate) to GDP (guanosine diphosphate). This inhibits *ras* activity, an activity involved in cell proliferation and centrally implicated in many cancers. Thus, the NF1 gene may function like a tumor suppressor gene, analogous to the retinoblastoma gene, with loss of activity predisposing to proliferation and malignancy. This would explain many of the clinical findings in NF1 patients and place this gene in a critical position relative to cancer research.—J. Johnson, M.D.

Prenatal Prediction of Risk of the Fetal Hydantoin Syndrome
Buehler BA, Delimont D, van Waes M, Finnell RH (Univ of Nebraska; Washington State Univ, Pullman)
N Engl J Med 322:1567–1572, 1990   2–3

A relationship between maternal epilepsy, anticonvulsant drugs, and an increased incidence of congenital abnormalities has been suspected for at least 25 years. It is becoming increasingly apparent that anticonvulsant drugs that are metabolized to form toxic oxidative metabolites pose the highest teratogenic risk to the developing fetus. This indicates that it is the rate of detoxification of the reactive epoxide into an inactive metabolite that determines an embryo's susceptibility to birth defects brought about by anticonvulsant drugs.

The above hypothesis was examined by measuring microsomal epoxide hydrolase activity in amniocytes to predict whether infants exposed in utero to hydantoin anticonvulsant drugs are at risk for the structural or developmental anomalies related to fetal hydantoin syndrome. Before the fetuses at risk could be identified, it was necessary to measure epoxide hydrolase activity in a randomly selected sample of amniocytes from 100 pregnant women during gestation weeks 14 through 16. The values for the samples ranged from a low of 8% of the standard to a high of 116% of the standard; the values were distributed as presented in Figure 2–1. Enzyme activity was also measured in fibroblasts from the 12 children with fetal hydantoin syndrome and amniocytes from the 4 fetuses in whom the syndrome was subsequently

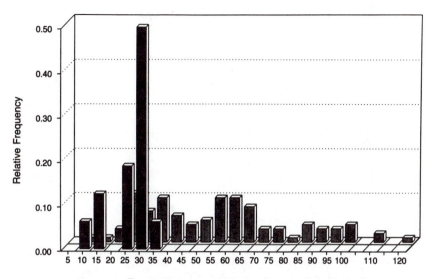

Epoxide Hydrolase Activity (% of standard)

Fig 2–1.—Distribution of epoxide hydrolase activity in 100 random samples of amniocytes (*shaded bars*) and in fibroblasts (12 samples) or amniocytes (4 samples) from infants determined retrospectively or prospectively to have the fetal hydantoin syndrome (*dark bars*). The enzyme activity in the samples from patients with the fetal hydantoin syndrome was less than 35% of the standard, whereas it ranged from 8% to 120% of the standard in the random samples of amniocytes. (Courtesy of Buehler BA, Delimont D, van Waes M, et al: *N Engl J Med* 322:1567–1572, 1990.)

diagnosed. Studies of 3 infants from whom both amniocytes and fibroblasts were taken indicated that the enzymatic activity was similar in the 2 tissue groups, differing by no more than 2% within individual patients. In this second series, too few samples were available to estimate statistically if there was a normal distribution of values. However, in the affected children, the range of enzymatic activity was quite limited; the lowest value was 9.6% of the standard, and the range extended only to 30% of the standard.

In a prospective study of 19 pregnancies monitored by amniocentesis, an adverse outcome was predicted for 4 fetuses on the basis of low enzyme activity, less than 30% of the standard. In all 4 instances the mother was receiving phenytoin monotherapy, and postnatally the infants had clinical findings compatible with fetal hydantoin syndrome. The 15 fetuses with enzyme activity greater than 30% of the standard were not determined to be at risk. All 15 neonates lacked any characteristic features of fetal hydantoin syndrome.

These preliminary results suggest that it is possible to identify fetuses at increased risk for phenytoin-induced congenital malformations by measuring the activity of epoxide hydrolase in amniocytes. At present, it is premature to attribute all the phenytoin-induced congenital abnormalities to the presence of toxic oxidative metabolites in the fetus. However, it does seem that measurement of the enzyme involved with the biotransformation of the epoxide to a less toxic metabolite can be used as a helpful biomarker of fetuses at high risk for fetal hydantoin syndrome.

▶ Cynthia F. Bearer, M.D. Ph.D., neonatologist and Director of Pediatric Environmental Health at Children's Hospital Oakland, California, provides her commentary on this selection:

▶ A teratogenic role for the arene oxide metabolites of the hydantoins has been hypothesized for some time. Buehler et al. examined this theory further by studying the association between epoxide hydrolase activity in fetal cells and the fetal hydantoin phenotype. In an initial study of 100 random samples of amniocytes they found a trimodal distribution of epoxide hydrolase activity, suggesting this enzyme follows an autosomal codominant inheritance pattern. Amniocytes from 19 women treated with phenytoin were examined in the second trimester of pregnancy for epoxide hydrolase activity and the offspring were examined for characteristics of fetal hydantoin syndrome. The 4 affected infants had low epoxide hydrolase activity. These were the only infants with low epoxide hydrolase activity. Although the data presented appear to be convincing, independent confirmation and longitudinal follow-up of all exposed infants in the study is necessary before the assay should be routinely used as a diagnostic test. Will long-term neurodevelopmental outcomes match the craniofacial phenotypes? In other words, is the same mechanism also responsible for the neurodevelopmental effects seen in fetal hydantoin syndrome? This may be inferred, perhaps, from other data on the natural history of this syndrome but this paper does not address that issue. Are fetuses with intermediate epoxide hydrolase activity at some risk if exposed to very high hydantoin levels?

Assuming confirmation of the Buehler et al. data, several inferences might be made: (1) that the arene oxide metabolite is a strong candidate for the active teratogen; and (2) that the risk of developing fetal hydantoin syndrome if exposed to phentoin prenatally may be limited to a relatively small subset of the population.

Some other teratogens may behave similarly. Clinically observable effects of thalidomide were seen in only 10% to 20% of fetuses exposed during the critical stage of development; a comparable figure for retinoic acid is about 20% of exposed infants. Fetal alcohol syndrome is seen in only 59 out of 1,000 live births to chronically alcoholic women. One can speculate that the variable expression of these phenotypes, too, could be influenced by genetically determined differences in the metabolism of these compounds. The implications of these findings could be enormous. Perhaps we can identify subpopulations at high risk for affected offspring for many prenatal exposures. The power of epidemiologic studies may be improved by focusing on a higher risk population. The biomechanical mechanism of teratogenesis might now be studied by following the fate of the toxic intermediate metabolites. Increased knowledge of the mechanism could lead to new interventions. Of course, some teratogenic agents may act directly without involving intermediary metabolites. In these cases, differences in pregnancy outcome might result from genetic variation involving other mechanisms, and different diagnostic approaches would be needed.

The potential for misuse of this information is also great. High risk women may be banned from work places or jobs because of potential exposures in the work environment. Insurance coverage for birth defects in the offspring of certain epileptic women could be questioned. Other situations for discrimination based on these findings exist.

Is prospective screening for high risk individuals desirable? If exposure to phenytoin will predictably result in a malformed infant, will one be able to prevent exposure? Is this true for other environmental teratogens? Or will this allow the development of new drugs that avoid those metabolic pathways or new drugs that block them? And finally, should everyone's genetic background for drug metabolism be determined? Will this knowledge improve the state of the nation's health?—C.F. Bearer, M.D. Ph.D.

Cervical Cystic Hygroma in the Fetus: Clinical Spectrum and Outcome
Langer JC, Fitzgerald PG, Desa D, Filly RA, Golbus MS, Adzick NS, Harrison MR (Univ of California, San Francisco; McMaster Univ, Hamilton, Ontario)
J Pediatr Surg 25:58–62, 1990   2–4

Most surgical studies describe cervical cystic hygroma as an isolated lesion. The fetal prognosis is excellent after surgical excision, nevertheless, the widespread use of prenatal sonography has suggested that the outcome of fetuses with cystic hygroma is almost universally fatal. Because of this wide discrepancy, the records of 29 cases of cervical cystic hygroma seen at 2 centers in a 4-year period were reviewed to study the clinical spectrum and outcome of cervical cystic hygroma.

Hygroma was diagnosed in 27 fetuses before 30 weeks' gestation. In 2 of the 27, both with Noonan's syndrome, the hygroma underwent spontaneous regression and the fetuses survived to term: 1 died at 2 weeks of age, and the other survived. The remaining 25 were aborted. Of these, 18 had associated chromosomal or structural anomalies (table), and 21 had hydrops fetalis and/or diffuse lymphangiomatosis. Karyotype analysis was successful in 17 fetuses: 9 were normal, 7 were 45X, and 1 was trisomy 21. Fetuses with normal chromosomes had a higher incidence of polyhydramnios, other structural anomalies, and consanguinity or previous abnormal pregnancies.

In 2 fetuses the hygroma was diagnosed after 30 weeks' gestation. One had normal sonogram at 17 weeks' gestation. In both fetuses the hygromas were lateral in location and not associated with hydrops or other anomalies. Both underwent surgical excision within 4 days of life and survived, although 1 required permanent tracheostomy because of extensive hypopharyngeal involvement.

Fetal cervical cystic hygromas commonly develop before 30 weeks' gestation and are usually associated with chromosomal or structural abnormalities. The prognosis is dismal in this group, and genetic counseling de-

Associated Anomalies in 29 Fetuses with Cervical Cystic Hygroma

None	11
Chromosomal anomalies	
45X	7
Trisomy 21	1
Structural anomalies	
Cardiac defect	6
Hydronephrosis	3
Neural tube defect	3
Cleft lip/palate	2
Multiple pterygium syndrome	2
Skeletal anomalies	1
Imperforate anus	1
Ambiguous genitalia	1

(Courtesy of Langer JC, Fitzgerald PC, Desa D, et al: *Pediatr Surg* 25:58–62, 1990.)

pends on the karyotype. A cystic hygroma can develop late in pregnancy, but the prognosis for this type is more favorable.

▶ This is a most helpful delineation of cystic hygroma in the fetus. Again, as in hydronephrosis in the fetus, it is necessary to know all possibilities to make a rational clinical decision. It is thought that the early lesions result from the failure at around 8 weeks' of the embryonic jugular lymph sacs to fuse with the venous system. To illustrate the variation in nature, Baccichetti described the spontaneous resolution of a cystic hygroma that was first noted at 13 weeks. The infant is well at 18 months with only a slight pterygium colli and is a 46XX normal female.—M.H. Klaus, M.D.

Reference

1. Baccichetti C, et al: *Perinat Progn* 10:399, 1990.

First Trimester Prenatal Treatment and Molecular Genetic Diagnosis of Congenital Adrenal Hyperplasia (21-Hydroxylase Deficiency)
Speiser PW, Laforgia N, Kato K, Pareira J, Khan R, Yang SY, Whorwood C, White PC, Elias S, Schriock Eliz, Schriock Eldon, Simpson JL, Taslimi M, Najjar J, May S, Mills G, Crawford C, New MI (New York Hosp–Cornell Med Ctr; Meml Sloan-Kettering Cancer Ctr; Univ of Tennessee, Memphis, Univ of Tennessee, Chattanooga; Vanderbilt Univ, Nashville)
J Clin Endocrinol Metab 70:838–848, 1990   2–5

In the female fetus, congenital adrenal hyperplasia caused by 21-hydroxylase deficiency results in genital ambiguity and may cause erroneous assignment of the newborn infant to the male sex. Prenatal diagnosis has been possible for 2 decades in pregnancies known to be at risk for congenital adrenal hyperplasia. Chorionic villus sampling (CVS) allows eval-

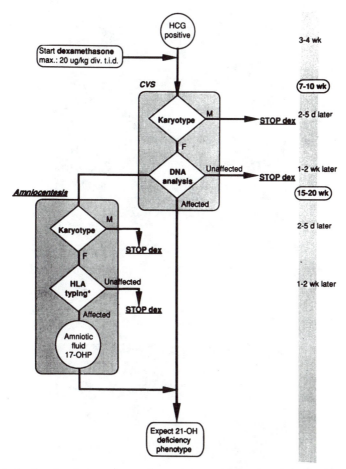

Fig 2–2.—Procedure for management of pregnancies at risk for congenital adrenal hyperplasia caused by 21-hydroxylase deficiency. (Courtesy of Speiser PW, Laforgia N, Kato K, et al: *J Clin Endocrinol Metab* 70:838–848, 1990.)

uation of the fetus at 8 to 10 weeks of gestation, early enough to begin treatment of the fetus with dexamethasone. This method of diagnosis and treatment was used in 49 pregnant women who had previously given birth to a child affected with congenital adrenal hyperplasia caused by 21-hydroxylase deficiency.

The women met with genetic counselors to consider their treatment options (Fig 2–2). It was recommended that dexamethasone therapy be started as soon as pregnancy was confirmed (4 weeks). If the fetus was male or unaffected, as later determined by CVS or amniocentesis, therapy would be discontinued. Analysis of chromosomal DNA extracted from cultured villus tissue or amniotic fluid specimens verified the suspected abnormality.

Of the women, 18 (37%) chose to undergo CVS and 31 (63%) under-

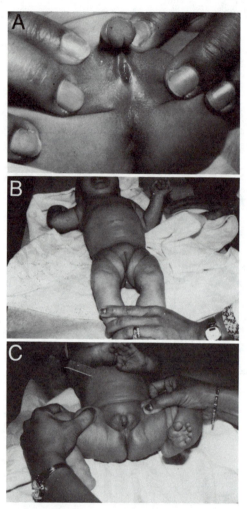

Fig 2–3.—Genitalia of prenatally untreated (**A**) and treated (**B1** and **B2**) sisters in family C with salt-wasting 21-hydroxylase deficiency. Note the presence of only mild clitoromegaly in the prenatally treated sibling. Although the firstborn child who was not treated prenatally had a urogenital sinus and requires multistage surgical correction, her sister has separate urethral and vaginal orifices. Mild virilization in the prenatally treated sibling may be attributable to suboptimal dexamethasone dosage from week 17 to term (Courtesy of Speiser PW, Laforgia N, Kato K, et al: *J Clin Endocrinol Metab* 70:838–848, 1990.)

went amniocentesis. Dexamethasone was started at an average gestational age of 7 weeks in the CVS group and 9 weeks in the amniocentesis group. In the amniocentesis group, 21-hydroxylase deficiency was found in 7 infants; only 2 (1 female) were treated prenatally. Parents of the female infant had refused treatment until 21 weeks of gestation, and the child was born with ambiguous genitalia. In the CVS group, 1 prenatally treated affected female was born with normal genitalia; another had a lesser degree of ambiguity than her older sister who was not prenatally treated (Fig 2–3).

A favorable outcome depends on starting dexamethasone as soon as possible in the first trimester, proper dosage, and noninterruption of therapy. Chorionic villus sampling is preferable to amniocentesis because it allows diagnosis at an earlier gestational date. In families known to be at risk, early diagnosis of 21-hydroxylase deficiency by CVS/molecular genetic techniques assures proper sex assignment at birth and reduces the need for postnatal genital surgery.

▶ Contributing this comment is Felix Conte, Ph.D., Professor of Pediatrics and Co-Director of the Pediatric Endocrine Unit at the University of California, San Francisco:

▶ The reports of David and Frost (1) and Evans et al. (2) first indicated that dexamethasone administered to pregnant women would cross the placenta, suppress the adrenal gland of the fetus, and thus diminish virilization of the external genitalia of the female fetus affected with P450c21 hydroxylase deficiency. Subsequent studies by Forest et al. (3) and Pang et al. (4) have attested to the feasibility of prenatal treatment of female infants affected with P450c21 hydroxylase deficiency. This report by Speiser et al. reviews and extends previous observations. As noted by Migeon (5) prenatal therapy may eliminate the need for plastic surgery on the external genitalia of affected females. However, the number of reported cases is limited and the effects on the external genitalia are variable. The morbidity of dexamethasone on the pregnant female as well as its long-term effects on the growth and development of the infant are yet to be determined in a large cohort of treated patients. Successful therapy must commence early in gestation before either accurate diagnosis or determination of fetal sex is possible. Hence 7/8 of the pregnancies in whom treatment is started will result in a nonaffected female or a male in whom no benefit will occur. Furthermore, prenatal diagnosis by amniocentesis is associated with a risk of fetal death of about 0.3%, and chorionic villus sampling, 0.8% (6).

Genetic counseling of the pregnant female at risk should involve a frank discussion of our current understanding of the risks and benefits of prenatal diagnosis and therapy. However, until more data are available, it would seem prudent to include patients who desire prenatal diagnosis and therapy in large multicenter studies so that the risk/benefit ratio to the mother and child can be ascertained and optimized.—F. Conte, Ph.D.

References

1. David M, Forest MG: *J Pediatr* 105:799, 1984.
2. Evans MI, et al: *JAMA* 253:1015, 1985.
3. Forest MG, et al: *Endocr Res* 15:277, 1989.
4. Pang S, et al: *N Engl J Med* 322:111, 1990.
5. Migeon CJ: *J Clin Endocrinol Metab* 70:836, 1990.
6. Rhoads GG, et al: *N Engl J Med* 320:609, 1989.

A Single Chorionic Gonadotropin Assay for Maternal Serum Screening for Down's Syndrome

Muller F, Boué A (INSERM U 73, Paris; Hôpital Ambroise Pare, Boulogne, France)
Prenatal Diag 10:389–398, 1990   2–6

Advanced maternal age increases risk of trisomy 21, yet 75% of Down's syndrome births are in women younger than age 35 years. While ultrasound may be used to detect Down's syndrome, sonographic signs may be detected as late as the 22nd week of pregnancy. A prenatal screening test on maternal serum was developed for Down's syndrome.

Using the HT 21 enzyme immunoassay, human chorionic gonadotropin (HCG) in maternal serum was measured in a prospective study of 9,040 women. Women with HCG values just below the cutoff level were screened by careful ultrasound. Amniocentesis was recommended in pregnancies where the HT 21 values were equal or above the 95th percentile. Maternal age was also calculated as a risk factor for Down's syndrome. Using this assay in a retrospective study of maternal sera sampled during pregnancy with Down's syndrome, the detection rate of trisomy 21 was about two-thirds (table).

Human chorionic gonadotropin is a promising maternal serum marker for screening pregnancies with increased risk of Down's syndrome. Maternal age was useful in evaluating the risk of trisomy 21. Careful follow-up screening is recommended by ultrasound for low values and by amniocentesis for high values of HCG.

▶ We have asked John Johnson, M.D., Associate Director of Medical Genetics at Children's Hospital Oakland, California, for his comments on this selection:

Human Chorionic Gonadotropin Levels in Pregnancies With Trisomy 21 (Women Aged Younger Than 38 Years)

hCG levels	Retrospective study		Prospective study	
	No	%	No	%
>99th percentile	18	36	5	31·25
95th–98th percentile	14	28	4	25
70th–94th percentile	18	36	7*	43·75
	50		16	

*Four trisomy 21 fetuses were diagnosed by an amniocentesis performed for (1) abnormal findings at ultrasonography (2 cases); (2) maternal age (37 years) associated with high HT 21 values (90–94th percentile). Three trisomy 21 fetuses were lifeborn: in a 20-year-old woman, the HT 21 value was at the 85th percentile; no abnormal finding was observed at ultrasonography performed at 20 weeks (an atrioventricular valve deficiency was diagnosed after birth); in a 37-year-old woman the HT 21 value was at the 85th percentile; no amniocentesis was performed; in a 24-year-old woman, the HT 21 value was at the 94th percentile; no abnormal finding was detected with ultrasonography.

(Courtesy of Muller F, Boué A: Prenatal Diag 10:389–398, 1990.)

▶ This is one of many studies directed toward developing a rational screen for pregnancies at risk for chromosomal anomalies, especially trisomy 21. The current screening process, offering amniocentesis to pregnant women over the age of 35, detects at most 25% of all trisomy 21 cases. A method is clearly required to detect this condition in younger women who are having the majority of babies with chromosomal anomalies.

In this study, standards for serum β-HCG in the second trimester were established retrospectively in 2,779 pregnancies known to have a normal outcome. Results in 50 pregnancies in older women who were found to have trisomy 21 fetuses were compared with this control group. As in other studies, the median value in trisomy 21 pregnancies was higher, about 2.4 multiples of the control median. This phase of the study established that 64% (32) of the fetuses with Down's syndrome could be detected if amniocentesis were performed on women with β-HCG values above the 95th percentile.

The significant results from this study are in the prospective component. β-HCG was measured in 9,040 pregnancies in women of all ages, and amniocentesis was recommended for those with values above the 95th percentile. In women of age 37 the less stringent cutoff of the 90th percentile was used. (The authors did not clarify whether less stringent criteria were used for older women, and they did not provide a rationale for this alteration.) Of significance is that high resolution ultrasound studies were offered to the group with values between the 90th and 95th percentiles. Sixteen Down's syndrome pregnancies occurred and 13 were detected using this protocol. As anticipated, β-HCG determinations above the 95th percentile identified 9 of the 16 (56%), with 2 more above the 90% percentile in 37-year-olds. Two others had abnormal ultrasounds with β-HCG values in the 90th to 95th percentiles. One of the 3 pregnancies with trisomy 21 would have been detected if the β-HCG value had been 1 percentile higher. As in other studies, low β-HCG values were found to indicate a risk of abnormal outcome, and 3 of 10 pregnancies with values at or below the 1st percentile were found to have abnormal ultrasounds and were affected with trisomy 18.

Important aspects of this study are that a large prospective group (9,040) was sampled, that women of all ages were screened, and that ultrasound was used effectively to augment the β-HCG testing. The prediction is that a population-based program with an amniocentesis rate of 5% might detect about 70% of Down's syndrome fetuses, which is a major improvement over a program (age-risk), which in California now screens about 3% of all pregnancies, detecting significantly less than half of all trisomy 21 affected fetuses. Whether β-HCG should be used as the *only* screening test is not addressed by this study. Many other studies indicate that a combination of MSAFP, β-HCG, and estriol is optimum, but detection rates have not been significantly better than 70%. Regardless of the ultimate choice of screening tests, a major change in public and health care perceptions is in order, as maternal age over 35 will no longer be the sole indication for amniocentesis, and indeed many women in this age group will be found to have insufficient risk to justify performance of this procedure.—J. Johnson, M.D.

Femur Length Shortening in the Detection of Down Syndrome: Is Prenatal Screening Feasible?

Nyberg DA, Resta RG, Hickok DE, Hollenbach KA, Luthy DA, Mahony BS (Swedish Hosp Med Ctr, Seattle; Univ of Washington Hosp, Seattle)
Am J Obstet Gynecol 162:1247–1252, 1990   2–7

Several studies suggest an association between short femur length and Down's syndrome. To investigate further, femur length and biparietal diameters were measured in 49 fetuses with Down's syndrome (trisomy 21) and 572 chromosomally normal fetuses before genetic amniocentesis between 15 and 20 menstrual weeks. The ratios of measured femur length/predicted femur length and biparietal diameter/femur length were calculated for each fetus to evaluate the potential utility of femur length shortening for the prenatal detection of Down's syndrome. The predicted femur length was calculated from a regression equation relating the biparietal diameter and femur length derived from a sample group of 384 consecutive fetuses with normal karyotypes.

With the regression equation derived from the normal sample cohort, short femur lengths (measured femur length/predicted femur length ratio ≤0.91) were significantly more frequent in fetuses with Down's syndrome (14.3%) compared with fetuses with normal karyotypes (6.1%). However, the maximum predictive value was only 0.93% for a high-risk population (prevalence of Down's syndrome, 1:250) and 0.33% for a low-risk population (prevalence of Down's syndrome, 1:700).

These findings support previous reports that fetuses with Down's syndrome demonstrate short femur lengths relative to the biparietal diameter than do fetuses with normal karyotypes. However, this study shows a much lower predictive value than originally suggested, and does not support short femur length as a screening test for Down's syndrome.

▶ This report as well as that of Shah et al. (1) does not find the measurement of the femur in early pregnancy a useful tool in detecting Down's syndrome. Shah et al. found that the biparietal diameter ratio had a sensitivity of only 18%. The major group for any test to detect consists of mothers less than 35 years of age who are carrying a Down's infant, because mothers over 35 account for only 25% of the total, and they usually have amniocentesis. In this study, the femur length identified only 14% of the fetuses with Down's syndrome. For those interested in another new test presently under study to detect Down's syndrome see Abstract 1–9.—M.H. Klaus, M.D.

Reference

1. Shah YG, et al: *Obstet Gynecol* 75:186, 1990.

Isolation of Fetal Trophoblast Cells From Peripheral Blood of Pregnant Women

Mueller UW, Hawes CS, Wright AE, Petropoulos A, DeBoni E, Firgaira FA, Mor-

ley AA, Turner DR, Jones WR (Flinders Univ of South Australia, Bedford Park, South Australia)
Lancet 336:197–200, 1990

2–8

A procedure that isolates fetal trophoblast cells from maternal peripheral blood by means of monoclonal antibodies of high specificity and affinity was developed and tested in 13 pregnant women. Peripheral blood samples were obtained from 12 women in early pregnancy (8–12 weeks) and 1 woman in late pregnancy (34 weeks). The 5 murine monoclonal antibodies that were used, FDO161G, FDO66Q, FDO338P, FDO78P, and FDO93P, showed high specificity and affinity for human syncytiotrophoblast and nonvillous cytotrophoblast cells, but not for any other cells or serum components in maternal blood.

Although the yield of trophoblast cells isolated from maternal blood was low, sufficient numbers were isolated to allow polymerase chain reaction (PCR) amplification of the Y-chromosome-specific DNA sequence. The fetal sex predicted by PCR analysis of these cells was in agreement with the sex of the fetus as determined by karyotyping of chorionic villous samples in 11 of 12 women in early pregnancy and with the sex of the infant on delivery in the woman studied in late pregnancy.

Fetal trophoblast cell isolation that is carried out during the first trimester of pregnancy allows noninvasive diagnosis of a wide range of single-gene disorders without posing a risk to the mother or fetus.

▶ This report describes a beginning but hopefully major step forward in prenatal diagnosis. When this technique is perfected it will permit the diagnosis of a wide range of inherited disorders in the first trimester without the risks of amniocentesis or chorionic villus sampling. It is dependent on the presence of a small number of fetal cytotrophoblasts invading the maternal circulation. Though the yield of fetal cells was low, amplification by PCR would permit identification of a range of single-cell disorders.—M.H. Klaus, M.D.

Measurement of Activity of Urea Resistant Neutrophil Alkaline Phosphatase as an Antenatal Screening Test for Down's Syndrome

Cuckle HS, Wald NJ, Goodburn SF, Sneddon J, Amess JAL, Dunn SC (Med Coll of St Bartholomew's Hosp, London)
Br Med J 301:1024–1026, 1990

2–9

Abnormally high or low concentrations of various substances can be found in serum from pregnant women carrying fetuses with Down's syndrome. The value of measuring maternal urea resistant neutrophil alkaline phosphatase activity as an antenatal screening test for Down's syndrome was assessed in 72 women with fetuses diagnosed by amniocentesis or chorionic villus sampling as having Down's syndrome and 156 women with normal fetuses. Blood samples were collected at 9 to 27 weeks of pregnancy.

The main outcome measure was activity of urea resistant neutrophil al-

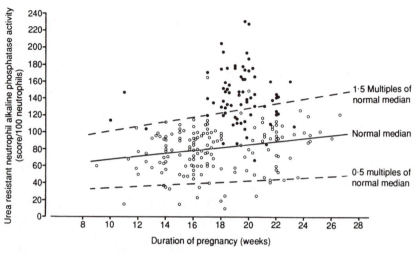

Fig 2–4.—Urea-resistant neutrophil alkaline phosphatase activity according to duration of pregnancy in 72 women whose fetuses had Down's syndrome *(filled circles)* and 156 controls *(open circles)*. (Courtesy of Cuckle HS, Wald NJ, Goodburn SF, et al: *Br Med J* 301:1024–1026, 1990.)

kaline phosphatase measured cytochemically. In the index patients, the median enzyme activity was 1.65 times the expected median for the controls at the same point in their pregnancy. A cutoff value identifying the 5% of controls with the highest activities yielded a detection rate of 79% (Fig 2–4).

Activity of urea resistant neutrophil alkaline phosphatase may be an effective antenatal screening technique for detecting fetuses with Down's syndrome. Its use in such screening may substantially improve the detection rate of this disorder. However, before it can be introduced into routine medical practice, it must be automated so that it can be used on a large scale and is less subjective.

▶ A new test is now under study to perhaps be added to measurement of alpha-fetoprotein, unconjugated estriol, and human chorionic gonadotrophin. Although promising, there are many questions to be answered. Most puzzling is why the urea resistance should remain long after the birth of the infant. Since many tests have failed when placed under close scrutiny the authors are appropriately cautious. More information earlier in pregnancy is needed on the performance of the test as well as the frequency distribution for women with and without Down's syndrome. Most importantly, the test must be made less subjective and should be automated.—M.H. Klaus, M.D.

Oral Contraception and Congenital Malformations in Offspring: A Review and Meta-Analaysis of the Prospective Studies
Bracken MB (Yale Univ)
Obstet Gynecol 76:552–557, 1990

The association between oral contraceptive (OC) use and risk of congenital malformations is not clear, possibly because most studies lack sufficient statistical power to detect significant effects. Using data from 12 prospective epidemiologic studies, meta-analysis was used to estimate the risk of congenital malformations from OC exposure in early pregnancy. The analysis was restricted to stillbirths and livebirths. Congenital heart defects and limb reduction defects were analyzed separately. Women who used OCs either during pregnancy or within 1 month of conception were compared to 3 nonexposure comparison groups, including women who conceived while using other forms of contraception, women who used OCS before their pregnancy, and women who had never used OCs.

Overall, 6,102 exposed and 83,167 unexposed women were studied. The typical relative risk from all 12 studies was 0.99 for all malformations; this risk was consistent whichever comparison group was used. The typical risk was 1.06 for congenital heart defects and 1.04 for limb reduction defects.

This meta-analysis shows a lack of association between OC use and risk of congenital malformations, which agrees with the results of most of the better-designed case-control studies.

▶ Offering comment on this article is Donna M. Fedorkow, Clinical Scholar at the Department of Obstetrics and Gynecology, McMaster University, Hamilton, Ontario.

▶ The importance of accurately identifying factors potentially teratogenic to the fetus is reflected in individual counseling as well as in the medicolegal realm. Cause and effect is an extremely difficult relationship to determine, particularly in the case of congenital anomalies. The birth of such a child often provokes a painstaking search to explain the event, often implicating actions or events in the absence of clearly defined risk.

The effect of periconceptual contraception on the development of congenital malformations is controversial. The majority of the studies fail to show clear risk. However, the studies have often been criticized for a sample size insufficient to show true risk, resulting in low power.

Meta-analysis provides a method to combine existing data considering quantitative and qualitative elements. It is a new class of publication, transgressing the limits of original research and traditional empiric reviews. The technique is particularly useful when there seems to be a disparity among the results of several studies or when the effect is too small to be accurately measured in a single study. The benefits and pitfalls of this technique are addressed by Goodman (1).

The technique of meta-analysis has been applied recently to assess the risk of birth defects with maternal OC use (above abstract) and spermicide use (2). Neither study demonstrated a significantly increased risk in major congenital anomalies in the offspring of exposed individuals. Although such studies are always at risk of bias in reporting, it would appear that periconceptual maternal

OC or spermicide exposure does not increase the risk of congenital anomalies.—D.M. Fedorkow

References

1. Goodman SN: *Ann Intern Med* 114:244, 1991.
2. Einarson TR, et al: *Am J Obstet Gynecol* 162:655, 1990.

A Case-Control Study of Maternal Smoking and Congenital Malformations

Van Den Eeden SK, Karagas MR, Daling JR, Vaughan TL (Univ of Washington; Fred Hutchinson Cancer Research Ctr, Seattle)
Pediatr Perinat Epidemiol 4:147–155, 1990   2–11

Tell me where is fancy bred
Or in the heart or in the head?
How begot, how nourished?
Reply, reply.—Shakespeare

To assess the association between maternal smoking during pregnancy and congenital malformations, a population-based case-control study was conducted using data from the Washington State Birth Records for 1984 to 1986. The smoking histories of 3,284 case mothers who had singleton livebirths with a recorded congenital malformation were compared to those of 4,500 randomly selected control mothers who had a singleton livebirth without a malformation. Case-control differences were examined using a stratified analysis after controlling for the confounding effects of maternal age and parity.

When all malformations were taken as a group, there was no significant association with maternal smoking; however, when specific malformations were analyzed, increased risks were observed for microcephalus, cleft defects, and club foot. There was no association between maternal smoking and Down's syndrome or any other malformation. The increased risk, however modest, of giving birth to a child with congenital malformations should encourage women not to smoke during pregnancy.

▶ Our bias against smoking has been more than adequately expressed in past issues of the YEAR BOOK OF NEONATAL AND PERINATAL MEDICINE (Abstract 11–13 of the 1990 YEAR BOOK; Abstracts 3–15 and 3–16 of the 1989 YEAR BOOK; Abstracts 3–15 and 3–16 of the 1987 YEAR BOOK). Maternal tobacco use has been incriminated in a number of adverse perinatal outcomes including stillbirth, growth retardation, sudden infant death, and respiratory infections. This is a fairly typical case-controlled epidemiologic approach to determine whether maternal smoking increases the risks for congenital malformations. The inherent limitations include the fact that no quantitative data regarding smoking were available and birth defects were obtained from birth certificates, implying that they would have to have appeared soon after birth. Additionally, only live births were considered. Thus, if cigarette smoking increased the number of le- thal malformations this would not be apparent from the data analysis. When all malformations were taken as a group there was no association with smoking, although there was an increased risk for a few specific lesions, including micro- cephaly, oral clefts, and club foot, and a reduced risk for Down's syndrome. The risks may be dose dependent, but this information was not available. We cannot strongly implicate smoking with the occurrence of birth defects; we can strongly recommend that tobacco intake during pregnancy be restricted to zero. But then again who will listen? Warning: Quitting smoking now greatly reduces serious risk to your health.—U.S. Surgeon General.—A.A. Fanaroff, M.B.B.Ch.

Cardiac Teratogenesis of Trichloroethylene and Dichloroethylene in a Mammalian Model
Dawson BV, Johnson PD, Goldberg SJ, Ulreich JB (Univ of Arizona)
J Am Coll Cardiol 16:1304–1309, 1990   2–12

The compounds trichloroethylene and dichloroethylene are among the most common water contaminants in the United States and abroad. Con- siderable information is available on trichloroethylene and closely related compounds that addresses short-term and long-term toxicity and general teratogenicity, and an earlier avian study demonstrated the cardiac ter- atogenesis of trichloroethylene. In this mammalian study, there was a dose-dependent relationship of selective cardiac teratogenesis with trichloroethylene and dichloroethylene.

Five groups, including a control group, were formed from 70 impreg- nated female rats. At the period of organ differentiation and development in the rat fetus, solutions were delivered into the gravid uterus from an intraperitoneal osmotic pump. A variety of cardiac defects were found in the groups administered trichloroethylene and dichloroethylene. Some congenital heart defects (3%) were found in the control group. However, 9% and 12.5% were found in the lower dose trichloroethylene and dichloroethylene groups, respectively. In the higher dose groups, 14% of the trichloroethylene and 21% of the dichloroethylene groups showed anomalies. Dichloroethylene was administered at a 10-fold lower concen- tration than trichloroethylene but appeared to be at least as teratogenic. Both agents appear to be specific cardiac teratogens because only 1 non- cardiac anomaly was found.

Because of the study design, extrapolation to human exposure may be inappropriate. However, a dose-dependent relationship was shown be- tween fetal exposure to trichloroethylene and dichloroethylene during or- ganogenesis and cardiac defects in mammals.

▶ The differences between animal and human studies are illuminated by this report. A relationship is established, beyond reasonable doubt, between trichlo- roethylene and dichloroethylene and cardiac malformations. Both the timing and the dosing are precise and they can be adjusted at the whim of the investigators. These chemical agents can and do cause cardiac lesions in rats. A dose relationship can be established and the 2 agents directly compared. To extrapolate these findings to humans takes a quantum leap, one that is impossible to make. In pregnancy neither the dose nor the duration of exposure to teratogens is precise. Furthermore there are many confounding variables clouding the picture. For example, in the fetus exposed to cocaine or its metabolites, the number of additional noxious agents, including alcohol, tobacco, marijuana, and other stimulants is rarely known. Not surprisingly, it is difficult to determine cause and effect and to separate genetic from environmental disturbances. It has been almost fortuitous that many of the syndromes attributable to medications or other chemical agents have been so well defined!

The heart is a tough organ; a marvellous mechanism that, mostly without repairs, will give valiant service up to a hundred years.—Dr. Willis Potts, Heart Surgeon

A.A. Fanaroff, M.B.B.Ch.

Prenatal Cocaine Exposure and Fetal Vascular Disruption
Hoyme HE, Jones KL, Dixon SD, Jewett T, Hanson JW, Robinson LK, Msall ME, Allanson JE (Univ of Arizona; Univ of California, San Diego; Univ of Iowa; State Univ of New York, Buffalo; Southwest Biomedical Research Inst, Scottsdale, Ariz)
Pediatrics 85:743–747, 1990   2–13

We will learn to think of outselves, our personalities, as an orchestra of chemical voices in our heads.—Dr. A.J. Mandell

Maternal cocaine use during pregnancy continues to increase. It has been proposed that vasoconstriction or hemorrhage might lead to fetal vascular disruption of the CNS or genitourinary system. Ten children born to cocaine abusers had structural defects apparently associated with vascular disruption. Four of the children were born before 36 weeks' gestation and 3 exhibited growth deficiency of postnatal onset. Six of the children had been exposed to drugs other than cocaine and 4 to cocaine alone.

Two infants had intracranial hemorrhage in the neonatal period and both later exhibited developmental delay. Three infants had nonduodenal intestinal atresia or infarction at the time of delivery. Seven children had limb reduction defects. Four had cardiac anomalies of various types. One child had congenital genitourinary anomalies. One was stillborn. There was a variety of other structural abnormalities, including hemangiomas, choanal stenosis, and single umbilical artery.

Women who conceive while abusing cocaine should know of the risk of embryonic or fetal vascular compromise. Maternal serum alpha-fetoprotein estimates and fetal ultrasonography may detect vascular disruptive events.

▶ The toll of cocaine use during pregnancy continues to mount. This series adds to the growing evidence that fetal vascular disruption resulting from cocaine abuse may result in structural abnormalities. The difficulty in establishing cocaine as a teratogen may relate to variability in dosage, timing, and route of cocaine exposure. Cocaine may alter morphogenesis by causing vasoconstriction or hemorrhage. The anatomical changes will be dependent on the timing and the organ involved. Intestinal vascular disruption could result in an atresia or necrotizing enterocolitis. Brain hemorrhage, cardiac, and genitourinary malformations have all been documented. Further support for these hypotheses are provided by Lipshultz et al. (1) who reported an increased rate of cardiac malformations among infants exposed to cocaine in utero (relative risk, 3.7; 95% confidence interval, 1.4–9.4) than among the cocaine negative comparison group (actual incidence, 65/1,000 vs. 18/1,000). These included structural cardiovascular malformations, ECG abnormalities, and possibly cardiopulmonary autonomic dysfunction. The precise risk of incidence of malformations attributable to cocaine is not yet available. Regrettably, the ongoing epidemic will no doubt provide ample opportunities to determine this risk from a large cohort. See also Abstracts 2–7, 3–8, and 3–9 from 1990 YEAR BOOK OF NEONATAL AND PERINATAL MEDICINE.—A.A. Fanaroff, M.B.B.Ch.

Reference

1. Lipshultz SE, et al: *J Pediatr* 118:44, 1991.

Screening for Carriers of Tay-Sachs Disease Among Ashkenazi Jews: A Comparison of DNA-Based and Enzyme-Based Tests
Triggs-Raine BL, Feigenbaum ASJ, Natowicz M, Skomorowski M-A, Schuster SM, Clarke JTR, Mahuran DJ, Kolodny EH, Gravel RA (Hosp for Sick Children, Toronto; EK Shriver Ctr, Waltham, Mass; Harvard Univ; Univ of Florida, Gainesville)
N Engl J Med 323:6–12, 1990   2–14

The possibility that DNA-based screening can be used for carriers of Tay-Sachs disease in Ashkenazic Jews was prompted by the recent elucidation of the molecular basis of the 3 hexosaminidase A (HEXA) mutations in this population: 2 mutations, a splice-junction mutation at the 5′ end of intron 12 and another at the 4 base pair insertion in exon 11, causing infantile Tay-Sachs disease, and a third mutation, a G-to-A nucleotide substitution in exon 7, accounting for the adult-onset form of the disease. The DNA samples from 62 Ashkenazic obligate carriers were examined for these mutation sites by means of DNA amplification with the polymerase chain reaction followed by polyacrylamide-gel electrophoresis. The DNA-based test was used in 216 Ashkenazic carriers identified by the enzyme-based test widely used for Screening for Tay-Sachs disease.

The 3 specific mutations accounted for all but 1 of the mutant alleles (98%) in the 62 Ashkenazic obligate carriers. Among the mutations causing the infantile disease, the insertion mutation accounted for 85% of the alleles and the splice-junction mutation accounted for 15%. Of the 216 Ashkenazic carriers identified by the enzyme test, 177 (82%) had 1 of the specific mutations by DNA analysis. Of these, 79% had the insertion mutation, 18% had the splice-junction mutation, and 3% had the less severe exon 7 mutation. The DNA analysis did not identify a mutant allele in the remaining 39 (18%) persons. These were considered probably false positive, although there remains some possibility of unidentified mutations. In addition, DNA analysis identified the carrier status in 1 of 152 persons defined as noncarriers by the enzyme-based test.

The DNA test is a useful supplement to currently used diagnostic tests to screen for carriers of Tay-Sachs disease. The DNA test allows precise definition of the carrier state for the known mutations, and is simple enough to be performed in small centers.

▶ Tay-Sachs disease is a rare but devastating disorder in the general population. The gene frequency for this disorder is 1 in 27 among Ashkenazic Jews, and 1 in 3,600 infants are affected (100 times greater than the rest of the population). Enzymatic screening has been established for the population at risk, resulting in a significant decline in the number of affected infants. The new gold standard for detecting this disorder is presented above. It is indeed remarkable to note "the simplicity of the DNA test will allow it to be performed in small centers without the rigorous quality control required for the enzyme assay." The rapidity with which the molecular biology technology has been converted from the research bench to the clinical arena is almost like a fairy tale. Although the enzyme assay and DNA test are equally sensitive, the positive predictive value of the DNA test is far superior. The 18% false positives identified by enzyme assay have not been adequately explained and are under investigation. The recommendation of the authors for "implementation of DNA testing in conjunction with enzyme screening for Tay-Sachs disease in Ashkenazi Jews" is well-justified. How far behind is the genetic engineering to correct this single gene defect?—A.A. Fanaroff, M.B.B.Ch.

Fetal Choroid Plexus Cysts: A Report of 100 Cases
Ostlere SJ, Irving HC, Lilford RJ (St James's Univ Hosp, Leeds, England)
Radiology 175:753–755, 1990   2–15

To determine the prevalence and significance of fetal choroid plexus cysts detected on screening ultrasound scans, an estimated 11,700 ultrasound scans performed over a 2½-year period were reviewed. Single cysts were found in 42 fetuses, bilateral cysts were found in 52, and multiple cysts were found in 6. The cysts varied considerably in size and shape.

In 95 cases follow-up scans were obtained at about 26 weeks' gestation. At this time all but 5 of the cysts had resolved, and 4 of these resolved by about 30 weeks' (the fifth case was not available for follow-up).

One fetus died at 23 weeks' gestation as a result of preeclamptic toxemia. A second pregnancy was terminated at 21 weeks after amniocentesis prompted by the presence of large bilateral choroid plexus cysts revealed trisomy 18. Ninety-five of the 98 live neonates were healthy, 3 had trisomy 18, and 1 had bilateral syndactyly of the second and third toes.

In addition to the cases presented here, there have been 18 reported cases of trisomy 18 and 2 cases of trisomy 21 associated with fetal choroid plexus cysts. Because these cysts are generally benign and resolve later during gestation, amniocentesis is not always indicated. In the present study all 3 cases of trisomy 18 had bilateral cysts with a maximum diameter of 1 cm or more. Such findings, together with other structural abnormalities and intrauterine growth retardation, suggest a high risk for chromosomal abnormalities.

▶ Last year we discussed a series of 38 cases of cysts of the choroid plexus and concluded that they resolved spontaneously or were of no clinical significance the vast majority of times. When associated with other malformations it is necessary to exclude chromosomal anomalies, notably trisomy 18 (1). To this experience we now add 100 more subjects, identified in a busy scanning unit in Leeds, England. More doesn't necessarily make us any smarter. The natural history of choroid cysts as noted in these 100 patients is almost identical with that of Benacerraf. The algorithm outlined above is the logical approach to avoid unnecessary invasive procedures on the fetus.—A.A. Fanaroff, M.B.B.Ch.

Reference

1. 1990 Year Book of Neonatal and Perinatal Medicine, Abstract 7–6.

Are Choroid Plexus Cysts an Indication for Second-Trimester Amniocentesis?
Benacerraf BR, Harlow B, Frigoletto FD Jr (Harvard Univ)
Am J Obstet Gynecol 162:1001–1006, 1990   2–16

Most choroid plexus cysts seen in the second-trimester fetus are benign, but occasionally these cysts have been associated with aneuploidy, particularly trisomy 18. To determine whether the association of choroid plexus cysts with trisomy 18 is sufficiently high to warrant amniocentesis, the incidence of choroid plexus cysts and other ultrasonographic abnormalities was evaluated in 26 consecutive fetuses of 13.5 to 36 weeks' gestation with trisomy 18.

Twenty of the 26 fetuses (77%) had major sonographic abnormalities suggestive of aneuploidy. Among the 17 fetuses between 15 and 20 weeks' gestation only 5 (30%) had choroid plexus cysts. Six of the 26 fetuses had no sonographic anomalies suggestive of an abnormal karyotype.

If 30% of the 6 fetuses with no other sonographic abnormalities have choroid plexus cysts, 1.8 fetuses with trisomy 18 would have choroid plexus cysts without other sonographic findings. The incidence of choroid plexus cysts in all second-trimester fetuses is reportedly 1%. Given an estimated incidence of trisomy 18 of 3 per 10,000 births, it is calculated that a total presumptive sample of 86,667 patients would be needed to generate the 26 cases of trisomy 18. In this hypothetical sample of 86,641 (86,667 − 26) fetuses without trisomy 18, 858 (0.99%) would have choroid plexus cysts. Thus, there would be 1 fetus with trisomy 18 for every 477 normal fetuses with choroid plexus cysts and no other sonographic abnormality.

Because the risk of losing a pregnancy from amniocentesis is about 1 per 200 cases, 2 normal fetuses would be lost for each fetus with trisomy 18 identified if amniocentesis were done to seek trisomy 18 in all second-trimester fetuses with choroid plexus cysts. This exceeds the risk currently accepted for prenatal diagnostic procedures.

▶ We continue the controversy concerning the relationship between cysts of the choroid plexus and trisomy 18 that began in the 1990 YEAR BOOK OF NEONATAL AND PERINATAL MEDICINE; this time with a solution. Though my associate observed last year that the controversy was not resolved, his conclusion "that in most instances a cyst of fetal choroid plexus is a normal variant" is correct. The calculations of these authors point the way to the clinical approach when a cyst is found on ultrasound.—M.H. Klaus, M.D.

3 Medical Complications of Pregnancy

Thromboxane A₂ Synthesis in Pregnancy-Induced Hypertension
Fitzgerald DJ, Rocki W, Murray R, Mayo G, FitzGerald GA (Vanderbilt Univ, Nashville)
Lancet 335:751–754, 1990   3–1

Pregnancy-induced hypertension that affects 5% to 15% of pregnancies causes significant fetal morbidity and mortality. Thromboxane A₂ may play an important causal role. Thromboxane A₂ biosynthesis is known to be higher in normal pregnancy than in nonpregnant women, but no one has reported whether thromboxane A₂ formation is higher in pregnancy complicated by hypertension. The biosynthesis of thromboxane A₂ in patients with pregnancy-induced hypertension was measured and compared with indexes of disease severity.

Eight women with moderate to severe pregnancy-induced hypertension and 6 normotensive pregnant women were studied. Urinary excretion of thromboxane B₂ metabolites as markers of thromboxane A₂ synthesis was measured at term. Excretion of 2,3-dinor-TxB₂ and 11-dehydro-TxB₂ was significantly higher in patients with hypertension. Thromboxane metabolite excretion was correlated with mean arterial blood pressure, plasma lactate dehydrogenase, and platelet count. Excretion of both metabolites rapidly dropped post partum and paralleled the resolution of clinical signs of hypertension.

In this series, increased thromboxane A₂ biosynthesis correlated with disease severity. It may therefore have a pathogenetic role in pregnancy-induced hypertension. A rationale is provided for the use of aspirin for treating and preventing pregnancy-induced hypertension.

▶ We have asked James M. Roberts, M.D., Professor of Obstetrics, Gynecology, and Reproductive Sciences and Senior Staff at the Cardiovascular Research Institute of the School of Medicine, University of California, San Francisco, to provide his insights on this selection:

▶ In this article the authors present interesting findings relevant to the pathogenesis and treatment of preeclampsia. They also remind us that thromboxane concentration measured in blood may be extremely misleading because of the release of thromboxane from platelets during the preparation of plasma. They

41

use state-of-the-art techniques to measure the urinary excretion of thromboxane metabolites to avoid this problem.

Their studies document that the production of thromboxane is increased in preeclampsia, supporting the hypothesis that activation of platelets is present in women with this disorder. Their suggestion that the weak correlation of these metabolites with several markers of the clinical severity of the disease indicates involvement of thromboxane as pathogenetically important is speculative. However, this hypothesis certainly fits with the apparent positive feedback present in the preeclamptic syndrome. Preeclamptic women never get better, only worse (with varying rates of progression), and the feed forward activation of platelets by thromboxane released secondary to platelet activation is consistent with this. The findings also provide a rationale for aspirin prophylaxis.

The authors, in previous work, have found similar increases of thromboxane metabolites in other clinical conditions not associated with increased blood pressure, which brings up 2 important points. It is unlikely that vasospasm is sufficient to activate platelets if it is not sufficient to increase blood pressure, and elevated thromboxane levels probably are not the explanation for increased blood pressure in preeclampsia.

The explanation for the platelet activation is intriguing. The authors propose activation within the placental circulation. An alternate explanation would be activation of platelets secondary to endothelial cell dysfunction in the systemic circulation. Several lines of evidence suggest endothelial cell injury before clinically relevant preeclampsia, which could be the cause (but equally likely the effect) of platelet activation.

The authors are to be congratulated on the selection criteria for the women diagnosed as having "pregnancy-induced hypertension." All patients were in their first pregnancy, had elevated uric acid, and had increased protein excretion. They were not just hypertensive, but rather satisfied the criteria urged by Chesley to enable us to truly understand the pregnancy-specific disorder of primarily first pregnancy that is more appropriately termed preeclampsia. Women with elevated blood pressure during pregnancy comprise a diverse group, and failure to rigorously define the preeclamptic subset probably explains the previous failure, cited by the authors, to demonstrate increased thromboxane metabolite excretion in "mild preeclampsia."

In summary, thromboxane metabolites are increased in preeclamptic women apparently unrelated to increased blood pressure, emphasizing that this disorder is more than simply "pregnancy-induced hypertension."—J.M. Roberts, M.D.

Doppler Ultrasound and Aspirin in Recognition and Prevention of Pregnancy-Induced Hypertension
McParland P, Pearce JM, Chamberlain GVP (St George's Hosp Med School, London)
Lancet 335:1552–1555, 1990   3–2

Doppler flow-velocity waveforms from the uteroplacental circulation in early pregnancy can effectively recognize a group of women at high risk of hypertensive disorders. Because pregnancy-induced hypertension is associated with an imbalance of the prostacyclin/thromboxane system, low-dose aspirin appears to be promising in preventing pregnancy-induced hypertension and its complications. In the screening of 1,226 nulliparous women with Doppler uteroplacental flow-velocity waveforms during early pregnancy, 148 (12%) were identified at high risk of pregnancy-induced hypertension. Of these, 100 were randomly assigned to receive either low-dose aspirin, 75 mg daily, or placebo from 24 weeks' gestation to determine whether low-dose aspirin could reduce the incidence and complications of hypertensive disorders of pregnancy.

The incidence of pregnancy-induced hypertension did not differ significantly between the aspirin and placebo groups (table). However, proteinuric hypertension and hypertension arising before 37 weeks' gestation occurred significantly less often in the aspirin group than in the placebo group. Fewer aspirin-treated women had low birth weight babies than placebo-treated women, but the difference was not significant. The only infant death in the aspirin-treated group was caused by a cord accident during labor, whereas all 3 infant deaths in the placebo group were caused by severe hypertensive disease. There were no maternal or neonatal side effects to low-dose aspirin.

The risk of pregnancy-induced hypertension can be substantially reduced by the administration of low-dose aspirin from 24 weeks' gesta-

	Pregnancy Outcomes			
	Placebo group	Aspirin group	95% CL (%)*	p
No (%) with				
Pregnancy-induced hypertension	13 *(25%)*	6 *(13%)*	−3 to 28	NS
Proteinuric hypertension	10 *(19%)*	1 *(2%)*	6 to 29	<0·02
Onset of hypertension before 37 wk	9 *(17%)*	0	7 to 27	<0·01
Mean (SD)				
Gestation at delivery (wk)	38·7 (3·9)	39·5 (2·1)	..	NS
Birthweight (g)	2954 (852)	3068 (555)	..	NS
No (%) of infants				
<2500 g	13 *(25%)*	7 *(15%)*	−5 to 25	NS
<1500 g	4 *(8%)*	0	0 to 15	NS
Below 5th centile	7 *(14%)*	7 *(14%)*	..	NS
Mean (SD) blood loss				
at delivery	358 (228)	289 (188)	..	NS
Perinatal deaths	3	1	..	NS

*95% CL = 95% confidence limits for difference in proportions.
†*Abbreviation:* NS, not significant.
(Courtesy of McParland P, Pearce JM, Chamberlain GVP: *Lancet* 335:1552–1555, 1990.)

tion. Doppler flow-velocity waveforms from the uteroplacental circulation is an effective and reproducible screening test that determines which women should receive low-dose aspirin.

▶ Low-dose aspirin therapy has been recommended for hypertensive disorders in pregnancy because they have been associated with an imbalance in the prostacyclin/thromboxane system (1). Prostacyclin, a potent vasodilator and stimulus to renal renin production, is enhanced in normal pregnancy. Prostacyclin biosynthesis normally increases during pregnancy but it is reduced throughout the course of gestation in women with pregnancy induced hypertension in favor of thromboxane (2). Aspirin in low doses inhibits thromboxane synthesis and restores the vascular responsiveness to angiotensin II. More than 1,000 women were screened to determine if abnormal Doppler ultrasound would predict pregnancy-induced hypertension. Of these, 148 women were deemed at risk and 100 were randomized to aspirin or placebo groups. Proteinuric hypertension and growth retardation were numerically but not significantly reduced with aspirin. When these data are added to the previously published experience with low-dose aspirin, a trend is established but no definite pattern has yet emerged. There have been far too few patients studied. The patients have been identified in a nonuniform manner so that some studies have included a significant percentage of women with preexisting hypertension. The ideal dose of aspirin is not known and there remains the possibility of vascular and hemorrhagic problems in the fetus and newborn. We applaud the authors plea for a collaborative study of the problem even though the acronym CLASP (Collaborative Trial of Low-Dose Aspirin in Pregnancy) did not grab me.

This report from London calls for a quote from Prince Charles, Duke of Wales:

Breathtaking success, is, like the celebrate Tower of Pisa, slightly off balance. It is frightening how dependent on drugs we are all becoming and how easy it is for doctors to prescribe them as the universal panacea for our ills.

A.A. Fanaroff, M.B.B.Ch.

References

1. 1990 Year Book of Neonatal and Perinatal Medicine, Abstract 3–2.
2. Fitzgerald DJ, et al: *Circulation* 75:956, 1987.

Early Doppler Ultrasound Screening in Prediction of Hypertensive Disorders of Pregnancy
Steel SA, Pearce JM, McParland P, Chamberlain GVP (St George's Hosp Med School, London)
Lancet 335:1548–1551, 1990   3–3

Doppler ultrasound screening offers a noninvasive means of detecting complicated pregnancies. In previous studies it was reported that pregnancies complicated by preeclampsia or intrauterine growth retardation show abnormal Doppler waveforms from the uteroplacental circulation. The possibility that such waveforms may be a means of predicting pregnancies complicated by preeclampsia and intrauterine growth retardation was studied in 1,198 nulliparous women who were screened at a median of 18 weeks' gestation.

Examinations were performed with 4 MHz continuous-wave Doppler ultrasound equipment. Women whose first examination showed abnormal waveforms underwent a second ultrasound examination at 24 weeks.

Results from 1,014 examinations were available for analysis. One hundred eighteen women (12%) had persistently abnormal waveforms in repeat ultrasound scans at 24 weeks' and were taken to have a positive test result. These women had a significantly higher rate of hypertension (25%) than women with normal Doppler waveforms (5%). Intrauterine growth retardation occurred in 7 women with abnormal waveforms, but in none of those with normal findings. Women with abnormal waveforms also had a significantly higher frequency of delivery by cesarean section.

Early recognition and treatment of pregnancy-induced hypertension would reduce mortality and morbidity in these high-risk cases. Although the predictive value of Doppler ultrasound screening for abnormal waveforms was poor, the sensitivity of the test was 63% for proteinuric hypertension and 100% for hypertension with associated intrauterine growth retardation. The test is inexpensive, easy to perform, and noninvasive.

▶ Hypertensive disorders with a host of different etiologies affect 10% to 20% of pregnant women. There are no tests available that accurately determine those women at greatest risk for the disorder. The rollover test is simple but has sensitivity ranges from 4% to 88%. Surprisingly, mild hypertension without proteinuria was again found to be beneficial and associated with larger infants. In contrast, hypertension with proteinuria augurs poorly for fetal growth. In the above study 2% to 3% of the nulliparous population was so identified. The Doppler waveforms identify the vast majority of women with severe hypertension but unfortunately yielded a high false positive rate. As this is not harmful perhaps other than psychologically and the test is neither invasive nor that expensive it seems worthy of further evaluation, remembering that the reliability of the Doppler is determined by the skill of the operator.

Good advice is one of those insults that ought to be forgiven.—Unknown

A.A. Fanaroff, M.B.B.Ch.

Can Prepregnancy Care of Diabetic Women Reduce the Risk of Abnormal Babies?
Steel JM, Johnstone FD, Hepburn DA, Smith AF (Royal Infirmary of Edinburgh; Univ of Edinburgh)
Br Med J 301:1070–1074, 1990

3–4

Diabetic women are at risk for having infants with congenital malformation. The chance of an abnormality in the baby is greater the higher the maternal blood glucose level during organogenesis. Whether a prepregnancy clinic for diabetic women could achieve tight glycemic con-

TABLE 1.—Clinical Characteristics of Attenders (No. = 143) and Nonattenders (No. = 96) at Prepregnancy Clinic for Diabetic Women

	Attenders	Non-attenders	p Value
Mean age (years) (SD)	27·5 (3·9) (n=143)	25·2 (4·6) (n=96)	< 0·001*
Mean weight at booking (kg) (SD)	63·5 (9·0) (n=137)	63·9 (10·8) (n=92)	NS*
No (%) married or in stable relationship	135 (94) (n=143)	72 (75) (n=96)	< 0·001[†]
No (%) primigravid	71 (50) (n=143)	58 (60) (n=96)	NS
No (%) smoking	33 (24) (n=137)	41 (45) (n=92)	< 0·005[†]
No (%) in social classes I–IIIa	52 (38) (n=137)	27 (29) (n=92)	NS
No (%) in social classes IIIb–V	85 (62) (n=137)	65 (71) (n=92)	

Note: Figures in brackets are numbers of women for whom data were available.
*Independent t test.
[†]Chi-square test.
(Courtesy of Steel JM, Johnstone FD, Hepburn DA, et al: Br Med J 301:1070–1074, 1990.)

TABLE 2.—Mean (± 1 SD) Hemoglobin A_1 Concentrations Before and During Pregnancy Among Attenders and Nonattenders at Prepregnancy Clinic for Diabetic Women

	Haemoglobin A_1 (%)	
	Attenders	Non-attenders
First attendance	11·9 (2·4) (n=118)	---
Booking	8·9 (1·5) (n=135)	10·9 (2·2) (n=69)
First trimester	8·4 (1·3) (n=135)	10·5 (2·0) (n=50)
Second trimester	7·8 (1·0) (n=134)	8·9 (1·6) (n=64)
Third trimester	7·6 (1·0) (n=134)	8·1 (1·1) (n=67)

Note: Figures in brackets are numbers of women for whom data were available.
(Courtesy of Steel JM, Johnstone FD, Hepburn DA, et al: *Br Med J* 301:1070–1074, 1990.)

trol in early pregnancy, thereby reducing the high incidence of major congenital malformation in the infants of these patients, was investigated.

One hundred forty-three insulin-dependent women attending the clinic and 96 insulin-dependent women not receiving the intervention were studied. Compared with the control group, the women attending the clinic had a lower hemoglobin A_1 concentration in the first trimester of pregnancy, a higher incidence of hypoglycemia in early pregnancy, and fewer infants with congenital abnormalities. Compared with the women attending the prepregnancy clinic, the women not given specific prepregnancy care had a relative risk of 7.4 of giving birth to babies with congenital abnormalities (Tables 1 and 2).

Tight control of the maternal blood glucose level in the early weeks of pregnancy can be achieved through a prepregnancy clinic approach. Such control is associated with a highly significant decrease in the risk of serious congenital anomalies in the infants. Hypoglycemic episodes apparently do not result in fetal malformation, even when these episodes occur in organogenesis.

▶ This is a major step forward in the care of diabetic women and confirms the extensive work of Fuhrmann (1), who demonstrated a reduction in the incidence of malformed babies with prepregnancy hospitalization and strict diabetic control. In addition, as this YEAR BOOK goes to press, the recent report by Kitzmiller et al. (2) solidifies the concept a bit more. They observed 1 major congenital anomaly in 84 infants (1.2%) of women treated before conception compared to 12 anomalies in 110 infants (10.9%) of mothers in the postconception group. There was initial concern that hypoglycemia associated with strict control may be injurious to the fetus because in some animal models, hypoglycemia resulted in an increase in malformations. There was no evidence for this concern in this or the Kitzmiller study. With the knowledge that strict control of diabetes beginning before conception markedly reduces the incidence of congenital malformation we must now dissiminate this information widely so that it becomes part of the common knowledge.—M.H. Klaus, M.D.

References

1. Fuhrmann K, et al: *Diabetic Care* 6:219, 1983.
2. Kitzmiller J, et al: *JAMA* 265:731, 1991.

Diabetes Mellitus During Pregnancy and the Risks for Specific Birth Defects: A Population-Based Case-Control Study
Becerra JE, Khoury MJ, Cordero JF, Erickson JD (Ctrs for Disease Control, Atlanta)
Pediatrics 85:1–9, 1989   3–5

The link between maternal diabetes mellitus and an overall increased risk of birth defects is well established. The present case-control study to evaluate the risks of specific malformations included 4,929 liveborn and stillborn infants with major malformations born over a 12-year period in a major metropolitan area. Also included was a matched group of 3,029 live infants who did not have birth defects. This group was matched to case infants by race, period of birth, and hospital of birth.

Maternal insulin-dependent diabetes mellitus was associated with 28 cases, for a relative risk of 7.9 compared with infants born to nondiabetic mothers. The relative risk for major CNS disorders was 15.5 and that for cardiovascular system defects was 18 (table). For all major disorders the absolute risk was 18.4; for CNS malformations it was 5.3 and for cardiovascular system malformations it was 8.5.

Mothers with gestational diabetes mellitus who required insulin in the third trimester were 20.6 times more likely than nondiabetic mothers to have infants with major defects of the cardiovascular system. Mothers with gestational diabetes who did not require insulin showed no such increased risk.

These results suggest a stronger association between maternal diabetes mellitus and birth defects than was previously thought. Gestational diabetes mellitus is implicated as a risk factor for major cardiovascular system defects. Strict metabolic control before conception and during early gestation can lower the incidence of birth defects among infants of diabetic mothers.

Primary prevention efforts to reduce perinatal mortality in the offspring of diabetic women should attempt to identify and educate those with established diabetes mellitus before they conceive. Women with established risk factors for gestational diabetes mellitus, risk factors similar to those for non–insulin-dependent diabetes mellitus, may benefit from outreach efforts before they become pregnant.

▶ Add another episode to the long-playing saga of the relationship between diabetes mellitus during pregnancy and birth defects. This is a retrospective, pop-

Risks for CNS, Cardiovascular System, and All Major Defects Among Infants of Diabetic Mothers, Atlanta Birth Defects Case-Control Study, 1988

Diabetic Group	Central Nervous System		Cardiovascular System		All Major Defects	
	RR	R%	RR	R%	RR	R%
All insulin users (n = 47)	7.4 (2.5, 21.8)	2.5	12.9 (4.8, 34.6)	6.1	5.2 (2.1, 13.2)	12.1
Insulin-dependent diabetes mellitus (n = 28)	15.5 (3.3, 73.8)	5.3	18.0 (3.9, 82.5)	8.5	7.9 (1.9, 33.5)	18.4
Non-insulin-dependent diabetic insulin users						
All (n = 19)	2.1 (0.3, 13.3)	0.7	9.7 (2.7, 35.3)	3.3	3.4 (1.0, 11.7)	7.9
Gestational diabetic (n = 12)	3.0 (0.2, 50.6)	1.0	20.6 (2.5, 168.5)	9.7	6.5 (0.8, 50.6)	15.1
Non-insulin users						
All (n = 30)	0.4 (0.1, 3.4)	0.1	1.8 (0.6, 4.9)	0.8	1.0 (0.5, 2.0)	2.3
Gestational diabetic (n = 16)	0	0	1.9 (0.5, 6.8)	0.9	0.8 (0.3, 2.1)	1.8

Abbreviations: RR, relative risk (compared with that of nondiabetic mothers); R%, absolute risk (per 100 live births).
Notes: Risks were adjusted for race, hospital, and year of birth, maternal education, maternal age, and maternal history of other chronic illnesses and alcohol intake during first trimester of pregnancy. Results in parentheses are 95% confidence intervals.
(Courtesy of Becerra JE, Khoury MJ, Cordero JF, et al: *Pediatrics* 85:1–9, 1990.)

ulation-based case study that, by definition, results in certain "limitations" or flaws. Data was gathered by history and not all charts were reviewed for confirmation. Furthermore, despite this excellent database, the absolute frequency of specific defects and exposure is low. It is a bit disconcerting to note that the rate of gestational diabetes was only 0.3%. Uniform screening with glucose loading suggests that rates are closer to 2% to 3%. The period under review

(1968–1980) was earlier than widespread population screening for carbohydrate intolerance in pregnancy. The etiology of the malformation, as noted in gestational diabetics, is speculative, as there is no information regarding glucose control in the first trimester of these subjects.

The association between diabetes and congenital malformations has been established beyond reasonable doubt. It remains to be proven that tight control of glucose early in pregnancy can reduce this figure. The prudent approach would appear to be to educate diabetics and manage them so that their glucose control is optimal before conception as well as throughout the pregnancy (1).—A.A. Fanaroff, M.B.B.Ch.

Reference

1. 1989 YEAR BOOK OF NEONATAL AND PERINATAL MEDICINE, Abstract 3–4.

Transplacental Passage of Insulin in Pregnant Women With Insulin-Dependent Diabetes Mellitus: Its Role in Fetal Macrosomia
Menon RK, Cohen RM, Sperling MA, Cutfield WS, Mimouni F, Khoury JC (Univ of Cincinnati; Children's Hosp of Pittsburgh)
N Engl J Med 323:309–315, 1990   3–6

The human placenta is impenetrable to free insulin; thus, the insulin in the fetus and in the amniotic fluid is considered to be entirely of fetal origin. In addition, the inability to detect radiolabeled insulin in the cord serum of neonates born to mothers with insulin-dependent diabetes mellitus (IDDM) who had been given radiolabeled insulin before delivery has been interpreted as evidence against the placental transfer of insulin-antibody complexes. Consequently, insulin given to a pregnant woman with IDDM is not considered to cross the placenta to the fetus and has not been considered an etiologic factor in diabetic fetopathy. However, the plasma half-life of intravenously administered insulin is at most 30 minutes, and a slow transfer of insulin may remain undetected by this technique.

In 1981 Bauman and Yalow detected animal insulin in the cord serum of 2 infants whose mothers with IDDM had received animal insulin and had anti-insulin antibodies in their serum. However, the clinical relevance of this finding, which was based on the use of an antibody that distinguished porcine and bovine from human insulin, has not been established. In the present study a method based on high performance liquid chromatography was used to quantitate insulin in small volumes (0.5–1.0 mL) of cord serum from 51 infants born to mothers with IDDM.

Only human insulin was detected in cord serum in 6 mothers given only human insulin. Among the other 45 infants, whose mothers had been given animal insulin during pregnancy, 28 (group 1) had mean levels of animal bovine or porcine) insulin of 707 pmol/L) that accounted for a mean of 27.4% of the total mean insulin concentration (2,393 pmol/L) measured in the cord serum. The cord-serum insulin concentration in the

Relationship Between Birth Weight and Cord-Serum Concentrations
of Animal, Human, and Total Insulin in 28 Infants With Detectable
Animal Insulin in Cord Serum

INSULIN	INFANTS WITH MACROSOMIA (N = 12)	CORRELATION (r) WITH BIRTH WEIGHT	INFANTS WITHOUT MACROSOMIA (N = 16)
	pmol/liter		*pmol/liter*
Animal insulin	1113±321*	0.39†	402±110
Human insulin	2726±599‡	0.43†	908±163
Total insulin	3839±840‡	0.47'§	1309±259

Note: Plus-minus values are means ± standard error. Macrosomia was defined as birth
weight of more than 2 SDs above mean. Birth weight was analyzed as number of SDs from
mean for gestational age.
*$P < .05$ for comparison with infants without macrosomia, by Wilcoxon rank-sum test.
†$P < .05$ by Spearman's rank-correlation coefficient for all 28 infants.
‡$P < .02$ for comparison with infants without macrosomia, by Wilcoxon rank-sum test.
§$P < .02$ by Spearman's rank-correlation coefficient for all 28 infants.
(Courtesy of Menon RK, Cohen RM, Sperling MA, et al: N Engl J Med 323:309–315,
1990.)

other 17 infants (group 2), in whom only human insulin was detected
(mean of 381 pmol/L), was only 15% of that detected in group 1.
There was a significant correlation between the maternal and the cord-
serum concentrations of anti-insulin antibody and the concentration of
animal insulin in the infant, indicating that the animal insulin was transferred as an insulin antibody complex. Twelve infants in group 1 had
macrosomia and 16 were of appropriate birth weight. The 12 infants
with macrosomia had significantly higher cord-serum concentrations of
animal, human, and total insulin than those without the condition (table).

Considerable amounts of antibody-bound insulin are transferred from
the mother to the fetus during pregnancy in some women with IDDM.
The degree of transfer is related to the maternal concentration of anti-
insulin antibody. The correlation between macrosomia and the concentrations of animal insulin in cord serum suggests that the transferred insulin has biologic activity and indicates that the formation of antibody to
insulin in the mother is a determining factor on fetal outcome that is independent of maternal levels of blood glucose.

▶ Satish Kalhan, M.D., Professor of Pediatrics, Rainbow Babies and Children's
Hospital, Case Western Reserve University School of Medicine, Cleveland,
comments as follows:

▶ This study by Menon et al. clearly demonstrates that significant amounts of
insulin administered to the pregnant mother get transferred to the fetus and
that antibodies to the insulin could function as carrier proteins for the transport
of insulin across the placenta. Actually, the carrier protein appears to protect to
some extent the insulin administered to the mother against the insulin-degrad-
ing enzymes present in the placenta.

The data in the present study raise some interesting questions. Why are these data different from previously published studies? The data in animal studies have been controversial, and probably some interspecies differences do exist regarding transport of peptides across the placenta. However, studies in normal pregnant women performed over 1 hour using radioactive labeled insulin have shown no transfer of insulin across the placenta, in early gestation or at term (1,2). The same is true for other peptides such as growth hormone and glucagon (3,4). In addition, Gruppuso et al. (5) recently demonstrated that in the normal rhesus monkey, radioactive iodine labeled proinsulin and C-peptide were also not transported from the mother to the fetus. Actually, there was a significant degradation of these hormones in the uteroplacental unit and immunoreactive fragments of these peptides were detected in the fetal circulation.

Administration of foreign (animal) insulin to diabetic subjects induces insulin antibodies, the majority of which are of the IgG type. Several studies have shown that the insulin antibody titers are of similar magnitude in both the mother and the infant, suggesting a passage of these antibodies across the placenta (6,7). Similar observation has been made in animal studies. However, the passage of these globulins is relatively slow. Thus, if these antibodies were to act as carrier proteins, the insulin bound to the antibodies will be transferred to the fetus slowly and will not be easily demonstrable in an acute experiment. This might explain the differences in the present study from the previous data.

The second and more important question raised by this study concerns diabetic fetopathy. Menon et al. found a significant correlation between infant macrosomia and the concentration of animal insulin in cord serum. Is this merely an association or a cause-and-effect relationship? As discussed by Schwartz (9) in an editorial accompanying the paper by Menon et al. the fetal and neonatal hyperinsulinemia in diabetic pregnancy is the result of excessive secretion of insulin by the fetus and is thus of endogenous origin. Even in the present study only 27% of the total insulin measured in the macrosomic infants was of animal origin. The remaining 73% was human insulin, possibly of fetal origin because the mothers of these infants were producing no or very little insulin. It should also be pointed out that the antibody-bound insulin is not necessarily biologically active; it is the free insulin that is responsible for the consequences observed in infants of diabetic mothers. Thus, the hyperinsulinism observed in the infants of diabetic mothers is primarily the result of excessive fetal secretions of insulin caused by stimulation by glucose and amino acids transferred to the fetus in prodigious amounts. The observed association in the present study may simply be a marker of the severity of maternal diabetes, i.e., women with long-standing diabetes are likely to be receiving insulin for a longer time and thus have higher titers of insulin antibodies. Finally, as stated by Schwartz, "Evidence accrued over the past 30 years supports the concept that the transfer of nutrients from the mother to fetus stimulates pancreatic insulin secretion in the fetus, with diverse metabolic effects. In the presence of maternal insulin antibodies, maternal or exogenous insulin may be carried to the fetus as well. The consequences of fetal hyperinsulinism are independent of the insulin source."—S. Kalhan, M.D.

References

1. Kalhan SC, et al: *J Clin Endocrinol Metab* 40:139, 1975.
2. Adam PAJ, et al: *Diabetes* 19:409, 1969.
3. King KC, et al: *Pediatrics* 48:534, 1971.
4. Adam PAJ, et al: *J Clin Endocrinol Metab* 34:772, 1982.
5. Gruppuso PA, et al: *J Clin Invest* 80:1132, 1987.
6. Thorell JI: *Acta Endocrinol* 52:255, 1966.
7. Spellacy WN, Goetz FC: *Lancet* 2:222, 1963.
8. Thorell JI: *Acta Endocrinol* 52:268, 1966.
9. Schwartz R: *N Engl J Med* 323:340, 1990.

Delayed Childbearing and the Outcome of Pregnancy

Berkowitz GS, Skovron ML, Lapinski RH, Berkowitz RL (Mount Sinai School of Medicine; Hosp for Joint Diseases, New York)
N Engl J Med 322:659–664, 1990   3–7

You don't object to an aged parent, I hope—Charles Dickens

There has been a trend among American women to delay childbearing until after age 30 years because they wish to first pursue educational and career goals. Previous studies of pregnancy complications and adverse pregnancy outcomes among older primiparous women have been inconclusive. Pregnancy complication rates, infant mortality, and infant birth weights for 3,917 primiparous women, aged 20 years or older who delivered a singleton infant during a 3-year period were compared.

Of the women, 58% were aged 30 years or older at the time of their first delivery. These women were more likely than the younger women to be white, to have attended college, and to have a history of infertility, spontaneous abortion, or induced abortion. Women aged 35 years

Association Between Maternal Age and Selected Complications of Pregnancy*

VARIABLE	MATERNAL AGE 30–34			MATERNAL AGE ≥35		
	UNADJUSTED ODDS RATIO†	ADJUSTED ODDS RATIO†	95% CI	UNADJUSTED ODDS RATIO†	ADJUSTED ODDS RATIO†	95% CI
Antepartum complications‡	1.2	1.1	0.9–1.4	2.1	2.0	1.6–2.5
Intrapartum complications§	1.2	1.2	0.99–1.5	1.4	1.4	1.1–1.8
Second stage of labor >2 hr	1.7	1.5	1.2–1.9	1.8	1.6	1.2–2.1
Cesarean-section delivery	1.3	1.3	1.1–1.5	1.9	1.8	1.5–2.2
1-Min Apgar <7	1.2	1.2	0.9–1.6	0.8	0.8	0.5–1.2
5-Min Apgar <7	1.2	1.3	0.6–2.7	0.4	0.5	0.1–1.6
Admission to newborn ICU	1.2	1.3	1.1–1.6	1.2	1.4	1.1–1.8

*CI denotes confidence interval; *ICU,* intensive care unit.
†Women aged 20–29 years served as the reference group.
‡Defined as the presence of gestational diabetes, pregnancy-induced hypertension, gestational bleeding, abruptio placentae, or placenta previa.
§Defined as the presence of hypertension, uterine bleeding, or fetal distress.
(Courtesy of Berkowitz GS, Skovron ML, Lapinski RH, et al: *N Engl J Med* 322:659–664, 1990.)

or older tended to have low birth weight and very low birth weight infants somewhat more often than younger women. The rate of preterm delivery before 37 weeks' gestation was not much higher among women aged 30 to 39 years than among women aged 20 to 29 years, and the rate of preterm delivery was actually slightly lower among women aged 40 years and older. The rate of delivery of infants who were small for gestational age was slightly lower among women aged 30 to 34 years and those aged 40 years or older compared with women aged 20 to 29 years. The rate among women aged 35–39 years was identical to that among women aged 20–29 years. The rates of specific antepartum and intrapartum complications were higher among older women (table).

Older primiparous women have higher rates of complications of pregnancy and delivery compared with younger primiparous women. However, except for a slightly increased risk of delivering a low birth weight infant among mothers aged 35 years or older, advancing maternal age at first birth does not appreciably increase the risk of an adverse outcome in singleton gestations.

▶ Childbearing is increasingly postponed as women enter college and the work force and develop careers outside the home. The above report presents an appraisal of delaying pregnancy as seen through the eyes of the private practitioner. The cohort is sociodemographically skewed to the upper-middle class with the patients predominantly white, married, and college-educated. The findings can therefore not necessarily be extrapolated to an unmatched sociodemographic group. Traditionally, with advancing age the frequency of low birth weight infants and pregnancy complications such as gestational diabetes, hypertension, and bleeding increase. There is also a greater incidence of fetal distress and need for delivery by cesarean section. This is a small cohort and not all of these complications were statistically significant. Furthermore, chromosomal anomalies, miscarriages, and malformations were not primary outcome variables. With these exclusions the conclusion that with the exception of low birth weight advancing maternal age "did not appreciably increase the risk of an adverse outcome in singleton gestations" is acceptable. It is worth noting that in this socioeconomic group the outlook for low birth weight babies is more favorable.

Spellacy (1) monitored a cohort of 511 women aged 40 years and older and compared them with women aged 20 to 30 years. When correcting for maternal weight and smoking the complication rates were not significantly different. Nonetheless, hypertension, macrosomia, and low Apgar scores were more likely among the heavier women. If you are the reassuring kind then these two reports should reassure those women contemplating delaying childbearing as well as their caretakers. Not all women age at the same pace, and age of course is relative. If childbearing is going to be postponed, for whatever reasons, then it is necessary to not abuse the body with cigarettes and to maintain ideal body weight.

How much more elder art thou than thy looks!—*Shakespeare, The Merchant of Venice*

A.A. Fanaroff, M.B.B.Ch.

Reference

1. Spellacy WN, et al: *Obstet Gynecol* 68:452, 1986.

Grand Multiparity: A Nationwide Survey
Samueloff A, Mor-Yosef S, Seidman DS, Rabinowitz R, Simon A, Schenker JG
(Hadassah Univ Hosp, Jerusalem)
Isr J Med Sci 25:625–629, 1989   3–8

Grand multiparity, defined as deliveries of 7 or more infants, is considered an obstetric hazard to both mother and fetus, even in modern obstetric practice. The obstetric performance of grand multipara (GMP) and the risks attributed to high parity were evaluated in the first nationwide survey on grand multiparity. Data on 22,814 deliveries of at least 26 weeks' gestation in 30 maternity wards in Israel over a 3-month period were reviewed.

Of the 22,679 evaluable deliveries, 1,542 (6.8%) were in GMP mothers. Compared with primiparae and multiparae, GMPs showed an increased incidence of antenatal complications including hypertension, diabetes, and preeclampsia (table), and all correlated significantly with maternal age. Malpresentation (Fig 3–1), meconium-stained amniotic fluid, large-for-date babies and multiple births were significantly more common in GMPs; none of these correlated with maternal age. The perinatal mortality rate, 16 per 1,000 births, was significantly increased in GMPs compared with the overall mortality rate. All deaths occurred in babies born to mothers aged older than 34 years. There was no correlation between maternal age and perinatal death. Grand multiparity remains a high risk factor, both for the mother and infant.

▶ It would appear that it is not so grand to be a grand multip. The risks are increased for both mother and fetus. These include hypertension, diabetes, multiple births, malpresentations, and cesarean sections together with mac-

---

Medical Disorders Complicating Pregnancy (Percent)

	Total population (n = 22,679)	Primi-parae (n = 4,851)	Multiparae (n = 16,286)	Grand multiparae (n = 1,542)	$P*$
Diabetes	1.3	0.9	1.4	2.2	< 0.05
Hypertension	1.6	2.2	1.3	3.5	< 0.001
Preeclampsia	2.2	4.0	1.6	2.9	NS

*Statistical analysis compared multiparas with grand multiparas only.
(Courtesy of Samueloff A, Mor-Yosef S, Seidman DS, et al: *Isr J Med Sci* 25:625–629, 1989.)

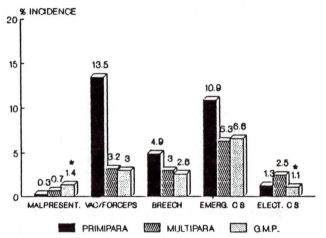

Fig 3–1.—Relationship between parity and malpresentation and interventions during delivery. *Asterisk* indicates *P* < .001 when comparing multiparas with grand multiparas; *CS*, cesarean section. (Courtesy of Samueloff A, Mor-Yosef S, Seidman DS, et al: *Isr J Med Sci* 25:625–629, 1989.)

rosomia and increased perinatal deaths. Adverse outcomes were associated particularly with advancing maternal age and lower socioeconomic status. This was an impressive, carefully documented, prospective, national study, conducted over a 3-month period. Over the years, the definition of grand multip has increased from 5 to 7 infants or more. Reports from a controlled, stable population in Jerusalem have raised questions as to whether grand multip parity confers greater risk on the mother and fetus (1–3). The national survey, however, lays to rest any doubts about the risks of grand multiparity.—A.A. Fanaroff, M.B.B.Ch.

References

1. Seidman DS, et al: *Int J Gynaecol Obstet* 25:1, 1987.
2. Eidelman AI, et al: *Am J Obstet Gynecol* 158:389, 1988.
3. Seidman DS, et al: *Am J Obstet Gynecol* 158:1034, 1988.

Routine Hospital Admission in Twin Pregnancy Between 26 and 30 Weeks' Gestation
MacLennan AH, Green RC, O'Shea R, Brookes C, Morris D (Univ of Adelaide; Queen Victoria Hosp, Adelaide; Flinders Med Ctr, South Australia)
Lancet 335:267–269, 1990   3–9

Traditionally, women with twin pregnancies are admitted to the hospital in the third trimester to reduce the frequency of complications. However, because most perinatal morbidity and mortality associated with delivery occur before 30 weeks' gestation, a prospective study was undertaken to assess the benefits of hospital admission in twin pregnancy between 26 and 30 weeks' gestation. In a multicenter study, 141 women with uncomplicated twin pregnancies were randomly assigned to either outpatient care or hospital admission between 26 and 30 weeks' gestation.

There were no significant differences in the frequencies of major maternal complications in pregnancy and labor between the 72 women assigned to outpatient care and 69 women admitted to the hospital. However, women admitted to the hospital routinely at 26 weeks' were 2.76 times more likely to be readmitted after 30 weeks' gestation than women assigned to outpatient care. Mean birth weights at birth and birth weights of twins by birth order did not differ significantly between groups, even after analyzing for intention to treat or treatment received. In the inpatient group, 22 infants were delivered before 32 weeks' gestation compared with 10 in the outpatient group. Except for small-for-dates infants, there was a trend toward greater frequency of preterm delivery, neonatal intensive care, and higher morbidity or mortality in the inpatient group. These data show that routine hospital admission of women with twin pregnancies from 26 weeks' gestation offers no benefit to mother or infants and should be abandoned.

▶ Despite little or no convincing data to support the practice of bed rest for twin gestations during the third trimester, such therapy has become commonplace around the globe. This Australian collaborative study was designed to study that practice and determine its effectiveness. Once again, under the harsh light of a randomized prospective controlled study, a negative result emerges. As bluntly stated by the authors, "There was no benefit of a hospital admission from 26 weeks' gestation." Routine admission at this time preferred neither the mother nor the fetuses. There are a few notable observations with regard to the study. First, although 11 centers participated, two thirds of the cases were contributed by 2 centers. Furthermore, many of the major problems were with the fetuses presented before 26 weeks' gestation, suggesting that if bed rest is to impact on perinatal morbidity in twin gestations, it must be implemented before 26 weeks' gestation. Also, the original power estimates required 188 twin gestations, but the interim analysis was convincing enough to terminate the enrollment early. It is always revealing to look at costs in other countries; note the hospitalization costs of $4000 a month, bargain basement rates, as compared to the United States. My abiding impression is that this topic will not yet be laid to rest.—A.A. Fanaroff, M.B.B.Ch.

Effect of Maternal Work Activity on Preterm Birth and Low Birth Weight
Teitelman AM, Welch LS, Hellenbrand KG, Bracken MB (Yale Univ; George Washington Univ, Washington, DC)
Am J Epidemiol 131:104–113, 1990   3–10

While physical activity during pregnancy does not necessarily cause adverse pregnancy outcomes, certain types of strenuous work and pro-

Association of Gestational Age and Rate of Preterm Delivery With Maternal Work
Activity, New Haven, Connecticut, 1980–1982

Work activity group	No.	Gestational age (weeks from LMP*)		% preterm	No.	RR*	95% CI*
		Mean	SD*				
Standing	182	37.9	2.9	7.7	14	2.84	1.34–6.00
Active	526	38.2	2.0	2.8	15	—†	—†
Sedentary	498	38.2	2.0	4.2	21	1.50	0.76–2.94
Total	1,206			4.2	50		

$F = 1.70$, df = 2, 1,204, $p = 0.184$

*Abbreviations: LMP, last menstrual period; SD, standard deviation; RR, relative risk; CI, confidence interval.
†Reference category.
(Courtesy of Teitelman AM, Welch LS, Hellenbrand KG, et al: Am J Epidemiol 131:104–113, 1990.)

longed standing have been associated with preterm delivery and lower birth weights.

In a sample of 1,026 women, the rate of preterm births among women with jobs requiring prolonged standing was 7.7% compared with 4.2% for those with sedentary jobs and 2.8% for those with active jobs (table). The odds of preterm delivery in women with a standing job were 2.72. With adjustments for variables of parity, smoking, education, caffeine and marijuana use, race, gestational age at interview, and marital status, there was a significant association between standing on the job and preterm birth. While the rate of low birth weight was also higher in the standing group than in the sedentary or active group, the association was not significant when other maternal factors were included.

Even after controlling for socioeconomic and lifestyle factors, there was a significant association of prolonged standing with gestational age. These results are consistent with previous reports. The low birth weight associated with prolonged standing in this study is not significant when controlled for other factors. Among employed women, there is evidence that work involving prolonged standing may increase the risk of preterm delivery but not the risk of low birth weight.

▶ The following comment is provided by Susan K. Cummins, M.D., M.P.H., Public Health Medical Officer, California Department of Health Services, Environmental Epidemiology and Toxicology Branch:

▶ This retrospective cohort study explores the relationship between work activity, preterm birth, and low birth weight in 1,206 working women. Investigators classified the mother's occupation reported early in pregnancy into 1 of 3 activity levels: standing, active, and sedentary. After adjustment for confounding factors, preterm delivery occurred 2.7 times more often in women in standing jobs compared to women in active jobs. No association between work activity and birth weight was found.

Several study design limitations may have resulted in a conservative estimate of the risk associated with standing at work during pregnancy. First, because no data on actual work activity among respondents was available, job titles were used to estimate work activity. Some job titles may have been misclassified into the wrong activity category. For example, dentists and dental assistants were classified into standing jobs even though most dentists and dental assistants sit when they treat patients. Since many job titles were included in the study, the impact of misclassification of a few titles is likely to be small. Second, as the authors acknowledge, no data were available on the duration of working during pregnancy. If women in standing jobs worked more in the last trimester, then this study may be assessing duration of work rather than work activity during pregnancy.

This is the first study in the United States to demonstrate an association betwen work activity and increased risk for preterm birth. Because preterm birth is a common serious adverse pregnancy outcome and most American women must work outside the home during pregnancy, the findings have important implications for public policy after safe working practices during pregnancy. Because of the impact of these results on public policy, future studies that assess individual work activity patterns and duration of working during pregnancy should be performed.— S.K. Cummins, M.D., M.P.H.

The Effect of Physical Activity During Pregnancy on Preterm Delivery and Birth Weight

Klebanoff MA, Shiono PH, Carey JC (Natl Inst of Child Health and Human Development, Bethesda, Md; Univ of Oklahoma)
Am J Obstet Gynecol 163:1450–1456, 1990   3–11

Some studies have linked physical activity with preterm delivery whereas other studies have found no association. The relationship between physical activity in both employment settings and nonemployment settings and pregnancy outcome was studied prospectively in 7,101 women.

Only prolonged periods of standing were associated with a modestly increased risk of preterm delivery at an adjusted odds ratio of 1.31. Heavy work and exercise were not associated with preterm delivery. The proportion of preterm infants did not differ among women in standing, active, or sedentary occupations. After controlling for confounding variables, physical activity was not associated with gestational age–adjusted birth weight.

Although previous studies have suggested a link between physical activity and pregnancy outcome, in this study only prolonged periods of standing slightly increased the risk of preterm delivery. Unmeasured socioeconomic differences may have accounted for the previously described associations. The role of activity restriction in high-risk pregnancies should be evaluated carefully.

Heavy Lifting During Pregnancy: A Hazard to the Fetus? A Prospective Study

Ahlborg G Jr, Bodin L, Hogstedt C (Örebro Med Ctr Hosp; Örebro County Council; Karolinska Hosp, Stockholm, Sweden)
Int J Epidemiol 19:90–97, 1990   3–12

It is a common belief that heavy physical exertion during pregnancy is hazardous to the fetus. Several epidemiologic studies also suggest that physical exertion is a risk factor for spontaneous abortion, preterm birth, and low birth weight. However, all these studies are retrospective and subject to recall bias. In a prospective study, 3,906 Swedish women who worked during pregnancy were studied to define the influence of heavy lifting during pregnancy on gestational age, birth weight, and risk of fetal death (spontaneous abortion or stillbirth). Information on exposure was collected on the women's first contact with the antenatal care center.

In general, women who reported heavy lifting did not have more unfavorable outcomes than other women, although the estimates varied between different occupations. For all occupations, the odds ratio was 1.11 for fetal death, 0.85 for preterm birth (<37 weeks' gestation), and 0.78 for low birth weight (<2500 g). However, among women who stopped working before the 32nd week of pregnancy, lifting of weights greater than 12 kg more than 50 times per week increased the risk of preterm birth, with an odds ratio of 1.71. Chemical exposure was also associated with increased risk of unfavorable outcome.

Contrary to popular belief, this prospective study indicates that heavy lifting during pregnancy does not increase the risk of fetal death, although there is an indication that heavy lifting may increase the risk of preterm birth among women who stop working before the 32nd week of pregnancy. It appears that preventive routines and regulations in Sweden may have helped reduce the possible risks from heavy lifting during pregnancy.

▶ Jeffrey B. Gould, M.D., M.P.H., Professor and chair of Maternal and Child Health at the School of Public Health, University of California, Berkeley, offers his comment on Abstracts 3–11 and 3–12:

▶ From an evolutionary/historical perspective, it is unlikely that high levels of physical activity during pregnancy would constitute a major hazard for the fetus. Speculation aside, the impact of work on the outcome of pregnancy is one of the more difficult areas of clinical inquiry. From a personal perspective work can represent a burden required for survival or a source of self-fulfillment, self-esteem, and social support (1). Working during pregnancy may self-select women whose health status allows them to continue working. This type of self-selection could account for the improved outcome (decreased preterm births) observed in women who did light work during pregnancy (2). Conversely, the finding that increased preterm birth occurred in women who did heavy lifting only if they stopped working before the 32nd week could also represent a selection phenomena (3). Both papers suggest that work during pregnancy is not a major source of risk for poor pregnancy outcome. These studies have 2 important strengths. The first is that they were prospective. By interviewing the pregnant women about their work and lifestyles before they gave birth the investigators were able to eliminate recall bias. By asking about other factors that adversely affect pregnancy and are more likely to occur in working women they were able to adjust for possible confounders. Indeed, after making careful adjustments for confounding variables Klebanoff and associates speculate that unmeasured socioeconomic differences rather than physical activity per se may have been the source of poor pregnancy outcome previously observed in working mothers (2). It is of some interest that a recent case control study of U.S. Army primigravidas demonstrated a 1.75 increased risk of preterm delivery in women with the highest physical activity levels (4). The authors suggest cautious interpretation of their provocative results because of missing data and limitations in their confounder analysis. For a straightforward, astute review of work during pregnancy I recommend Culpepper and Thompson's chapter in *New Perspectives on Prenatal Care* (1).—J.B. Gould, M.D., M.P.H.

References

1. Culpepper L, Thompson JE: Work during pregnancy, in Merkatz IR, Thompson JE (eds): *New Perspectives on Prenatal Care.* New York, Elsevier, 1990, pp 211–234.
2. Klebanoff MA, et al: *Am J Obstet Gynecol* 163:1450, 1990.
3. Ahlborg G Jr, et al: *Int J Epidemiol* 19:90, 1990.
4. Ramirez G, et al: *Am J Perinatol* 80:728, 1990.

Prediction of Risk for Preterm Delivery by Ultrasonographic Measurement of Cervical Length

Andersen HF, Nugent CE, Wanty SD, Hayashi RH (Univ of Michigan, Ann Arbor)

Am J Obstet Gynecol 163:859–867, 1990   3–13

Preterm delivery is said to be more frequent among women with premature cervical effacement. The value of endovaginal sonographic measurement of cervical length was examined in 178 women with singleton gestations and no cervical incompetence who were seen for routine obstetric ultrasonographic examination. One hundred thirteen patients were assessed by 30 weeks' gestation. The probe was manipulated so that the entire cervical canal could be visualized, and estimates of length were made using markers.

Progressive shortening of average cervical length was noted after 30 weeks' gestation. Although a majority of preterm deliveries occurred in patients with below-median length estimates by the endocervical method, abdominal ultrasonographic measurements did not correlate with preterm delivery. Logistic regression analysis showed a significant trend toward a higher risk of preterm birth as endovaginal ultrasonographic cervical length declined (Fig 3–2). An endovaginal ultrasonographic cervical

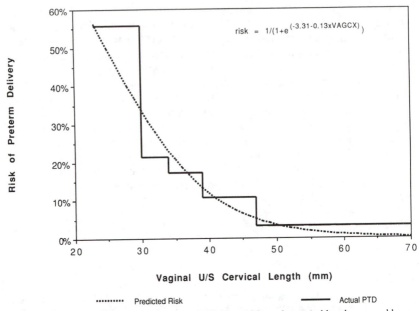

Fig 3–2.—Logistic regression analysis of risk of preterm delivery by cervical length measured by endovaginal ultrasonography. *Solid line,* actual preterm delivery rate; *broken line,* predicted risk by regression equation. (Courtesy of Andersen HF, Nugent CE, Wanty SD, et al: *Am J Obstet Gynecol* 163:859–867, 1990.)

measurement less than 39 mm was associated with a significantly increased risk of preterm delivery (25.0% vs. 6.7%) and detected 76% of preterm births.

There does seem to be a relationship between cervical shortening and preterm delivery, but no optimal cutoff point for predicting the risk is apparent.

▶ Diana Petitti, M.D., Associate Professor, Department of Family and Community Medicine, University of California, San Francisco, offers her insights (and 2 tables) to accompany this selection:

▶ In their population, Andersen et al. find a convincing association between endovaginal ultrasonographic measurement of cervical length and risk of preterm labor. The investigators identify the need for replication before their findings are accepted; this point cannot be emphasized too much. In other populations and in the hands of other examiners, the association may not hold up.

The authors discuss the potential usefulness of endovaginal ultrasonic measurement of cervical length as a screening test to identify women at high risk of preterm labor. Using the median as the cutoff point for labelling a women high risk, the sensitivity and specificity of this measurement as a "test" for preterm labor seem high—76% sensitivity and 59% specificity. However, at this level of sensitivity and specificity, the false positive rate is 78% and the accuracy (true positives plus true negatives) is only 54% in a population with a 15%

Table 1.—Sensitivity, Specificity, False Positive, False Negative and Accuracy Rates for Endovaginal Ultrasonic Measurement of Cervical Length When Cut-Off Point Is the Median

		Truth			
		Pre-term Labor	Not Pre-term	Total	
Test	< median	13	47	60	sensitivity=13/17=76% specificity=48/95=59% false positive rate =47/60=78%
	>= median	4	48	52	false negative rate=4/52=8% accuracy=13+48/112=54%
		17	95	112	

Table 2.—Sensitivity, Specificity, False Positive, False Negative, and Accuracy Rates for Endovaginal Ultrasonic Measurement of Cervical Length When Cut-Off Point Is the 25th Percentile

		Truth			
		Pre-term Labor	Not Pre-term	Total	
Test	< 25th	8	15	23	sensitivity=8/17=47% specificity=80/95=84% false positive rate =15/23=65%
	>= 25th	9	80	89	false negative rate=9/89=10% accuracy=8+80/112=79%
		17	95	112	

rate of preterm labor, the rate in the population studied (Table 1). Put another way, this measurement would label more than half of all women high risk, and more than three quarters of those labelled high risk would deliver normally. In a population with a lower rate of preterm labor, say 10%, the false positive rate would be 86%.

The rate of false positives can be reduced by changing the cutoff point for labelling women high risk from the median to the 25th percentile. This improvement is at the expense of sensitivity—the correct identification of the women who have preterm labor. In their population, only 8 of 17 women with preterm labor would be correctly identified as high risk using the 25th percentile of cervical length as the cutoff point (Table 2).

The relationship between short cervical length and preterm labor is of theoretical interest. Endovaginal ultrasonographic measurement of cervical length appears to have little promise as a general screening tool for preterm labor, because it has a high false positive rate when used at a cutoff point that makes it sensitive.—D. Petitti, M.D..

Randomized Prospective Trial Comparing Ultrasonography and Pelvic Examination for Preterm Labor Surveillance

Lorenz RP, Comstock CH, Bottoms SF, Marx SR (William Beaumont Hosp, Royal Oak, Mich; Hutzel Hosp, Detroit; Wayne State Univ, Detroit)
Am J Obstet Gynecol 162:1603–1610, 1990
3–14

The precocious maturity of the cervix is a significant risk factor for preterm birth. The effectiveness of cervical assessment by either ultrasonography or bimanual examination was evaluated in a program for preterm labor surveillance. All patients were seen weekly for patient education, review of symptoms, and cervical evaluation from 20 to 37 weeks' gestation. Patients at risk for preterm birth (57) were randomly assigned to either ultrasonographic evaluation or pelvic examination; the 2 patient groups did not differ in demographic or obstetric factors.

The overall rate of preterm delivery was 18%. Preterm labor was significantly more frequent in the ultrasonographic group than in the pelvic group (52% vs. 25%). Patients in the ultrasonographic group received tocolytic agents significantly more often than the pelvic group (52% vs. 25%). Infant birth weights, length of gestation, and neonatal morbidity or mortality did not differ significantly between groups.

These data show that patients at risk for preterm birth under surveillance by ultrasonographic assessment of the cervix fared no better than those followed by bimanual examination. Ultrasonography is a less effective tool for early intervention for patients at risk for preterm labor, and may even cause some problems, possibly increased uterine activity secondary to bladder distention required for the procedure.

▶ Notch another victory for the simple versus the complex, high technology approach to a problem. Although this is a prospective randomized trial with a small number of subjects enrolled, power analysis indicated an 80% chance of determining a 2.5 week prolongation of gestation in the ultrasonography group. Multiple outcome variables were studied without observed benefit. Therefore, the authors suggest that the actual power is greater than 80%. It is of little consequence that ultrasound was not superior to bimanual palpation. Repeated ultrasonography was not only not superior, but may, in some manner, have contributed to prematurity.

The distressing aspect of this report is the 18% rate of premature delivery. This is admittedly a high-risk group de novo. However, they are a closely monitored, compliant group of private patients, subjected to early tocolytic therapy. The reasonable expectation would be that the prematurity rate should diminish under these circumstances. The battle to determine those at risk for premature deliveries and the means to intervene on their behalf must be waged with ever-increasing intensity.

Round about what is, lies a whole mysterious world of might be.—Longfellow

A.A. Fanaroff, M.B.B.Ch.

Calcium Supplementation During Pregnancy May Reduce Preterm Delivery in High-Risk Populations

Villar J, Repke JT (Natl Inst of Child Health and Human Development, Bethesda, Md; Johns Hopkins Hosp)
Am J Obstet Gynecol 163:1124–1131, 1990   3–15

Calcium supplementation during pregnancy may lower smooth muscle contractility and tone, leading to lower blood pressure and a decrease risk of premature labor and delivery. This double-blind, placebo-controlled trial assessed the effect of calcium supplementation with 2 g daily of calcium carbonate in healthy parturients aged 17 and under. Most were nulliparous. Eighty-four calcium recipients were compared with 78 women given placebo.

Calcium was given for a mean of about 14 weeks. Dietary calcium intake was comparable in the 2 groups of women. Calcium-treated women had fewer preterm deliveries and fewer low birth weight infants than placebo recipients. These findings persisted after adjusting for compliance with treatment, urinary tract infection, and chlamydial infection.

These findings suggest that this simple intervention be considered for high-risk populations. The effect of calcium supplementation is possibly mediated by changes in the renin-angiotensin system and its interaction with pregnancy-induced hypertension.

▶ When this group went back to the drawing board to find a remedy for the unacceptable prematurity rate, few would have predicted that the suggested remedy would literally be to eat the chalk. Other antidotes had yielded disappointing results and the grass roots programs so successful in France had not led to paydirt in the United States (1). This prospective randomized blinded study has proven calcium supplementation superior to a placebo in preventing prematurity. Although the results were a statistician's delight they must be tempered by the knowledge that this is only the first blush of success. Calcium supplementation must be subjected to a broader multicenter study to confirm its efficacy and determine its mechanism of action. There is a ray of light among the gloom associated with the depressing prematurity rate. The therapy is cheap, readily available, nontoxic, and an essential component of the diet. We look forward to the confirmatory studies and hope that they demonstrate the same outcomes.

The truth is rarely pure, and never simple.—Oscar Wilde

A.A. Fanaroff, M.B.B.Ch.

Reference

1. 1987 YEAR BOOK OF NEONATAL AND PERINATAL MEDICINE, Abstract 3–22.

Risk Factors for Preterm Premature Rupture of Fetal Membranes: A Multicenter Case-Control Study
Harger JH, Hsing AW, Tuomala RE, Gibbs RS, Mead PB, Eschenbach DA, Knox GE, Polk BF (Univ of Pittsburgh; Johns Hopkins Univ; Harvard Univ; Univ of Texas at San Antonio; Univ of Vermont; et al)
Am J Obstet Gynecol 163:130–137, 1990   3–16

Previous studies of risk factors in preterm premature rupture of membranes have been small, uncontrolled, or not specifically focused on risk factors. The role of 41 potential risk factors in a case-control study conducted at 6 tertiary perinatal centers in the United States was reported. The 341 women with preterm membrane rupture at 20 to 36 weeks' gestation were matched with 253 controls for maternal age, gestatonal age, parity, clinic or private patient status, and previous mode of delivery.

Multiple logistic regression analysis showed that 3 variables were independent risk factors for preterm premature membrane rupture: antepartum vaginal bleeding in more than 1 trimester, current cigarette smoking, and previous preterm delivery. Women who still smoked were more than twice as likely to be affected, and those with previous preterm delivery had a 2.5-fold relative risk.

Intense efforts are needed to persuade pregnant women to stop smoking, especially those with a past history of preterm premature rupture of membranes. Close attention also is needed when vaginal bleeding occurs during pregnancy.

▶ It should be apparent to the readers that I have a bias toward selecting multicenter case-control studies and for that matter any well-designed, prospective randomized trials. I seem to wait in vain for earth-shattering information to be discerned from one of these studies. This study took place in 1982/1983 and included diverse populations so that the results would be applicable to a broad spectrum of situations and populations. Extensive data were gathered and a comprehensive analysis was performed. One is left wondering, however, why the analysis took so long and the publication only appeared in 1990? The usual suspects, antepartum vaginal bleeding in more than 1 trimester (odds ratio, 7.4), cigarette smoking (odds ratio, 2.1) and previous preterm delivery (odds ratio, 2.5) emerged from the logistical regression analysis onto the leader board. These were the factors already established in previous studies and no new insights into the problem have really been provided. The deleterious effects of cigarette smoking have been features in the YEAR BOOKS over the past few years (1–3). The message to the pregnant population that cigarettes are bad has not penetrated. Obstetricians are already alerted to women who bleed at any time during pregnancy and previous premature delivery already prompts the team to expect trouble. Further massaging of this data is fruitless. Perhaps the next multicenter case-controlled study will yield a better crop!

There is nothing else but grace and measure,
Richness, quietness and pleasure.— Charles Baudelaire

A.A. Fanaroff, M.B.B.Ch.

References

1. 1990 YEAR BOOK OF NEONATAL AND PERINATAL MEDICINE, Abstract 11–3.
2. 1989 YEAR BOOK OF NEONATAL AND PERINATAL MEDICINE, Abstracts 3–15 and 3–16.
3. 1987 YEAR BOOK OF NEONATAL AND PERINATAL MEDICINE, Abstracts 3–15 and 3–16.

Neonatal Outcome After Prolonged Preterm Rupture of the Membranes

Rotschild A, Ling EW, Puterman ML, Farquharson D (Univ of British Columbia, British Columbia's Children's Hosp, Vancouver)
Am J Obstet Gynecol 162:46–52, 1990

3–17

Prolonged preterm rupture of the membranes is associated with pulmonary hypoplasia and skeletal compression deformities. Because current management protocols for premature membrane rupture dictate a conservative and expectant approach unless evidence of maternal or fetal infection dictates otherwise, the association of oligohydramnios and pulmonary hypoplasia with prolonged premature rupture of membranes becomes increasingly important. Eighty-eight neonates who were born after rupture of the membranes of 7 days or more and onset before 29 weeks' gestation were evaluated to determine the relative importance of perinatal risk factors in predicting pulmonary hypoplasia and severe skeletal deformities.

Pulmonary hypoplasia was present in 14 of the 88 infants (16%). Mean gestational age of the 14 was 26.2 weeks. This group also had high mortality (71%) and higher incidence of skeletal deformities (65%), air leaks (64%), and persistent pulmonary hypertension (43%) (table). There was no pulmonary hypoplasia in any infant with rupture of membranes that occurred after 26 weeks' gestation. Logistic regression analysis showed that gestational age at onset of membrane rupture had a significant effect on the odds that pulmonary hypoplasia would occur in the

Clinical Profile of Infants Born After Rupture of Membranes of 7 Days or More That Occurred Before 29 Weeks' Gestation

	No pulmonary hypoplasia (n = 74)	Pulmonary hypoplasia (n = 14)
Gestational age at birth (wk)*	28.2 ± 2.16 (24-34)	26.2 ± 2.14 (24-31)
Birth weight (gm)*	1191 ± 362 (640-2280)	903 ± 278 (580-1590)
Gestational age at ROM (wk)*	25.1 ± 2.68 (15-28)	20.9 ± 3.17 (16-26)
ROM (days)*	22.4 ± 18.5 (7-126)	38.4 ± 20.9 (8-67)
Oligohydramnios		
Severe	26 (35%)	7 (50%)
Moderate	20 (27%)	5 (36%)
Deformities		
Severe	0 (0%)	5 (36%)
Moderate	9 (12%)	4 (29%)
Pneumothoraces	11 (15%)	9 (64%)
Persistent pulmonary hypertension of the newborn	8 (11%)	6 (43%)
Maternal amnionitis	35 (47%)	8 (57%)
Neonatal infection	4 (5%)	0 (0%)
Small for gestational age	6 (8%)	1 (7%)
Died	8 (11%)	10 (71%)

*Values are mean ± standard deviation (range).
(Courtesy of Rotschild A, Ling EW, Puterman ML, et al: *Am J Obstet Gynecol* 162:46–52, 1990.)

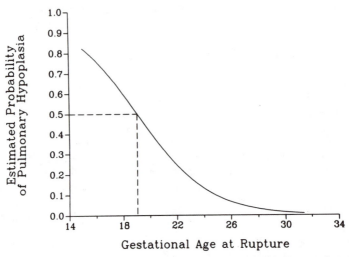

Fig 3–3.—Relationship between gestational age at rupture of membranes, duration of rupture, and pulmonary hypoplasia in 88 infants. (Courtesy of Rotschild A, Ling EW, Puterman ML, et al: *Am J Obstet Gynecol* 162:46–52, 1990.)

neonate, whereas the duration of membrane rupture and degree of oligohydramnios did not. The odds of pulmonary hypoplasia could be estimated on the basis of gestational age at membrane rupture, i.e., the probability of pulmonary hypoplasia at 19 weeks' gestation was .5, compared with only .01 at 31.1 weeks' gestation (Fig 3–3).

There was a strong correlation between the presence of pulmonary hypoplasia and severity of skeletal deformities in neonates. The severity of skeletal deformities was associated significantly with severity of oligohydramnios and duration of membrane rupture, but not with gestational age at onset of membrane rupture.

Gestational age at onset of rupture of membranes is the best single predictor of pulmonary hypoplasia. The stage of lung development may be an important factor in management and outcome of premature rupture of membranes.

▶ Preterm premature rupture of membranes, which complicates 1% of pregnancies, was subjected to meta-analysis in the 1990 NEONATAL AND PERINATAL YEAR BOOK (1). The analysis focused on respiratory distress syndrome. Premature rupture of membranes is featured again this time, emphasizing the problem of pulmonary hypoplasia. Premature rupture of membranes before 26 weeks' gestation would appear to call for another roll of the doom and gloom drum as there is considerable risk for the development of pulmonary hypoplasia. Beyond 26 weeks' the risks for pulmonary hypoplasia are trivial, but if the membranes give way before this time with loss of amniotic fluid, pulmonary development may be arrested. Pulmonary hypoplasia may be strongly suspected in utero if the chest circumference falls below the 5th percentile (sensitivity 88%, specificity 96%) (2). See also Abstract 4–12.—A.A. Fanaroff, M.B.B.Ch.

References

1. 1990 YEAR BOOK OF NEONATAL AND PERINATAL MEDICINE, Abstract 5–2.
2. 1989 YEAR BOOK OF NEONATAL AND PERINATAL MEDICINE, Abstract 1–22.

Pregnancy and Epilepsy
Bag S, Behari M, Ahuja GK, Karmarkar MG (All India Inst of Med Sciences, New Delhi, India)
J Neurol 236:311–313, 1990   3–18

Remember to cure the patient as well as the disease—A. Barach

A comprehensive study of epilepsy and pregnancy showed a doubling of overall risk of complications of pregnancy, labor, and postpartum hemorrhage in women with seizures. Low birth weight, infant mortality rate, and neonatal seizures were also increased in the children of epileptic women.

In a prospective study, 30 pregnant epileptic women were followed to determine how seizures and pregnancy affect each other. Estrogen can lower anticonvulsant drug levels by induction of hepatic enzyme activity, thereby increasing seizure frequency. The correlation of serum hormone and anticonvulsant drug levels with seizure frequency, pregnancy complications, occurrence of status epilepticus, and teratogenicity was also stated.

Seizure frequency increased in 14 of 30 patients, decreased in 1 patient, and remained unchanged in 15. Patients with increased seizure frequency had significantly higher estrogen and lower levels of progesterone and anticonvulsant drugs compared with those with no change in seizures.

Two patients had spontaneous abortions and 2 patients had status epilepticus. Those patients had high serum estrogen levels. One infant of a patient receiving carbamazepine and diphenylhydantoin had a ventricular septal defect.

Patients with an increased seizure frequency have significantly higher estrogen levels and lower progesterone and anticonvulsant drug levels than those without an increase in seizures. As suggested in other studies, the proconvulsant action of estrogen and the anticonvulsant action of progesterone may be contributing factors.

► Seizures before, during, or immediately after pregnancy increase the hazards for both the mother and offspring. Epilepsy complicates 0.3% to 0.5% of all pregnancies with previous seizure disorders, accounting for the minority of convulsions. The most comprehensive information on this disorder was derived from the Collaborative Perinatal Project in which 54,000 pregnant women were followed until their children were 7 years old (1). Complications of pregnancy, labor, and postpartum hemorrhage were doubled in women with seizures, and low birth weight, seizures, and infant mortality rate were increased in the offspring. There is, of course, the added hazard of birth defects related to the anticonvulsants (2,3). The more anticonvulsants used the greater the risk to the fetus. Agents such as valproic acid and hydantoin produce recognizable patterns of malformation. The present study was designed to correlate the frequency of seizures with hormonal changes during pregnancy. It is limited in scope (only 30 patients were followed), but the primary hypothesis is supported by the findings of increased seizures associated with elevated estrogen levels, and lower progesterone and serum anticonvulsant levels. Control of seizures during pregnancy requires close supervision, patient compliance, and careful drug monitoring.—A.A. Fanaroff, M.B.B.Ch.

References

1. Nelson KB, Ellenberg JH: *Neurology* 32:1247, 1982.
2. 1987 Year Book of Neonatal and Perinatal Medicine, Abstract 2–11.
3. 1990 Year Book of Neonatal and Perinatal Medicine, Abstract 2–12.

Intrauterine Growth Is Related to Gestational Pulmonary Function in Pregnant Asthmatic Women
Schatz M, Zeiger RS, Hoffman CP, Kaiser-Permanente Asthma and Pregnancy Study Group (Kaiser-Permanente Med Ctr, San Diego)
Chest 98:389–392, 1990   3–19

Asthmatic mothers reportedly have relatively low weight infants. Relative maternal hypoxia in normal women living at high altitudes reduces birth weights. The relationship of gestational lung function to birth weight in 352 pregnant women with documented asthma was studied. All had singleton births at 20 weeks' gestation or later.

Lower maternal forced expiratory volume in 1 second (FEV_1) during pregnancy was associated with a greater risk of lower birth weight. An FEV_1 of 90% of predicted normal was the most discriminating value; women with lower values were 2.5 times likelier to have an infant with a low ponderal index. Smoking was associated with lower birth weight but not with ponderal index.

It is especially important for asthmatic women to stop smoking when pregnant. Attempts should be made to optimize lung function during pregnancy. Raising the FEV_1 to at least 90% of predicted normal is a reasonable goal.

▶ Several small surprises in this large study of asthmatic women. First, there was a correlation ($P < .04$) between infant birth weight and mean percent predicted FEV_1 during pregnancy but it was small (r = .11) and independent of the severity of asthma. Second, asthma did not increase the incidence of prematurity or low birth weight infants (<2,500 g). Overall, asthma in mothers appears to have only a minimal effect on the growth of the fetus.—M.H. Klaus, M.D.

Estimation of the Risk of Thrombocytopenia in the Offspring of Pregnant Women With Presumed Immune Thrombocytopenic Purpura
Samuels P, Bussel JB, Braitman LE, Tomaski A, Druzin ML, Mennuti MT, Cines DB (Univ of Pennsylvania; Cornell Univ, New York)
N Engl J Med 323:229–235, 1990

3–20

Physicians still debate the optimal management of immune thrombocytopenic purpura during pregnancy. The risk of severe neonatal thrombocytopenia remains uncertain. The risk of neonatal thrombocytopenia and hemorrhage was estimated in infants born to mothers with immune thrombocytopenic purpura or presumed immune thrombocytopenic purpura. Whether platelet-antibody testing and maternal history of the condition are useful in identifying neonates at risk for thrombocytopenia were determined.

Pregnancy outcome in 162 women was studied. Two material features predicted a low risk of severe neonatal thrombocytopenia: the absence of a history of immune thrombocytopenic purpura before pregnancy and the absence of circulating platelet antibodies in women with a history of the condition. Eighteen 88 (20%) of the neonates born to women with a history of immune thrombocytopenic purpura had severe thrombocytopenia compared with none of the 74 born to women who first had thrombocytopenia during pregnancy. Eighteen of the 70 (26%) neonates born to women with a history of immune thrombocytopenic purpura with circulating platelet antibodies had severe thrombocytopenia. None of the babies born to women with a positive history but without circulating antibodies had this condition. Thus, the absence of a history of immune thrombocytopenic purpura or the presence of negative results on circulating-antibody tests in pregnant women means that the risk of severe neonatal thrombocytopenia in their infants is minimal.

▶ The guidelines for the management of pregnancies complicated by maternal idiopathic thrombocytopenia continue to evolve. There remain many options with regard to antenatal and intrapartum assessment and treatment. These include maternal antenatal steroid or intravenous immunoglobulin administration, fetal platelet counts before or during labor, and delivery by cesarean section. Highlights, if not quite clinical pearls, emerge from this publication as follows. There is only weak correlation between levels of maternal IgG, IgM, and C3 antiglobulin tests and neonatal platelet counts. Additionally, no single maternal platelet count serves as a threshold to identify thrombocytopenic fetuses at birth. All newborns with significantly low platelet counts on the day of delivery were born to mothers with an onset of immune thrombocytopenia documented before pregnancy. Although only 20% of fetuses will be affected, the risk for the fetus in subsequent pregnancies approximates 85%. There is minimal risk to the fetus of the mother who is first diagnosed during the current pregnancy. With regard to delivery, if circulating platelet antibodies are detected in pregnant women with a previous diagnosis of immune thrombocytopenia, then fetal platelet counts must be ascertained or delivery by cesarean section is recommended. The goals of minimizing invasive diagnostic procedures on the fetus, without rendering undue risk, can be accomplished taking the above data into consideration (1,2).

This life so short, the craft so long to learn.—Hippocrates

A.A. Fanaroff, M.B.B.Ch

References

1. 1989 YEAR BOOK OF NEONATAL AND PERINATAL MEDICINE, Abstract 1–3.
2. 1990 YEAR BOOK OF NEONATAL AND PERINATAL MEDICINE, Abstract 13–7.

Fetal Platelet Counts in Thrombocytopenic Pregnancy
Kaplan C, Daffos F, Forestier F, Tertian G, Catherine N, Pons JC, Tchernia G
(Inst National de Transfusion Sanguine, Paris; Institut de Puériculture, Paris;
Hôpital Beclère, Clamart)
Lancet 336:979–982, 1990   3–21

Unlike scalp sampling, percutaneous umbilical blood sampling (PUBS) can be performed, and repeated if necessary, during pregnancy without risk of precipitating labor. The fetal and maternal obstetric management of maternal chronic immune thrombocytopenia (ITP) is not clear. Fetal platelet counts were assessed by PUBS in 64 pregnancies in 62 women with maternal thrombocytopenia.

In 33 pregnancies associated with maternal chronic ITP, thrombocytopenia was present at term in 11 fetuses, including 4 with severe thrombocytopenia (plate count $<50 \times 10^9/l$). In the other 31 pregnancies, associated with symptomless maternal thrombocytoepnia (platelet count $<150 \times 10^9/l$) as an incidental finding, thrombocytopenia was present in 4 fetuses, including 1 with severe thrombocytopenia. In both groups, neither maternal platelet count nor antiplatelet antibodies correlated with fetal status. There was no apparent benefit of maternal corticosteroid therapy or intravenous immunoglobulin treatment. There was a good correlation between neonatal platelet counts and those obtained by PUBS. There were no maternal or fetal complications during PUBS.

Percutaneous umbilical blood sampling is a safe procedure and provides accurate platelet counts in thrombocytopenic pregnancies. All pregnant women with a history of ITP and women with moderate to severe thrombocytopenia of unknown origin, especially if detected early in pregnancy, should undergo near-term PUBS because fetuses in both groups are at risk for thrombocytopenia. Late PUBS is advocated to avoid the harzards of fetal scalp sampling and reduce the number of cesarean sections in thrombocytopenic women.

▶ How to manage these infants continues to be an enigma. Maternal indices do not help predict what was happening in the fetus, and for the fetus of a woman with known ITP neither intravenous gamma globulin nor maternal steroids was effective in altering the course. The authors believe that early-in-gestation cord sampling is dangerous to the fetus, and they recommend that it be limited to a very small population of women who are undergoing therapeutic trials or are being managed by a group very skilled in fetal cord sampling. To reduce the rate of cesarean sections in these mothers they suggest that near term a platelet count on the fetus be determined from a cord sample. Though there are no sure ways to prevent bleeding in these infants the authors' approach to the problem is reasonable.—M.H. Klaus, M.D.

Chronic Renal Disease and Pregnancy Outcome

Cunningham FG, Cox SM, Harstad TW, Mason RA, Pritchard JA (Univ of Texas Southwestern Med Ctr at Dallas)
Am J Obstet Gynecol 163:453–459, 1990   3–22

From 1971 through 1988, 37 women whose pregnancies were complicated by chronic renal insufficiency were followed prospectively. Of these, 26 had moderate renal insufficiency and 11 had severe renal insufficiency. The maternal, fetal, and perinatal outcomes in these women were examined.

Common maternal complications included anemia, chronic hypertension, and preeclampsia. Renal function deteriorated in 5 patients with moderate renal insufficiency and in 1 patient with severe renal insufficiency. These patients were followed for a mean of 5 years after delivery; all were chronically hypertensive and 4 required dialysis at a mean of 30 months after delivery. In addition, of 7 patients with stable renal function during pregnancy, 6 showed deterioration of renal function at a mean of 39 months after delivery. Blood volume expansion in women with moderate renal disease was normal, whereas women with severe disease had significantly attenuated expansion. Serial creatinine clearances did not increase during pregnancy in half the women with moderate insufficiency and none with severe renal disease.

There were 30 liveborn infants, and 6 pregnancies either aborted spontaneously or were electively terminated before 26 weeks' gestation. The only perinatal mortality was limited to 1 third-trimester fetal death. Preterm delivery complicated 13 of 32 (40%) pregnancies. Compared with women with severe renal insufficiency, those with moderate renal insufficiency were more likely to have live births (88% vs. 64%) and to have a lower incidence of fetal growth retardation (35% vs. 43%) and preterm delivery (30% vs. 86%). Mean birth weight in the moderate renal disease group was 2,500 g and in the severe renal disease group, it was 1,520 g. Birth weights correlated inversely with maternal serum creatinine concentration (Fig 3–4).

Pregnancy in women with moderate to severe renal insufficiency is commonly complicated by chronic hypertension, preeclampsia, and anemia. Perinatal complications include midpregnancy losses and low birth weight from preterm delivery, fetal growth retardation, or both. Despite

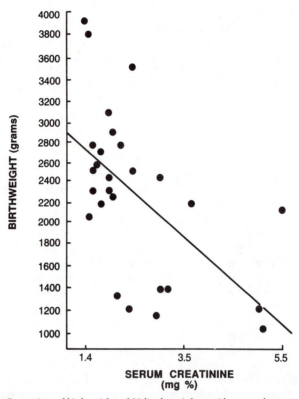

Fig 3–4.—Comparison of birth weights of 29 live-born infants with maternal serum creatinine concentrations (Spearman correlation coefficient = −.6252; P = .001). (Courtesy of Cunningham FG, Cox SM, Harstad TW, et al: *Am J Obstet Gynecol* 163:453–459, 1990.)

the high incidence of maternal morbidity, adverse perinatal outcome is not prohibitive.

▶ This report is useful to review when caring for patients with chronic renal disease. Though the infants of mothers with moderate disease (creatine 1.5 to 2.5 mg/dL) do reasonably well with a survival rate of 85%, a significant number of mothers in both the moderate and severe groups progress to renal failure requiring dialysis within a few years. Preeclampsia was also a common problem for women with chronic hypertension. Sadly, there is as yet no magic treatment for these women.—M.H. Klaus, M.D.

Vascular Malformations and Pregnancy
Sadasivan B, Malik GM, Lee C, Ausman JI (Henry Ford Hosp, Detroit)
Surg Neurol 33:305–313, 1990   3–23

The presence of a ruptured or unruptured arteriovenous malformation complicates the management of pregnancy. Pregnancy also affects the natural history of this malformation, making hemorrhage more likely.

Of 240 patients with cerebral vascular malformations seen between 1975 and 1989, 16 were pregnant. Eleven women had hemorrhage, 4 had seizures, and 1 had hydrocephalus. No maternal or fetal deaths occurred in the group with seizure or hydrocephalus. Among those with hemorrhage, 2 women and 1 fetus died. In the group with seizure or hydrocephalus, pregnancy was brought to term and obstetric indications were used to determine the method and time of delivery. The woman with hydrocephalus was treated by shunting, and the women with seizures were treated with medication. Antiepileptic drug levels were closely monitored to ensure therapeutic levels.

Vascular malformation is the most common cause of subarachnoid hemorrhage in pregnant women. The risk of rebleeding in the same pregnancy is approximately 27%. Emergency surgery is warranted if an arteriovenous malformation ruptures during pregnancy and the woman's condition deteriorates. In stable patients, pregnancy can be brought to term. The arteriovenous malformation can then be electively excised through a craniotomy.

▶ It is difficult with available data to decide when to do elective surgery to excise an arteriovenous malformation. It is also unclear whether labor increases the risk of hemorrhage. Since a third of pregnant women have markedly elevated cerebrospinal fluid pressures during labor, the authors believe it is probably safer to deliver by elective cesarean section. This report was included as a reference because rupture of a vascular malformation during pregnancy is the third most frequent nonobstetric cause for maternal death.—M.H. Klaus, M.D.

Perinatal Outcome of Forty-Nine Pregnancies Complicated by Acardiac Twinning
Moore TR, Gale S, Benirschke K (Univ of California, San Diego)
Am J Obstet Gynecol 163:907–912, 1990   3–24

Acardiac twinning affects 1 in 100 monozygotic twin pregnancies and 1 in 35,000 pregnancies overall. An acardiac twin requires the normal or "pump" twin to provide circulation for both. Pulsed Doppler examination has shown reversed flow through the umbilical artery of the acardiac twin. Acardiac twinning is associated with almost 50% mortality caused by prematurity and the occurrence of hydramnios and congestive heart failure in the pump-twin. This study comprises a database of 49 perinatal outcomes for pregnancies with acardiac twinning.

Outcome is associated with a favorable twin-weight ratio with the normal twin larger (Fig 3–5). Frequently, however, the acardiac twin may be equal size or larger than the normal twin. A high ratio of acardiac to normal twin weight was associated with higher risk of preterm delivery and other complications in the pump-twin. In cases of twin-weight ratios

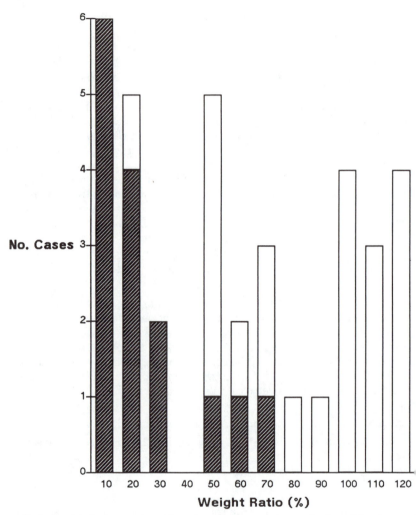

Fig 3–5.—Acardiac/pump-twin weight ratio and occurrence of congestive heart failure in pump twin. *Open bars* are cases with pump-twin congestive heart failure. Weight ratio is acardiac weight expressed as percentage of pump-twin weight. (Courtesy of Moore TR, Gale S, Benirschke K: *Am J Obstet Gynecol* 163:907–912, 1990.)

of greater than 50%, the frequencies of hydramnios, pump-twin congestive heart failure, and prematurity were 44%, 25%, and 94% compared with 18%, 0%, and 35% when the ratio was less than 50%.

Because half of acardiac twinning cases result in fetal death, optimal management may be aided by the prognostic measure of twin-weight ratio. Forecasting problems with preterm delivery, hydramnios, and congestive heart failure in the pump-twin may be helpful in counseling patients and managing cases.

▶ Though this is an uncommon problem it is valuable to inspect this report closely to determine how the high mortality rate can be possibly reduced, especially when the acardiac twin is large and close in weight to the viable twin. To improve mortality it is necessary to not mistake the acardiac twin for a twin who has died. Pulsed Doppler should be checked if these conditions are suspected to check for reverse flow through the umbilical artery. If the acardiac mass is relatively small (less than 25% of normal twin weight) the authors suggest conservative management. The special skills available in some units for fetal surgical interventions such as umbilical ligation should be strongly considered when the acardiac twin is large.—M.H. Klaus, M.D.

Foreign-Born and US-Born Black Women: Differences in Health Behaviors and Birth Outcomes
Cabral H, Fried LE, Levenson S, Amaro H, Zuckerman B (Boston Univ)
Am J Public Health 80:70–72, 1990   3–25

In the United States black neonates are at high risk of low birth weight and increased perinatal mortality, but the rate of low birth weight among foreign-born black women is two-thirds that of black women born in the United States. From a sample of 1,226 women who attended prenatal clinics of Boston City Hospital, 201 foreign-born and 616 U.S. born black women were studied to determine health behaviors and birth outcome.

Foreign-born black women had better prepregnancy nutritional status and more prenatal care visits than those born in the United States. In addition, they were less likely to smoke cigarettes, drink alcohol, or use street drugs during pregnancy. Infants of foreign-born black women had greater intrauterine growth, even after controlling for factors known to affect fetal growth.

Low-income black women in this community are not a homogeneous group in terms of prenatal risk and birth outcome. The findings suggest that culture and ethnicity should be considered when studying the relationship between maternal prenatal health behaviors and birth outcomes.

▶ This report does not solve the continuing puzzle of why black mothers have an increased perinatal mortality rate and prematurity rate but it does give some hints. Even after correcting for the older age, better education, greater number of prenatal visits, and less alcohol, marijuana, cocaine, and opiate use during pregnancy, the foreign-born women had heavier babies. Is it possibly related to malnutrition in mothers and grandmothers of these women? Studies of chronic starvation continued over several generations in animals with short gestations reveal that it requires many generations of adequate nutrition to achieve premalnutrition birth weights. Is it possible that black mothers will require several generations of adequate nutrition to decrease perinatal mortality?—M.H. Klaus, M.D.

The Association of Maternal Floor Infarction of the Placenta With Adverse Perinatal Outcome

Andres RL, Kuyper W, Resnik R, Piacquadio KM, Benirschke K (Univ of California, San Diego)
Am J Obstet Gynecol 163:935–938, 1990   3–26

Maternal floor infarction of the placenta is fairly rare. On gross examination, this disorder is characterized by a thickened gray-yellow maternal floor of the placenta with histologic evidence of massive fibrin deposition involving the decidua basalis and contiguous villi. The lesion, thought to be recurrent, has been linked to fetal death, preterm delivery, and intrauterine growth retardation. The association of this disorder with adverse perinatal outcomes was further investigated.

Forty-eight women had maternal floor infarction a total of 60 times. Fetal death occurred in 24 (40%) of the 60 cases. Of 36 liveborn infants, 21 (58.3%) were preterm. Fifty-four percent of the 35 liveborn infants for whom a birth weight was known showed evidence of intrauterine growth retardation. Of the 41 multiparous women in this series, 5 had documented recurrences. A review of the reproductive histories of the 48 women (196 pregnancies) revealed a significant incidence of fetal death, intrauterine growth retardation, and preterm death in 24.1%, 31.3%, and 35.4% of pregnancies, respectively.

The association between maternal floor infarction and fetal death emphasizes the importance of a placental examination in all cases of fetal death and intrauterine growth retardation. Because there is a risk of recurrence, the identification of maternal floor infarction should alert clinicians to the potential for fetal death, preterm birth, and growth retardation in later pregnancies.

▶ Commentary on this selection is provided by R.A. Williams, M.D., Chairman, Pathology Department, Children's Hospital Oakland, and Associate Professor of Pathology, University of California, San Francisco.

▶ This article clearly identifies the importance of recognizing maternal floor infarction of the placenta with its very frequent associations of fetal demise, premature birth, and intrauterine growth retardation, not only to provide an explanation of an unfavorable outcome of a particular pregnancy, but also because of the significant risk of recurrence of this condition in subsequent pregnancies. Unfortunately, not all obstetric hospitals have the policy of routinely examining all placentas from pregnancies with fetal demise, premature birth, or intrauterine growth retardation (1). It is also unfortunate that maternal floor infarction of the placenta is not widely recognized by pathologists, with the exception of those having special training or experience in perinatal pathology, and the condition is often overlooked or ignored even when the placenta is examined. Placental examination is essential in patients whose pregnancies have been complicated by these conditions so that appropriate antepartum management of subsequent pregnancies can improve their chances for a favorable outcome.— R.A. Williams, M.D.

Reference

1. Boyd PA, in Keeling JW (ed): *Fetal and Neonatal Pathology.* London, Springer-Verlag, 1987, p 45.

Hyperammonemia in Women With a Mutation at the Ornithine Carbamoyltransferase Locus: A Cause of Postpartum Coma

Arn PH, Hauser ER, Thomas GH, Herman G, Hess D, Brusilow SW (Nemours Children's Clin, Jacksonville, Fla; Johns Hopkins Univ; John F Kennedy Inst, Baltimore; Baylor Univ, Houston; Med Coll of Georgia, Augusta)
N Engl J Med 322:1652–1655, 1990   3–27

Ornithine carbamoyltransferase deficiency is an X-linked disorder of urea synthesis. The clinical and biochemical consequences of heterozygosity in women have not been studied systematically. The cases of 5 apparently healthy women who went into coma and who proved to be carriers of a mutation at the ornithine carbomyltransferase locus are described. In addition, plasma ammonium, amino acid, and urea levels in 16 additional asymptomatic women who are carriers of a mutant ornithine carbamoyltransferase allele were compared to those of 18 normal women of similar age.

Six episodes of coma occurred in 5 apparently healthy women who

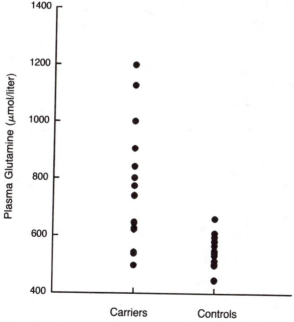

Fig 3–6.—Plasma glutamine levels in 16 controls and in 16 women with a mutation at the ornithine carbamoyltransferase locus. (Courtesy of Arn PH, Hauser ER, Thomas GH, et al: *N Engl J Med* 322:1652–1655, 1990.)

proved to be carriers of a mutant ornithine carbamoyltransferase allele. Four of the episodes occurred 3 to 8 days postpartum. The other 2 episodes occurred in women who had not recently given birth and were not associated with a clearly defined precipitating event. All 5 women had 1 or more signs and symptoms characteristic of the hyperammonemia that occurs in men affected by ornithine carbamoyltransferase deficiency, including nausea, vomiting, lethargy, confusion, ataxia, seizures, decorticate and decerebrate posturing, and cerebral edema. Two women had respiratory alkalosis. Hyperammonemia promptly decreased in 3 women treated with intravenous sodium benzoate, sodium phenylacetate, and arginine hydrochloride. Two women died.

Compared with noncarriers, asymptomatic carriers of the mutant allele had significantly increased plasma glutamine and ammonium levels (Fig 3–6) and lower plasma arginine and citrulline levels.

Female carriers of a mutant ornithine carbamoyltransferase allele are at risk for episodes of hyperammonemic coma. The relationship between the biochemical abnormalities and the risk of hyperammonemia and the effect of these biochemical abnormalities on the fetus are not known.

▶ J.J. Irias, M.D., Director of Endocrinology at Children's Hospital Oakland, California, provides the following comment.

▶ Two of the 5 symptomatic patients described here initially received a psychiatric diagnosis (postpartum depression; postpartum emotional adjustment). This underscores the fact that presenting findings for such conditions are not highly specific and that eternal vigilance is the price of early (or even correct) diagnosis. Examples of pitfalls for the unwary have included postpartum thyroid dysfunction (1–3) and drug toxicity (4).

In light of the present report, the clinician evaluating a puerpera whose symptoms have been assigned an emotional cause needs to be alert for signs of cerebral cortical dysfunction. A request for blood ammonia levels (or ammonium, if you want to be pKy) may need to come sooner rather than later if such signs are noted because treatment is obviously efficacious if provided promptly.

Awareness of this possibility is important, even though the condition would probably be quite unlikely in the absence of suggestive family or past medical history. Dr. Brusilow (personal communication) thinks that 1 in 25,000 women may carry 1 or the other mutation of the gene for ornithine carbamoyltransferase. If the findings in the 16 women studied are representative, two thirds, or a little more than 1 in 40,000 women, might exhibit a high plasma glutamine concentration; but only a (probably small) fraction of that group would be at risk for a clinically significant metabolic derangement.—J.J. Irias, M.D.

References

1. Amino N, et al: *N Engl J Med* 306:849, 1982.
2. Stewart DE, et al: *Am J Psychiatry* 145:1579, 1988.
3. Gerstein HC: *Arch Intern Med* 150:1397, 1990.
4. Iffy L, et al: *Obstet Gynecol* 73:475, 1989.

Effects of Clonidine on Breathing Movements and Electrocortical Activity in the Fetal Lamb
Bamford OS, Hawkins RL, Blanco CE (Univ of Maryland Hosp, Baltimore)
Am J Obstet Gynecol 163:661–668, 1990   3–28

Clonidine, an α_2-adrenergic agonist, has been used extensively as an antihypertensive during pregnancy, but there are few data on its effects on the fetus. The effects of high central concentrations of clonidine were studied in chronically prepared fetal lambs in utero. Clonidine was infused into a fetal lateral cerebral ventricle for up to 24 hours at 128 to 135 days' gestation. In control studies, artificial cerebrospinal fluid was infused. Fetal breathing, nuchal electromyogram, electrocortical activity, arterial pressure, heart rate, and arterial blood gases were recorded.

Clonidine infusion significantly reduced the incidence and episode duration of fetal breathing for the duration of the infusion period. Prolonged postinfusion hyperpnea also occurred. Clonidine infusion altered the normal regular cycling of fetal electrocortical activity states. The incidence and episode duration of high-voltage electrocortical activity were significantly reduced during clonidine infusion, and the incidence of high-voltage electrocortical activity remained significantly low over the 10-hour postinfusion period. Clonidine infusion was associated with an inhibition of nuchal muscle activity and a fall in heart rate but fetal arterial pressure and blood gases were not affected.

These findings confirm previous reports that clonidine effectively inhibits fetal breathing by a direct action on the brain stem. Because fetal breathing promotes lung development, long-term use of clonidine during pregnancy could slow pulmonary development. Until further information is available, clonidine should be used with caution during pregnancy.

▶ Offering his thoughts on this selection is David J. Durand, M.D., neonatologist at Children's Hospital Oakland, California.

▶ This study confirms 2 known factors. The first is that fetal breathing is controlled by a complex balance of factors, not all of which are active in the infant or adult. It now appears that central noradrenergic mechanisms have a potent effect on control of breathing in the fetus, unlike in the newborn where they have no effect.

The second is that medications administered to the pregnant mother may have potent and unsuspected effects on the fetus. We are continually reminded that the fetus is an unusual creature, and that extrapolating from the pharmacology of drugs in the adult to the fetus is a hazardous enterprise.—D.J. Durand, M.D.

Inconsistencies in Clinical Decisions in Obstetrics
Barrett JFR, Jarvis GJ, MacDonald HN, Buchan PC, Tyrrell SN, Lilford RJ (St James's Univ Hosp, Leeds, England)
Lancet 336:549–551, 1990   3–29

Proportion (Percent) of Cesarean Sections for Various
Indications in 1975, 1980, and 1985

Indication for caesarean section	1975	1980	1985
Emergency sections			
Fetal distress	27	37	56
FTP	34	26	16·3
Cord prolapse	8·6	7·7	2·8
Other	30·4	29·3	24·9
Elective sections			
Previous section	31	40·3	36·6
Breech	15	9·7	25·8
CPD	21·3	8·6	9·4
Placenta praevia	10	5·7	7·7
Other	22·7	35·7	20·5

Abbreviations: FTP, failure to progress; *CPD*, cephalopelvic disproportion.
(Courtesy of Barrett JFR, Jarvis GJ, MacDonald HN, et al: *Lancet* 336:549–551, 1990.)

From 1975 to 1985, the incidence of cesarean section increased dramatically from 5% to 13.6% in an English teaching hospital, with fetal distress accounting for most of these procedures (table). A retrospective audit of a sample of these cesarean sections was undertaken to determine whether audit may reduce the intrapartum section rate. The records of 50 patients who underwent emergency intrapartum cesarean section for fetal distress were reviewed by 1 professor, 3 health service consultants, and 1 senior registrar training in perinatology. Of these, the records of 40 patients were reviewed again at intervals of 3 months to 3 years by the assessors. Interobserver and intraobserver consistency in management decision were measured.

At least 4 of the 5 assessors indicated that 30% of the cesarean operations were unnecessary. The assessors were unanimous in agreeing or disagreeing with the original decision in only 28% of patients. In patients in whom the auditors disagreed with the actual management, the auditors recommended fetal pH measurements instead of immediate section in 38% of patients. When faced with identical information at a different time, the auditors were inconsistent in 25% of patients.

The most important findings in this study were the wide interobserver and intraobserver inconsistencies in decisions of management in obstetrics. Attempts to reduce an increasing cesarean section rate by audit must begin with a self-audit on the part of the assessors. These findings may have clinical implications for medical jurisprudence.

▶ The words of the song, "Who takes care of the caretaker while the caretaker is busy taking care," echoed through my mind as I perused this manuscript. I was not surprised by the initial finding of the panel that there was an excessive number of operative deliveries. Nor should I have been surprised by the fact that the perinatal trainee was most critical of the decisions to operate and disagreed 52% of the time. I was not, however, prepared for the inconsistency of the panelists, so that when presented with the same scenario they arrived at the same conclusion only between 60% and 82.5% of the time. These were in general very experienced personnel; the issue under consideration was not complex and I anticipated more internal consistency. As fetal distress was the main indication for cesarean section we must conclude that the criteria for defining fetal distress are fuzzy and precise definitions are urgently needed. As chart audits play a major role in litigation, the implications of this audit should have far-reaching consequences in the medicolegal arena. How consistent are these so-called medical experts? We can only speculate! Strikingly, at the time of re-review 3 cases were under litigation in the United Kingdom, a relatively nonlitiginous society. I shudder to think how many more would be snaking their way through the courts in the United States.

We do not wish to be better than we are, but more fully what we are.—V.S. Pritchett

A.A. Fanaroff, M.B.B.Ch.

Evaluation of Birth Defect Histories Obtained Through Maternal Interviews
Rasmussen SA, Mulinare J, Khoury MJ, Maloney EK (Univ of Florida, Gainesville; Ctr for Environmental Health and Injury Control, Ctrs for Disease Control, Atlanta; Computer Services Corp, Huntsville)
Am J Hum Genet 46:478–485, 1990   3–30

Studies on the genetic epidemiology of birth defects often rely on family history information provided by parents or other family members. To determine the accuracy of this information, the sensitivity, specificity, and positive predictive value (PPV) of mothers' responses regarding the presence of birth defects in their offspring were evaluated relative to data from the Atlanta Birth Defects Case-Control study. Mothers of 4,929 infants with major structural defects listed in the Metropolitan Atlanta Congenital Defects Program registry for 1968 to 1980 and mothers of 3,029 normal infants were interviewed via telephone as to whether their infants had birth defects or health problems diagnosed during the first year of life. Maternal responses were then compared with information abstracted from medical records.

The overall sensitivity, specificity, and PPVs of maternal responses on birth defect histories were 61%, 98%, and 47%, respectively. Factors that affected the mothers' ability to recall the presence and type of birth defects were maternal race, maternal education, maternal age, and length of time between birth and interview. Mothers who were white, 25 years of age or older, college educated, and/or whose infants were born during the earlier years of the study were most likely to correctly report the presence of a major defect. Type of birth defect was the most important determinant in the sensitivity of maternal responses. The information obtained from mothers about birth defects in their offspring may cause errors in studies of familial aggregation of birth defects if it is not properly invalidated.

▶ It is surprising what is not remembered. How selective our memory is for difficult events. The malformations that were not recalled were more often less serious, treated shortly after birth with good results, or discovered in a stillborn infant. It is hard to believe that if only the mother was questioned without exploring the medical records 21% of infants with major birth defects were missed. It would be useful to explore why this discrepancy occurred. Was it maternal denial, repression, or an inability to understand what the physician described? We should ask all parents to tell back to us what we have told them.—M.H. Klaus, M.D.

Maternal Depressive Symptoms During Pregnancy, and Newborn Irritability
Zuckerman B, Bauchner H, Parker S, Cabral H (Boston Univ)
J Dev Behav Pediatr 11:190–194, 1990   3–31

As early as 3 months postpartum, maternal depression is associated with less optimal infant behaviors and mother-infant interactions. Whether maternal depression during pregnancy contributes to neonatal neurobehavioral function and results in less optimal interactions seen in

---

Relationship Between Behavioral Variables and CES-D* Score

	N[†]	Mean CES–D Score (SD)	p Value
Consolability			
Unconsolable (score = 0,1)	91	23.1 (11.7)	
Consolable (score = 2)	828	18.2 (10.4)	0.001
Crying			
Absent/weak (score = 0,1)	71	18.2 (9.3)	
Normal (score = 2)	935	18.4 (10.6)	0.01
Excessive (score = 3)	91	21.9 (12.4)	
Alertness			
Poorly alert (score = 0,1)	225	19.3 (10.2)	
Alert (score = 2)	853	18.5 (10.8)	0.36

*Abbreviation: CES-D, Center for Epidemiologic Studies-Depression Scale.
†Ns vary for the different items because not all items completed for all infants.
(Courtesy of Zuckerman B, Bauchner H, Parker S, et al: *J Dev Behav Pediatr* 11:190–194, 1990.)

early life was determined. The study population consisted of 1,123 mothers and their term infants.

The Center for Epidemiologic Studies-Depression (CES-D) questionnaire for depressive symptoms was administered to the women during pregnancy. Infants were assessed by a pediatrician blind to the maternal CES-D scores. Higher maternal CES-D scores were associated with newborn unconsolability and excessive crying (table). Mothers with CES-D scores in the 90th percentile were 2.6 times more likely to have unconsolable newborns compared with women with CES-D scores at the 10th percentile.

Neurobehavioral functioning in the newborn could be affected by maternal depression in 2 ways. Maternal hormonal changes associated with depression could affect the newborn directly. Poor maternal health behaviors could also adversely affect newborn behavior more than women with CES-D scores in the 10th percentile. In this study, when poor maternal health factors were controlled, the relationship between CES-D score and newborn unconsolability and excessive crying remained the same.

Even before birth, a cycle of depressive symptoms in pregnancy may lead to infant irritability that leads to maternal depression.

▶ The question raised by this report is, what is the mechanism by which maternal emotions are transmitted to the fetus? The authors suggest 3 alternatives; first, a confounding variable not measured; second, maternal hormones such as catecholamines that would be transmitted across the placenta from mother to infant; and last, the early interaction of the depressed mother with her infant on the first day of life before the neonatal assessment. A clue may come from the work of Sontag at the Fell Institute in Yellow Springs, Ohio, who over 40 years ago noted that anxious women near term had fetuses with increased movement and a significantly increased fetal heart rate when compared to fetuses of nonanxious women.—M.H. Klaus, M.D.

The Validation of the Edinburgh Post-Natal Depression Scale on a Community Sample

Murray L, Carothers AD (Univ of Cambridge, England; Med Research Council Human Genetics Unit, Edinburgh)
Br J Psychiatry 157:288–290, 1990   3–32

Postnatal depression may exist in as many as 10% to 15% of women after childbirth, but it is often undetected. To address this problem a recently developed 10-item self-report questionnaire, the Edinburgh Postnatal Depression Scale (EPDS), was mailed to 702 women from the Cambridge City area when their infants were aged 6 weeks. An attempt was made to validate the use of the EPDS in a large representative sample. Ninety-two percent (646) of the women completed the questionnaire and agreed to continue the study. Those with scores of 13 or above and a sampling of those with scores below 12 were interviewed by a psychiatrist or psychologist who did not know the EPDS score at the time of the interview. After the interview any episodes of depression were classified as major or minor.

The results of this study were summarized in a table of EPDS thresholds and their corresponding values of specificity, sensitivity, and positive predictive value, based on logistic regression analysis. For example, a threshold of 12.5 correctly identified more than 80% of mothers with major depression and about 50% of those with minor depression, and it produced a sample in which about two thirds of the women were depressed.

These data give values for sensitivity and positive predictive value that are lower than those in 2 previous studies. It is believed that the previous findings were overestimates and that the results reported here give accurate guidelines for health care workers.

▶ Postnatal depression as a topic for discussion and medical detection has sadly been neglected by U.S. caretakers, leaving families and mothers to fend for themselves. Postnatal depression is separated from the baby blues that occur shortly after birth in the majority of women and the much rarer postnatal psychosis occurring in 1 of 1,000 births. About 11% to 15% of women suffer from postpartum depression 6 to 20 weeks after delivery, with symptoms of difficulty with sleeping and eating, crying periods, and often multiple difficulties with parenting. It is most important to recognize early because the depression can usually be quickly treated and the major disturbances in child development prevented.

This depression scale requires only a few minutes to fill out and appears ideal for a pediatric office. Using this simple tool, the physician can quickly assess the most important environmental aspect of an infant's life. If he finds a patient with postnatal depression it can be corrected with psychologic help. Usually, only 5 to 6 visits are required and drug therapy is usually not the first line of treatment.—M.H. Klaus, M.D.

The Prevalence of Illicit-Drug or Alcohol Use During Pregnancy and Discrepancies in Mandatory Reporting in Pinellas County, Florida
Chasnoff IJ, Landress HJ, Barrett ME (Northwestern Univ, Chicago; Operation PAR, St Petersburg, Fla; Addictions Research Inst of Illinois, Chicago)
N Engl J Med 322:1202–1208, 1990   3–33

Earlier estimates of the frequency with which illicit drugs and alcohol were used by pregnant women have been dependent on information collected in hospital-based populations before, at the time of, or after delivery. Furthermore, the majority of hospitals involved in such studies have served urban populations comprising mostly minority-group individuals of relatively low socioeconomic status.

A population-based study of the prevalence of illicit drug and alcohol use was carried out in pregnant women receiving prenatal care in Pinellas County, Florida, either at public health clinics or in private obstetric offices. Pinellas County is an urbanized area with a population of 860,000.

Its population has increased approximately 18% per year since the 1980 census. The minority population increased 25% during the same period. About 27% of all county residents are aged 65 years or older, 55% are between 18 and 64, and 18% are 17 or younger.

In March 1987 a statewide policy was adopted in Florida that necessitated the reporting of births to women who used drugs or alcohol during pregnancy. Hospitals were required to notify local health departments when such instances were suspected.

To determine the prevalence of substance abuse by pregnant women, urine samples were collected from 380 women enrolled in prenatal care at any of the 5 public health clinics in Pinellas County and from 335 women at any of 12 private obstetric offices in the county. A total of 715 urine specimens were collected at the first prenatal visits. There were significant differences in racial distribution and socioeconomic status between the public and private patients (table). The mean ages of the 2 groups of women were also significantly different; public health patients had a mean age of 22.6 years, whereas private patients had a mean age of 26.6 years.

Of the 715 women, 14.8% had positive results on toxicologic screening of urine for alcohol, cannabinoids, cocaine, or opiates. When alcohol was eliminated from the analysis, 13.3% of the urine specimens were positive for an illicit drug. There was no significant difference in the prev-

Demographic Characteristics and Drug-Use Patterns of Pregnant Women, According to Type of Health Care Provider

CHARACTERISTIC	PUBLIC CLINIC (N = 380)	PRIVATE OBSTETRICIAN (N = 335)	TOTAL (N = 715)
		number (percent)	
Race*			
Non-Hispanic white	198 (52.1)	301 (89.9)	499 (69.8)
Black	168 (44.2)	31 (9.3)	199 (27.8)
Hispanic	3 (0.8)	0 (0)	3 (0.4)
Asian	11 (2.9)	3 (0.9)	14 (2.0)
Socioeconomic status*†			
Low (<$12,000)	202 (53.2)	72 (21.5)	274 (38.3)
Middle ($12,000–25,000)	150 (39.5)	238 (71.0)	388 (54.3)
High (>$25,000)	28 (7.4)	25 (7.5)	53 (7.4)
Drugs identified in urine			
Alcohol	2 (0.5)	5 (1.5)	7 (1.0)
Cannabinoids	47 (12.4)	38 (11.3)	85 (11.9)
Cocaine‡	19 (5.0)	5 (1.5)	24 (3.4)
Opiates	1 (0.3)	1 (0.3)	2 (0.3)
Any of the above	62 (16.3)	44 (13.1)	106 (14.8)

*P < .0001 for the comparison between public and private patients, by chi-square analysis.

†The median annual family income in the ZIP code area where the woman lived was used as an indicator of socioeconomic status.

‡P < .01 for the comparison between public and private patients, by chi-square analysis.
(Courtesy of Chasnoff IJ, Landress HJ, Barrett ME: *N Engl J Med* 322:1202–1208, 1990.)

alence of positive results between public and private patients. The frequency of a positive result was similar among white and black women, although black women more frequently had evidence of cocaine use and white women more often revealed the use of cannabinoids. Despite the similar rates of substance abuse among the 2 groups, black women were reported to health authorities at about 10 times the rate for white women, and poor women were reported more often than women of higher socioeconomic status.

The use of illicit drugs is common among pregnant women regardless of race and socioeconomic status. If legally mandated reporting of substance abuse is to be free from racial or economic bias, it must be based on objective medical standards.

▶ This report is included to emphasize that the use of illicit drugs during pregnancy is widespread throughout our society in both poor and middle class women. Though poor women are more frequently reported to be using drugs, there is a similar proportion of private and obstetric clinic patients on drugs. Any campaign to reduce drug use must therefore involve the entire population.—M.H. Klaus, M.D.

4 Antepartum Fetal Surveillance

Ultrasound Screening and Perinatal Mortality: Controlled Trial of Systematic One-Stage Screening in Pregnancy (The Helsinki Ultrasound Trial)
Saari-Kemppainen A, Karjalainen O, Ylöstalo P, Heinonen OP (Helsinki Univ Central Hosp; Univ of Helsinki)
Lancet 336:387–391, 1990

4–1

Ultrasound screening has an important role in obstetric practice in assessing gestational age, monitoring fetal growth, confirming the site of the placenta, and detecting multiple gestations and major fetal anomalies. However, there is no agreement over the benefit of routine ultrasound screening. The benefit of systematic ultrasound screening of all pregnancies was compared with that of screening only selected patients.

During a 19-month study period, 95% of all pregnant women in the greater Helsinki area was recruited into the study. Of the 9,310 women who agreed to participate, 4,691 were randomly assigned to ultrasound screening between the 16th and 20th gestational weeks and 4,619 to follow-up only. Screened and nonscreened women received identical antenatal care, which included ultrasound examinations according to established practice. Before scheduled ultrasound screening, 11 women discovered that they were not pregnant, 549 miscarried, and 47 had induced abortions. Another 318 women did not attend their scheduled screening. There were 4,353 deliveries in the screening group, 72 of them twins, and 4,309 in the control group, 76 of them twins.

Screened women made fewer visits to the antenatal outpatient clinic than did control women. The number of labor inductions and the mean birth weights in the 2 groups were similar. Ultrasound screening corrected the expected delivery date by 10 or more days in 11.5% of the women. In the ultrasound screening group, all twin pregnancies were detected before the 21st gestational week, whereas only 76.3% of twin pregnancies were detected early in the control group.

Perinatal mortality in the screened group was 4.6/1,000 compared with a 9.0/1,000 mortality in the control group. The 49.2% reduction in perinatal mortality was mainly attributable to improved early detection of major congenital malformations, which led to pregnancy termination before the 25th gestational week. None of the women in the control group had induced abortion after an ultrasound finding of congenital malformation.

Ultrasound screening improved the management of pregnancy and was beneficial to neonates. Early screening saved women from later outpatient hospital visits and also decreased the antenatal use of hospital beds. The most important benefit of ultrasound screening was the early detection of half of all serious congenital malformations.

▶ The ultrasound screening studies reported to date have yielded conflicting data, with improved diagnosis of malformations, growth retardation, and multiple gestation, a benefit for postdatism, and reduced labor inductions, but with increased hospitalizations and no clear evidence of reduced perinatal mortality or improved outcome for twin gestations (1). The prevailing belief was that insufficient numbers had been evaluated and that a larger trial would establish whether routine ultrasound would reduce perinatal mortality. Remarkably, 95% of all pregnant women in the greater Helsinki area were enrolled, thus providing an ample sample size. The aim of the trial was to test whether "strictly timed, systematic screening of all pregnancies would reveal any benefits (or adverse effects) under circumstances in which one can neither prevent nor limit participants in a controlled clinical trial from having ultrasonography when desired." The trial did demonstrate benefits largely related to earlier diagnosis of multiple gestations and congenital anomalies. The perinatal mortality rate was significantly lower in the group screened with ultrasound, largely a result of the induced abortions for the malformations. Earlier and more accurate diagnosis of twin gestation and placenta previa together with reduced number of antenatal visits and antenatal hospital bed days were added benefits. There were no significant adverse effects. In Finland congenital malformations are the major cause of perinatal death (2). Therefore, routine screening can be endorsed. To extrapolate these findings to all other populations is too big a jump and remains a logistical nightmare. Not the least of the problems is to have enough personnel trained to accurately read the sonograms.—A.A. Fanaroff, M.B.B.Ch.

References

1. 1989 YEAR BOOK OF NEONATAL AND PERINATAL MEDICINE, Abstracts 3–21 and 3–30.
2. Eik-Nes SH, et al: *Lancet* 1:1347, 1984.

Absence of Need for Amniocentesis in Patients With Elevated Levels of Maternal Serum Alpha-Fetoprotein and Normal Ultrasonographic Examinations

Nadel AS, Green JK, Holmes LB, Frigoletto FD Jr, Benacerraf BR (Brigham and Women's Hosp, Boston; Harvard Med School)

N Engl J Med 323:557–561, 1990   4–2

We doctors know
a hopeless case if-listen: there's a hell
of a good universe next door; lets go—ee cummings

At present routine obstetric care includes screening for raised levels of maternal serum alpha-fetoprotein between 15 and 18 weeks after the last menstrual period. If the levels are elevated in 2 samples after adjustment for weight and race, and ultrasound examinations do not suggest an explanation, such as incorrect estimation of gestational age, multiple gestation, fetal death, or definite congenital anomaly, amniocentesis for measurement of the levels of alpha-fetoprotein and acetylcholinesterase in amniotic fluid is routinely recommended to exclude anomalies possibly missed by sonography.

The ultrasound findings in 51 consecutive fetuses with spina bifida, encephalocele, gastroschisis, or omphalocele that were delivered or aborted at 1 hospital were reviewed to evaluate the diagnostic accuracy of ultrasonography. In all instances the mothers had had a sonogram at 1 facility between 16 and 24 weeks after the last menstrual period. This information was used to calculate the probability of an affected fetus in a woman with a given level of maternal serum alpha-fetoprotein and normal sonographic results.

Table 1 shows the observed prevalence of the anomalies. These data are based on 87,584 pregnancies over a 12-year period and include liveborn infants, stillborn infants, and fetuses aborted in the second trimester. The total prevalence of spina bifida, encephalocele, omphalocele, and gastroschisis was .11%. Table 2 shows the calculated probability of these anomalies in fetuses of mothers with different maternal serum alpha-fetoprotein values. The probability of detecting an anomaly after a normal level 1 scan is shown for each maternal serum level of alpha-fetoprotein, corrected only for gestational age, fetal death, multiple gestation, and anencephaly. Table 2 also shows how these probabilities are influenced by a normal level 2 ultrasound study, assuming that the sensitivity of the technique is 94%, the lower limit of the 95% confidence interval for the present data.

The congenital anomalies identified by an alpha-fetoprotein screening program are unusual. Because there is considerable overlap between maternal serum alpha-fetoprotein values in normal pregnancies and in pregnancies complicated by an anomaly, the probability that a patient with a raised maternal level of serum alpha-fetoprotein is carrying an affected fetus is low. In the present study there was a 1.1% probability that the

TABLE 1.—Prevalence of Selected Anomalies
in 87,584 Pregnancies

ANOMALY	NO. OF CASES	PREVALENCE (%)
Spina bifida	45	0.05
Encephalocele	15	0.02
Gastroschisis	11	0.01
Omphalocele	25	0.03
Total	96	0.11

(Courtesy of Nadel AS, Green JK, Holmes LB, et al: *N Engl J Med* 323:557–561, 1990.)

TABLE 2.—Probability of Spina Bifida,
Encephalocele, Gastroschisis, or Omphalocele Before
and After Level 2 Ultrasound Scan

MATERNAL SERUM ALPHA-FETOPROTEIN*	PROBABILITY OF ANOMALY	
	BEFORE LEVEL 2 SCAN	AFTER NORMAL LEVEL 2 SCAN
	percent	
2.0	0.2	0.01
2.5	0.5	0.03
3.0	1.1	0.07
3.5	2.5	0.15
4.0	4.9	0.31

Note: According to maternal serum alphafetoprotein values.
*Expressed as multiples of median value.
(Courtesy of Nadel AS, Green JK, Holmes LB, et al: *N Engl J Med* 323:557–561, 1990.)

fetus of a woman with a maternal serum level of alpha-fetoprotein of 3 times the median was affected by a malformation associated with elevated levels of alpha-fetoprotein other than anencephaly.

It is suggested that women with raised maternal serum levels of alpha-fetoprotein be referred to institutions that are capable of performing level 2 ultrasonography. If the level 2 scan identifies an abnormal fetus, appropriate counseling should be provided.

▶ The saga of neural tube defects parallels the development of the field of neonatal/perinatal medicine. We have come full cycle from the time when every new patient was a surprise in the delivery room to an incredibly sophisticated and reliable screening program. Those with abnormal screens can be evaluated ultrasonographically and the diagnosis confirmed or refuted. This report demonstrates the refinement of the algorithm in the detection of neural tube defects. Amniocentesis has been eliminated in many instances because of the dependability of the ultrasound. A recent editorial in the *New England Journal of Medicine* by John Hobbins from Yale (1) eloquently summarizes the status of neural tube defects:

Although it will probably never be possible to eradicate neural tube defects, progress has been made in diminishing their incidence, identifying and characterizing the defects, counseling families who choose to continue a pregnancy, and decreasing morbidity by optimizing management at the time of delivery. The triumph for perinatal medicine has all been the result of beautifully integrated epidemiologic studies, prospective screening trials, rapid improvement in ultrasound imaging, implementation of rapidly evolving techniques of prenatal diagnosis, and better preoperative and postoperative care of mother and baby.—John Hobbins

See also reference 2.—A.A. Fanaroff, M.B.B.Ch.

References

1. Hobbins J: *N Engl J Med* 324:690, 1991.
2. 1990 YEAR BOOK OF NEONATAL AND PERINATAL MEDICINE, Abstracts 2–8, 2–9, and 2–10.

Fetal Heart Rate Responses to Maternal Exercise, Increased Maternal Temperature and Maternal Circadian Variation
Tuffnell DJ, Buchan PC, Albert D, Tyndale-Biscoe S (St James' Univ Hosp, Leeds, England)
J Obstet Gynaecol 10:387–391, 1990   4–3

An attempt was made to determine fetal heart rate responses to various physiologic stress states in 70 women at 35 to 40 weeks' gestation. Twenty fetuses were considered small for gestational age. Exercise consisted of walking up and down a flight of 30 stairs for 10 minutes. Some of the women were assessed before and after a 20-minute bath in water at 40° C. To assess maternal and fetal circadian variation, heart rate was recorded for 5 minutes each hour one 24 hours in 15 women. Twenty healthy term neonates were monitored for 24 hours within 2 days of birth.

In the exercise group 50 patients had infants who were of normal birth weight and 20 patients had small infants. Normal fetuses generally had a rise in heart rate and increased variability in heart rate during maternal exercise. These changes were not evident in small fetuses, although 4 had decelerations. Maternal heart rate rose in all groups.

In the warm bath group 31 patients had infants who were of normal birth weight and 11 patients had small infants. Normal fetuses had a rise in heart rate during the warm bath, whereas small fetuses did not. In 3 cases decelerations occurred.

A circadian variation was present in the mother and fetus but absent in the neonate.

Small fetuses have variable responses to maternal exercise and a rise in maternal body temperature, possibly reflecting impaired uteroplacental circulation. It seems wise to avoid exercise when growth retardation is a factor.

▶ This report confirms the presence of a circadian rhythm in the mother and fetus, but not in the newborn. It is implied that the mother imposes her circadian variation on the fetus and the fetal rhythm can be modified by suppressing its adrenal gland. Elevation of maternal temperature with a hot bath or exercise resulted in an increase in fetal heart rate, if the fetus was healthy and growing normally. The growth-retarded fetus was neither up to exercise nor enjoyed a relaxing warm bath, often manifesting bradycardia. The authors postulate that slowing of the fetal heart rate denoted fetal distress, but Artal (1) did not arrive at the same conclusion. Technical difficulties may account for some of the documented slowing. The implication that maternal exercise should be curtailed if the fetus is undergrown is reasonable. I was convinced that an increase in fetal heart rate with maternal exercise was a sign of fetal well-being. The burning question regarding the benefits of exercise during pregnancy was not addressed, perhaps next time. Moderate amounts of aerobic exercise are recommended, bearing in mind that the fetus can be stressed or distressed by overexertion of the mother.

Man should not try to avoid stress any more than he would shun food, love or exercise.—Hans Selye

A.A. Fanaroff, M.B.B.Ch.

Reference

1. Artal R, et al: *Lancet* 2:258, 1984.

The Effects of Acute Uterine Ischemia on Fetal Circulation
Calvert SA, Widness JA, Oh W, Stonestreet BS (Women and Infants Hosp of Rhode Island, Providence; Brown Univ)
Pediatr Res 27:552–556, 1990   4–4

Acute maternal hemorrhage is associated with increased perinatal morbidity and mortality. The effects of acute maternal hemorrhage on fetal oxygenation and organ blood flow were evaluated in chronically instrumented fetal sheep. Nine pregnant sheep (114–128 days' gestation), phlebotomized from the iliac artery at the point of origin of the uterine artery, were bled until maternal blood pressure was 60% of control value. Measurements were taken at baseline, after hemorrhage, and immediately and 2 hours after replacement of maternal blood. Fetal organ blood flow was measured by radionuclide-labeled microspheres.

Maternal bleeding resulted in a significant reduction in uterine blood flow. In the fetus, maternal hemorrhage resulted in hypoxemia, acidemia, decreased oxygen content, and a significant increase in blood flow to the high priority organs such as the brain, heart, and adrenal glands, but not to the kidneys, gastrointestinal tract, or carcass. Rapid replacement of maternal blood restored all parameters to baseline values.

The data indicate that acute maternal hemorrhage reduces uterine blood flow and causes fetal hypoxemia and acidemia with a secondary increase in blood flow to high priority organs. These effects are reversed with rapid replacement of maternal blood.

▶ The impetus for this beautifully executed pathophysiologic exercise was the observation that pregnancies complicated by third trimester bleeding were more likely to result in periventricular leukomalacia in the neonate. A controlled model of maternal hemorrhage was created in chronically instrumented sheep. Based on previous studies the alterations in organ blood flow and fetal acid-base status were eminently predictable and restoration of blood volume to the ewe restored all parameters to prehemorrhagic levels. I leave this study impressed with the barrage of physiologic data accumulated but unable to make any association between bleeding in the ewe and leukomalacia in the neonate. Did I miss something?

Logic must take care of itself.— Ludwig Wittgenstein

A.A. Fanaroff, M.B.B.Ch.

Is Intrauterine Growth Retardation With Normal Umbilical Artery Blood Flow a Benign Condition?
Burke G, Stuart B, Crowley P, Scanaill SN, Drumm J (Coombe Lying-In Hosp, Dublin)
Br Med J 300:1044–1045, 1990   4–5

Intrauterine growth retardation is a significant cause of perinatal death. There is no reliable method to establish whether an appropriately nourished fetus is small because of placental insufficiency or because of genetic and racial factors. In both instances the fetus is classified as growth retarded. Women with small but healthy fetuses may be hospitalized unnecessarily and undergo unnecessary intervention, including cesarean section. Doppler studies of the umbilical artery reportedly can identify a group of growth retarded infants at increased risk of intrapartum hypoxia. Although no correlation has been observed between the size of the fetus and hypoxia or acidosis, the absence of end-diastolic blood flow appears to be a good indication of asphyxia in growth-retarded fetuses.

One hundred seventy-nine women with singleton pregnancies were studied to determine if intrauterine growth retardation associated with normal umbilical artery blood flow is a benign condition. If the fetal abdominal circumference, measured by ultrasonography, was below the 5th centile for gestation, growth retardation was diagnosed. Of the 179 fetuses, 124 had normal umbilical artery velocity waveforms; 44 fetuses had type 2 flow and 11 had type 3. There were 2 midtrimester abortions of fetuses with type 3 flow; 1 was born alive but weighed less than 500 g and could not be resuscitated. Of 166 infants born after 34 weeks' gestation, 63 of 122 with normal flow and 33 of 44 with abnormal flow had a birth weight below the 5th centile. The table presents the relative risks of each outcome for abnormal flow (types 2 and 3) compared with normal flow (type 1).

Intrauterine growth retardation associated with normal umbilical blood flow is a different entity from that associated with abnormal flow. Normal flow is generally benign and abnormal flow is associated with a serious risk of adverse outcome.

► The presence of decreased umbilical artery blood flow in a growth-retarded fetus significantly decreases the chances of a good outcome, whereas growth retardation with adequate flow appears to be a rather benign condition. In a previous report by Nicolaides (1) 6 weeks of chronic oxygen administration to

Incidence (per 1,000 fetuses) of Adverse Outline With Normal and Abnormal Umbilical Artery Blood Flow

	Normal flow	Abnormal flow	Relative risk (95% CI)
Mid-trimester abortion		36.4	
Perinatal deaths	32.3	109.1	3.4 (1.0 to 11.5)
Mid-trimester abortions and perinatal deaths	32.3	145.5	4.5 (1.4 to 14.3)
Perinatal deaths (corrected for major congenital anomalies)		54.5	
Babies with cerebral irritation	8.1	18.2	2.3 (0.1 to 36.1)
Preterm delivery	48	418	8.6 (5.6 to 13.3)
Emergency Caesarean section for fetal distress (excluding stillbirths and elective sections)	38	222	5.8 (1.8 – 19.1)

(Courtesy of Burke G, Stuart B, Crowley P, et al: *Br Med J* 300:1044–1045, 1990.)

mothers with decreased umbilical blood flow appeared to be helpful in 5 se-verely affected infants. Further study of this heroic therapy would be helpful.— M.H. Klaus, M.D.

Reference

1. 1988 YEAR BOOK OF NEONATAL AND PERINATAL MEDICINE, Abstract 1–1.

Effect of the Pretest Probability of Intrauterine Growth Retardation on the Predictiveness of Sonographic Estimated Fetal Weight in Detecting IUGR: A Clinical Application of Bayes' Theorem
Simon NV, Surosky BA, Shearer DM, Levisky JS (York Hosp; York Coll of Penn-sylvania, York, Penn)
J Clin Ultrasound 18:145–153, 1990   4–6

A series of 405 women having singleton pregnancies, who underwent fetal age estimation by measuring crown-rump length, were classified into 4 risk categories for intrauterine growth retardation (IUGR). Retardation was defined as a neonatal weight below the 10th centile of the age-depen-dent birth weight distribution curve. All these women delivered a live in-fant at or after 34 weeks' gestation and within 1 week of an ultrasound study.

The incidence of IUGR ranged from 3.5% for very low risk infants to 88% for the highest risk group (table). The risk of a birth weight below the 2.5th percentile increased with the incidence of risk factors for IUGR. Severe IUGR was very unlikely in the very low risk group. A high pretest probability of IUGR warranted close surveillance of fetal well-being, even if the estimated fetal weight was within the 10th to 90th percentile range.

Ultrasonographic findings should be interpreted in the context of the pretest probability of IUGR. Close surveillance or timely interruption of pregnancy is warranted when the estimated fetal weight is below the 10th percentile and there is a reasonable probability of severe growth retarda-tion.

▶ Knowledge, skill, judgment, and experience together with intuition are com-puted by practitioners in arriving at major clinical decisions. These ingredients have been admixed in this report. Most of you waved good-bye to theorems after high school or college at the latest. At the conclusion of this manuscript I believe that there will be few staunch advocates for Bayes' theorem. It is based on the use of intuition and experience, personal or from published data, to improve positive and negative test results, in this case the prediction of IUGR. Confused? So was I, so I turned to the concluding statement. There is a study underway to test this theorem prospective, and then use it in a com-puter-expert system. I can hardly wait for the results.

Sample of 405 Women With Singleton Pregnancies Who Delivered Within 7 Days of an Ultrasound Scan, Classified into 4 Categories of Risk for IUGR.

Group	Pretest Risk of IUGR	N	Neonatal Weight Outcome					Mean Birth Weight (±SD)
			BW < 10th Percentile		BW < 2.5th Percentile		Percent of IUGR with BW < 2.5th Percentile	
		N	N	%	N	%	%	g
I	Very low	229	8	3.5	0	—	0	3490±338
II	Low	34	7	20.6	2	5.9	28.6	3101±446
III	Intermediate	117	58	49.6	28	23.9	48.3	2794±615
IV	High	25	22	88.0	19	76.0	86.4	2218±614
Total		405	95	23.5	49	12.1	51.6	3177±662

Abbreviations: N, number of patients; BW, birth weight.
(Courtesy of Simon NV, Surosky BA, Shearer DM, et al: *J Clin Ultrasound* 18:145–153, 1990.)

The appearance of a single great genius is more than equivalent to the birth of a hundred mediocrities.—Cesare Lombardo

A.A. Fanaroff, M.B.B.Ch.

Amniotic Fluid Glucose Concentration: A Rapid and Simple Method for the Detection of Intraamniotic Infection in Preterm Labor
Romero J, Jimenez C, Lohda AK, Nores J, Hanaoka S, Avila C, Callahan R, Mazor M, Hobbins JC, Diamond MP (Yale Univ)
Am J Obstet Gynecol 163:968–974, 1990   4–7

Intra-amniotic infection appears to be associated with preterm labor and delivery. Early diagnosis is desirable. The value of amniotic fluid glucose concentrations in the rapid diagnosis of intra-amniotic infection was investigated.

One hundred sixty-eight patients with preterm labor and intact membranes underwent amniocenteses. Amniotic fluid was cultured for aerobic and anaerobic bacteria and *Mycoplasma* species. Results were positive in

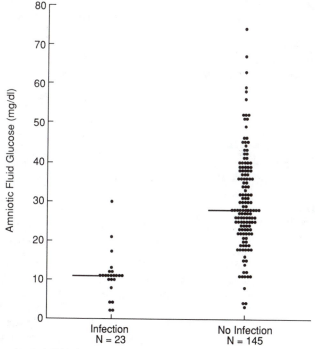

Fig 4–1.—Amniotic fluid glucose concentrations in the study population. The median amniotic fluid glucose concentration in patients with intra-amniotic infection was significantly lower in patients with negative amniotic fluid cultures (median, 11 mg/dL; range, 2–30 mg/dL vs. median, 28 mg/dL; range, 3–74 mg/dL, respectively; *P* < .0001). (Courtesy of Romero R, Jimenez C, Lohda AK, et al: *Am J Obstet Gynecol* 163:968–974, 1990.)

13.6% of 168 amniotic fluid cultures. Women whose amniotic fluid cultures were positive for microorganisms had significantly lower median amniotic fluid glucose levels than those with negative amniotic fluid cultures. Amniotic fluid glucose levels below 14 mg/dL had a sensitivity of 86.9%, a specificity of 91.7%, a positive predictive value of 62.5%, and a negative predictive value of 97.8% in detecting positive amniotic fluid culture (Fig 4–1).

Amniotic fluid glucose determination is a sensitive test for detecting intra-amniotic infection in women with preterm labor and intact membranes. Amniotic fluid glucose determination is also fast, simple, and inexpensive.

▶ One of the first questions raised by this report is why is the glucose level lowered with infection. In the spinal fluid, leukocytes in association with bacteria consume glucose, thereby lowering glucose levels. Most probably an inflammatory host response is associated with a reduced glucose concentration in amniotic fluid since there were 6 women in this report who had negative cultures for microorganisms but had a reduced glucose level. They did, however, have an acute inflammatory lesion of the placenta. In diagnosing amniotic fluid infection a low glucose level will probably be most useful in conjunction with a gram stain, white blood cell count and differential, and a culture—not too different than how we presently handle spinal fluids.—M.H. Klaus, M.D.

Fetal Assessment Based on Fetal Biophysical Profile Scoring. III: Positive Predictive Accuracy of the Very Abnormal Test (Biophysical Profile Score = 0)
Manning FA, Harman CR, Morrison I, Menticoglou S (Univ of Manitoba, Winnipeg)
Am J Obstet Gynecol 162:398–402, 1990   4–8

Fetal biophysical profile scoring (BPS) allows recognition of the fetal risk as well as categorization of degree of risk. The relationship between complete absence of all components of the fetal BPS (BPS = 0) and adverse perinatal outcome, as measured by indices of morbidity and mortality, was evaluated in the 29,958 referred high-risk patients during a 106-month study.

Of 29 (.0968%) fetuses that had a very abnormal BPS of 0 at a mean gestational age of 31.5 weeks, 14 (48.3%) died, as early as 30 minutes to as late as 7 days after the last test; 11 of these deaths were stillborn. Of the 18 (62%) fetuses born alive, all had at least 1 abnormal marker of perinatal morbidity. Among these survivors, 83% had intrauterine growth retardation, 83% were admitted to the neonatal intensive care unit, and 33% each had either low 5-minute Apgar scores or umbilical vein acidosis. Despite aggressive and intermediate intervention, 3 neonates died of asphyxia-related causes. With mortality and morbidity as end points, the positive predictve accuracy of a BPS of 0 was 100%.

These data indicate that a BPS of 0 should be considered a true perinatal emergency justifying intervention by delivery when there is a prospect of extrauterine survival.

▶ This report could be considered a form of quality check for the BPS. If a score of 0 is not going to predict morbidity and mortality, then the scoring system is worthless. There is already a large body of evidence to prove that it has some value (1). To refresh the uninitiated, a BPS of 0 means that during the 30 minutes of observation there has been no evidence of fetal flexor tone (opening and closing hand), no episodes of fetal breathing of at least 30 seconds' duration, fewer than 3 gross body movements, no pocket of amniotic fluid that exceeds 2 cm, and a nonreactive nonstress test (<2 accelerations of fetal heart rate for 15 sec >15 beats/min). In other words this fetus is either severely compromised or in a very, very deep sleep. The high mortality and morbidity encountered among these select few infants who were documented with such a score further validate the scoring system. There is some confusion as to how rapid a response is necessary for a score of 0. One fetus died within 30 minutes of detection, others survived over a week in utero. Conservative management is appropriately recommended for the grossly immature fetus and for multiple pregnancies in which the companion fetus had a normal score but was immature at less than 32 weeks'. Intrauterine transfusion may be curative for the anemic sensitized fetus.

There is considerable free association in the discussion of this manuscript with an attempt to establish a unifying concept to account for the low scores. Asphyxia, anemia, malformations, and infections don't usually easily fit into single concepts, and there are some ragged edges to some of the hypotheses. It is worth noting that not all stillbirths will be preceded by a BPS of 0. Specifically, if there is a normal volume of amniotic fluid there is automatically a score of 2. It is fair to conclude that a BPS score of 0 is rare but constitutes a perinatal emergency. In planning the course of intervention the maturity, estimated size, and number of fetuses, and the presence or absence of malformations or alloimmunization, will all be taken into consideration.

We are all in the gutter, but some of us are looking at the stars.—*Oscar Wilde*

A.A. Fanaroff, M.B.B.Ch.

Reference

1. 1990 YEAR BOOK OF NEONATAL AND PERINATAL MEDICINE, Abustracts 4–9 and 4–10.

Fetal Assessment Based on Fetal Biophysical Profile Scoring. IV: An Analysis of Perinatal Morbidity and Mortality
Manning FA, Harman CR, Morrison I, Menticoglou SM, Lange IR, Johnson JM (Univ of Manitoba, Winnipeg)
Am J Obstet Gynecol 162:703–709, 1990

4–9

Antepartum surveillance of fetal biophysical activities and responses to stress in utero offers a means of assessing relative perinatal risk. This fetal biophysical scoring provides a survey of 5 discrete biophysical variables. The relationship between the last biophysical profile score (BPS) and markers of perinatal morbidity and mortality was prospectively evaluated in a large referred population of high-risk pregnancies.

Of the 26,780 referred high-risk fetuses, 913 (3.41%) had a last BPS of 6 or less. There was a highly significant inverse linear correlation between the last test score and fetal distress, admission to a neonatal intensive care unit, intrauterine growth retardation, 5-minute Apgar score less than 7, and umbilical cord pH less than 7.20 (Fig 4–2). Combinations of these variables also had a highly significant inverse linear correlation with the last test score, but not for the incidence of meconium staining and major anomaly (Fig 4–3). There was also a highly significant inverse exponential relationship between the last BPS and perinatal mortality, both

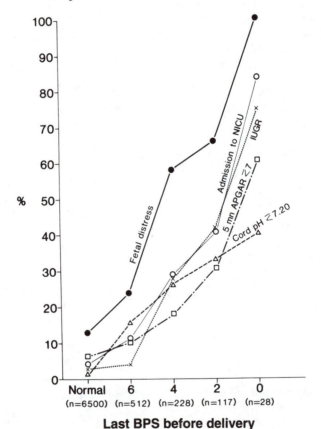

Last BPS before delivery

Fig 4–2.—Relationship between perinatal morbidity measured by 5 outcome variables and last biophysical profile scoring result before delivery. A significant inverse linear correlation is observed for each variable. (Courtesy of Manning FA, Harman CR, Morrison I, et al: *Am J Obstet Gynecol* 162:703–709, 1990.)

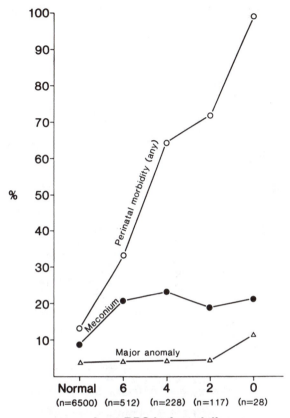

Last BPS before delivery

Fig 4–3.—Relationship between any perinatal morbidity, defined by the presence of either fetal distress, admission to neonatal intensive care unit, interauterine growth retardation, 5-minute Apgar score less than 7, and umbilical vein pH less than 7.20, either alone or in any combination. A highly significant inverse linear correlation is observed. In contrast, no relationship between meconium staining of amniotic fluid or the presence of major anomaly was observed. (Courtesy of Manning FA, Harman CR, Morrison I, et al: *Am J Obstet Gynecol* 162:703–709, 1990.)

by gross and corrected category and by gross and stillbirth and neonatal category (Fig 4–4).

Biophysical profile scoring provides an accurate fetal risk assessment, as well as insight into the extent of fetal compromise. There is a progressive risk of adverse perinatal outcome as the fetal BPS deteriorates.

▶ The BPS or modifications thereof (1) has become the gold standard for evaluating fetal well-being. As the cumulative experience increases, so does the reliability. The above statistical analysis is based on a monster database that includes 65,627 fetal BPS results compiled from 26,780 referred high-risk fetuses. These numbers should stand up to even the most critical reviews. I was a little perplexed by the lack of correlation between meconium-stained amniotic fluid and the biophysical profile. I should not be, as we all recognize that the

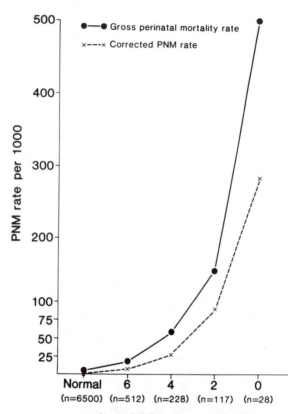

Last BPS before delivery

Fig 4–4.—Relationship between perinatal mortality, either total or corrected for major anomaly, and the last BPS result. This relationship is exponential and yields a highly significant inverse correlation with $\log_{10}$ conversion. (Courtesy of Manning FA, Harman CR, Morrison I, et al: *Am J Obstet Gynecol* 162:703–709, 1990.)

presence of meconium does not necessarily indicate fetal distress or compromise. Would that we could tell more reliably when it does.

Genius all over the world stands hand in hand, and one shock of recognition runs the whole circle round.—Herman Melville

A.A. Fanaroff, M.B.B.Ch.

Reference

1. 1990 YEAR BOOK OF NEONATAL AND PERINATAL MEDICINE, Abstract 4–9.

Does Reduction of Amniotic Fluid Affect Fetal Movements?
Sival DA, Visser GHA, Prechtl HFR (Univ Hosp, Groningen, The Netherlands)
Early Hum Dev 23:233–246, 1990   4–10

The study of fetal motility in oligohydramnios is of special interest. If mechanical restriction affects movement quality, such a factor should be considered when movement is assessed in the compromised fetus for diagnostic purposes. In a longitudinal study, the effect of the amount of amniotic fluid on the form of fetal general movement was studied in 19 pregnancies complicated by premature rupture of the amniotic membranes at 15 to 29 weeks' gestation. Before birth, general movements were studied at weekly intervals by continuous real-time ultrasound observation 1 hour in duration under standardized conditions. Eleven infants were studied in the early postnatal period using video recordings of their spontaneous movements.

Moderate reduction of amniotic fluid was associated with a decrease in the amplitude of general movements, but a more severe reduction of amniotic fluid was also associated with a decrease in the speed of general movements. The same quality of general movements was observed during repeated measurements in the majority of cases. Breech presentation was associated with small amplitude and low velocity in 90% of cases, whereas the presence of chorioamnionitis did not affect general movements. Postnatally, there was a tendency to retain the same amplitude and speed of movements as before birth and to normalize between 1 and 5 weeks. The fast components of movement, such as startles and twitches, were not affected by reduction in aminotic fluid volume.

Reduction in amniotic fluid causes an alteration of fetal general movement consisting of low speed and small amplitude. These changes continue after birth, indicating a short lasting carry-over effect on the functional properties of the motor system. These findings are important for the qualitative assessment of motor behavior in pregnancies complicated by premature rupture of membranes or intrauterine growth retardation. The latter is associated with abnormal general movements of monotonous slow character with reduced force and amplitude. It is the forcefulness of the motility and the presence of fast components that distinguish motor behavior in severe oligohydramnios from the growth-retarded fetus.

▶ These investigators are using 2 new tools to evaluate qualitatively and semiquantitatively fetal and postnatal movement behavior. As recently noted by Prechtl there is a continuity of movement between intrauterine and extrauterine life. This report uses the same qualitative approach discussed in another report by Ferrari (Abstract 7–1) and reveals some of its potential. A fascinating sideline is that several infants discussed in this paper were noted to have abnormal movements using the qualitative analysis and were later found to have abnormal neurologic development.—M.H. Klaus, M.D.

Fetal Breathing Movements in Pregnancies Complicated by Premature Membrane Rupture in the Second Trimester

Blott M, Greenough A, Nicolaides KH (Kings' College Hosp, London)
Early Hum Dev 21:41–48, 1990   4–11

In an earlier study it was found that in some pregnancies complicated by premature and prolonged membrane rupture (PPROM), fetal breathing movements (FBMs) were absent. In these cases the perinatal outcome was poor because of abnormal lung growth. In the present study the fetal breathing activity was assessed in 40 pregnancies complicated by oligohydramnios in the second trimester because of PPROM.

Patients underwent ultrasound scanning at referral and at 1- or 2-week intervals until delivery. A 30-minute real-time ultrasound examination was performed and fetal chest wall movements were recorded. The scan time was extended to 60 minutes if no FBMs were present. Patients were retrospectively classified according to whether FBMs were absent at all examinations, present at all examinations, or intermittent, i.e., absent at some examinations but present at others.

The PPROM occurred significantly earlier in the 12 patients with absent FBMs. All infants in this group died either in utero or in the neonatal period because of pulmonary hypoplasia. All infants survived in the group of 17 with FBMs always present. Six infants in the intermittent group survived, and 5 died either from pulmonary hypoplasia or from neonatal sepsis.

In pregnancies complicated by PPROM the persistent absence of FBMs was strongly associated with perinatal death caused by pulmonary hypoplasia. The mechanisms that inhibit FBMs are not known. Pulmonary hypoplasia in PPROM can only be predicted confidently after serial ultrasound examinations have all shown an absence of FBMs.

▶ We return again to predicting the presence of fetal pulmonary hypoplasia by assessing FBMs. Though it has been suggested that the presence of FBMs was not helpful in differentiating who will survive, the results might depend on the authors' definition of FBM. These authors defined fetal breathing as being present if a continuous period of chest wall movements lasted at least 60 seconds, with a breath-to-breath interval of 6 seconds or less. If no breathing movements were present during the span of 30 minutes the time was extended to 60 minutes. This definition results in a reasonable separation. As noted in the 1989 YEAR BOOK (1) fetal chest wall dimensions assessed from ultrasound are also helpful in determining the viability of the infant at birth (2). The next step is to seal the leak.—M.H. Klaus, M.D.

References

1. 1989 YEAR BOOK OF NEONATAL AND PERINATAL MEDICINE, Abstract 1–22.
2. Nimrod C et al: *Am J Obstet Gynecol* 158:277, 1988.

The Ultrasonographic Assessment of the Fetal Thorax and Fetal Breathing Movements in the Prediction of Pulmonary Hypoplasia
Blott M, Greenough A, Nicolaides KH, Campbell S (King's Coll School of Medicine and Dentistry, London)
Early Hum Dev 21:143–151, 1990   4–12

Neonatal death caused by pulmonary hypoplasia may result from oligohydramnios because of premature and prolonged rupture of the membranes (PPROM). The absence of fetal breathing movements (FBMs) and a reduced thoracic circumference have been suggested as useful markers in prenatal prediction of pulmonary hypoplasia. A normal range of fetal thoracic measurements was established for comparison to FBMs and thoracic measurements in the prenatal diagnosis of pulmonary hypoplasia.

In 20 pregnant women with oligohydramnios caused by PPROM, the presence or absence of FBMs was assessed. Fetal internal thoracic and cardiac circumferences were also measured, and the internal thoracic and lung areas were calculated. The 15 infants with FBMs survived. The 5 infants with absent FBMs died in the neonatal period of pulmonary hypoplasia.

In normal pregnancies, there is a linear growth in internal thoracic circumference and lung area with gestational age. Three of the fetuses who had pulmonary hypoplasia and 1 fetus who did not were below the 2.5th centile of a reference range from 76 normal pregnancies. The lung areas were also below the 2.5th centile of the reference range in 3 fetuses who had pulmonary hypoplasia and 2 fetuses who survived.

Although both thoracic and lung measurements tended to be lower in infants who had pulmonary hypoplasia, the only accurate predictor in the second trimester for pulmonary hypoplasia was the absence of FBMs. Accurate detection of fetal abnormalities in the second trimester will allow intervention.

▶ The normal amniotic epithelial layer is 8 to 12 mμ thick and metabolically extremely active. Hebertson (1) observed via transmission electron microscopy that with oligohydramnios the cells are less thick, microvilli are reduced in number and bizarre in shape, and there is squamous metaplasia present. The abnormal membranes then become part of the vicious cycle as they are unable to reconstitute the amniotic fluid. Pulmonary hypoplasia may be associated with both oligohydramnios or polyhydramnios, i.e., diaphragmatic hernia (see Abstract 5–1). Oligohydramnios may result in lung hypoplasia both as a direct result of fetal thoracic compression and indirectly through inhibition of fetal breathing. Terminology and definitions are critical in comparing studies. The authors defined oligohydramnios as the absence of a pocket of amniotic fluid less than 1 cm in diameter measured in 2 planes. Calculations of fetal lung area were based on measurements of transverse section of fetal thorax during apnea at the level of the four chamber view of the heart, and the reproducibility revealed a coefficient of variation of less than 6%. Fetal breathing movements were considered positive if at least 1 breath occurred every 6 seconds, lasting for at least a minute. Sustained FBMs appear necessary for lung development and are indicators of fetal well-being. In normal pregnancies linear growth of the internal thoracic circumference and lung area was established with advancing gestational age. These will be useful reference data for future investigators.

The data from this study is different from previous reports. Nimrod (2), for example, predicted pulmonary hypoplasia from thoracic measurement. Blott on the other hand found that the absence of sustained FBM in the second trimester was the most reliable predictor. Moessinger found fetal breathing, defined as 3 breaths in 6 seconds, in infants dying with pulmonary hypoplasia. Blott argues that sustained breathing movements are the key. Time will tell who is correct.

This report adds insight into the perplexing problem of pulmonary hypoplasia associated with oligohydramnios and validates the importance of FBMs. If these preliminary findings are substantiated, then the clinicians will have a useful predictor of pulmonary hypoplasia, which is of inestimable value both for counseling the family and planning the management of the infant. The overwhelming tendency has been to preach doom and gloom with the onset of oligohydramnios in the second trimester. This report offers hope and presents a rational approach to following the pregnancy and when to intervene. See also Abstract 3–17.—A.A. Fanaroff, M.B.B.Ch.

References

1. Hebertson RM, et al: *Obstet Gynecol* 68:74, 1986.
2. Nimrod C, et al: *Obstet Gynecol* 68:495, 1986.

The Effect of Caput Succedaneum on Oxygen Saturation Measurements
Johnson N, Johnson VA, Bannister J, Lilford RJ (St James's Univ Hosp, Leeds, England)
Br J Obstet Gynaecol 97:493–498, 1990   4–13

Fetal oxygen saturation can be measured noninvasively by transcutaneous techniques with reflectance oximetry. Probes can be attached to flat surfaces, providing an inexpensive, accurate, and rapid method of monitoring the intrapartum fetus. To study the effect of caput or edema on reflectance pulse oximetry, 30 newborns were examined.

A mean reduction of 15% in oxygen saturation was seen in infants with caput (Fig 4–5). However, the reading by reflectance oximetry on the presenting part was lower than the oxygen saturation of the fetus as a whole. The effect of caput and edema in producing low readings may be a result of the increased extracellular fluid and may be explained by the physics of spectrophotometry.

Wide-angle light-sensitive probes have allowed noninvasive transcutaneous fetal monitoring. However, because readings from a presenting part that develops edema may be lower than the fetus as a whole, obstetricians should use caution in interpreting and using these results.

▶ Though pulse oximeters are accurate, sturdy, and not expensive they do not record accurately over edematous tissue. Six hours after birth when the edema had disappeared the difference between the oxygen saturation recorded over the caput and temporal region was less than 3%. Whether the inaccurate oxygen saturation over the caput is secondary to interference in the measurement from the edema or the values are truly lowered is not known. The authors believe both factors may be at work. In either case the device could be very inaccurate during labor.—M.H. Klaus, M.D.

PULSE OXIMETRY

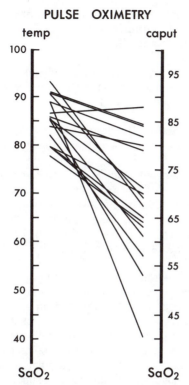

Fig 4–5.—The mean oxygen saturation recorded at birth over the caput and over the temporal region; $t = 5.3$; $P < .001$. (Courtesy of Johnson N, Johnson VA, Bannister J, et al: *Br J Obstet Gynaecol* 97:493–498, 1990.)

A Randomized Trial of Nurse-Midwifery Prenatal Care to Reduce Low Birth Weight

Heins HC Jr, Nance NW, McCarthy BJ, Efird CM (Med Univ of South Carolina, Charleston; Div of Reproductive Health, Centers for Disease Control, Atlanta; South Carolina Dept of Health and Environmental Control, Columbia)
Obstet Gynecol 75:341–345, 1990   4–14

Standard high-risk prenatal care by obstetricians was compared with nurse-midwife care in a controlled trial at 5 regional centers having state health department clinics. A total of 1,436 women at high risk of a low birth weight infant were studied. The nurse-midwives educated patients to recognize preterm labor, counseled them in terms of activity level, and delivered advice on stress reduction, social support, and nutrition. The 2 groups were comparable in race, educational and marital status, age, gravidity, and risk scores.

About one fifth of each group had low birth weight infants, and there was no significant reduction in very low birth weight infants. Births before 37 and 33 weeks' gestation occurred in similar proportions of the 2 groups. Of black women with high risk scores at the start of pregnancy, 2.6% in the intervention group and 6.7% of those seen by physicians had very low birth weight infants.

There was no particular advantage or disadvantage with nurse midwifery intervention in this study. Nurse-midwives could care for certain groups of high-risk women, and facilitate the coverage of a population that presently is underserved.

▶ This is not a pretty picture. The dismal success in reducing prematurity, together with the consequences of extremely premature delivery, are well-illustrated by this report. Once again, a prospective, multicenter, randomized, controlled trial draws a blank. The study is well-conceived, well-planned, and efficiently executed. The hypothesis was sound and the background data suggested the intervention should be effective. However, the results failed to support the premise that there would be a reduction in the incidence of low birth weight infants. With a rate of 20.5% in the control group, there was a wide margin for improvement. Lest I appear too pessimistic, there were positive aspects to this trial.

First, it is regional, rather than local, and of significant size, so that firm conclusions can be drawn. Second, the quality of care rendered by the midwives for the high-risk group appeared to be more than satisfactory. Third, the incidence of extreme prematurity was reduced in a subset of the population. It is, however, prudent to question the deployment of major resources across the country, using the above strategy, to decrease the prematurity rate.

At this point in time, I believe it is fair to comment that programs designed to reduce prematurity require reevaluation (see Abstract 3–15). Prematurity reduction must be a high priority among our health care programs.—A.A. Fanaroff, M.B.B.Ch.

5 Labor and Delivery

Randomized Investigation of Magnesium Sulfate for Prevention of Preterm Birth

Cox SM, Sherman ML, Leveno KJ (Univ of Texas Southwestern Med Ctr, Dallas)

Am J Obstet Gynecol 163:767–772, 1990   5–1

Magnesium sulfate is frequently used as a tocolytic agent, but no large randomized investigations comparing this therapy with untreated control subjects have been reported. To address this, 156 women with preterm labor between 24 and 34 weeks' gestation were randomly assigned to receive either intravenous magnesium sulfate or no tocolytic therapy. Magnesium sulfate was given as a 4 g loading dose, followed by a 2 g/hr infusion for 24 hours. The infusion rate was increased to 3 g/hr depending on uterine contractions.

Of the 76 women treated with magnesium sulfate, 62% received the maximum dose of 3 g/hr. Mean serum magnesium concentration was 5.5 mEq/L. Compared with 80 control pregnancies, magnesium sulfate tocolysis had no significant effect on duration of gestation, birth weight, neonatal morbidity, and perinatal mortality. Magnesium infusions were discontinued in 8 women because of toxicity. Magnesium sulfate infusions resulting in maximum serum magnesium concentrations of 5.5 mEq/L are ineffective in preventing preterm birth.

▶ Anne Regenstein, Fellow in Fetal Maternal Medicine at the University of California, San Francisco, and James M. Roberts, Ph.D., Professor of Obstetrics, Gynecology, and Reproductive Sciences, Senior Staff, Cardiovascular Research Institute, School of Medicine, University of California, San Francisco, offer their commentary:

▶ In this prospective, unblinded, randomized study comparing a 24-hour treatment of magnesium sulfate to placebo no benefit of this therapy was seen. Previous clinical and in vitro studies have suggested the efficacy of magnesium sulfate for tocolysis. The authors' conclusion that clinically safe infusions of magnesium sulfate are ineffective when used to prevent preterm birth needs to be qualified. At most they can state that no statistically significant difference was noted in the 156 pregnancies they studied. There was a trend in the magnesium sulfate treatment group to a heavier birth weight and a greater gestational age at delivery. A power analysis of their results reveals that their sample size was sufficient to detect an 8-day difference in time gained in utero or a 260 g difference in birth weight ($\alpha = 0.05$ and $\beta = 0.20$). Any benefits smaller than this would have gone undetected. A 2-day delay in delivery may be beneficial as this is the minimal delay one needs to allow betamethasone effectiveness. It would have been interesting if the authors had analyzed their data using the definition of successful tocolysis as prolongation of pregnancy for at least 48 hours.—A. Regenstein, Fellow, and J.M. Roberts, Ph.D.

Effects of Electronic Fetal-Heart-Rate Monitoring, As Compared With Periodic Auscultation, on the Neurologic Development of Premature Infants
Shy KK, Luthy DA, Bennett FC, Whitfield M, Larson EB, van Belle G, Hughes JP, Wilson JA, Stenchever MA (Univ of Washington; Grace Hosp, Vancouver)
N Engl J Med 322:588–593, 1990   5–2

In a multicenter, randomized clinical trial the early neurologic development was assessed in 93 prematurely born infants whose heart rates were monitored electronically during delivery. The findings were compared with those in 96 prematurely born infants whose heart rates were periodically monitored by auscultation. All infants had birth weights of 1,750 g or less and all had cephalic presentation. Fetal heart rates in the electronic group were classified as reassuring, nonreassuring, or abnormal; those in the auscultation group were classified as reassuring or abnormal.

The pH of blood from the scalps of fetuses with nonreassuring or abnormal heart rates was sampled. Infants were studied at 4, 8, and 18 months. Mental and psychomotor development was assessed by the Bayley Scales of Infant Development, and the Movement Assessment of Infants index was used at 4- and 8-month examinations. Each infant had a neurologic examination at 18 months.

At 18 months the mean mental development scores were 100.5 in the

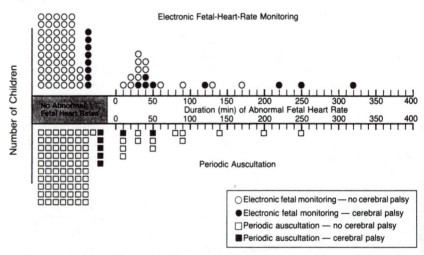

Fig 5–1.—Duration of abnormal fetal heart rates during intrapartum surveillance with electronic fetal monitoring or periodic auscultation among infants with and without cerebral palsy. *Asterisk* indicates child born after the decision was made during labor not to intervene with cesarean section because of fetal indications. (Courtesy of Shy KK, Luthy DA, Bennett FC, et al: *N Engl J Med* 322:588–593, 1990.)

electronically monitored group and 104.9 in the periodic auscultation group. Mean psychomotor development scores in the 2 groups were 94.0 and 98.3, respectively. Twenty percent of patients in the electronically monitored group had cerebral palsy versus 8% in the auscultation group. In the electronically monitored group only, the risk of cerebral palsy increased with the duration of abnormal fetal heart rate patterns (Fig 5–1). The median time to delivery after the diagnosis of abnormal heart rate patterns was 104 minutes in the electronically monitored group and 60 minutes in the auscultation group.

Electronic fetal heart rate monitoring does not lead to improved neurologic development in children born prematurely. It may be less effective than a structured program of periodic auscultation. In this series there was an unanticipated 2.9-fold increase in the odds of having cerebral palsy in the electronically monitored group. Low scores on the Bayley scales were also more common in the electronically monitored group.

▶ Though the median weights in the 2 groups are similar there is no data presented that the gestational ages of the very young infants were similar in each group. Though electronic fetal monitoring came in with a flurry with great expectations of reducing CNS damage only the early nonrandomized trials suggested an improved neonatal outcome. Though the courts have somehow blessed electronic fetal monitoring none of the 8 randomized trials favor its use. I wonder how the routine use of this procedure can somehow be reduced. What amount of data will be required to stop using this procedure routinely?—M.H. Klaus, M.D.

Prophylactic Intrapartum Amnioinfusion: A Randomized Clinical Trial
Strong TH Jr, Hetzler G, Sarno AP, Paul RH (Univ of Southern California; Los Angeles County/Univ of Southern California Med Ctr, Los Angeles)
Am J Obstet Gynecol 162:1370–1375, 1990   5–3

Intrapartum amnioinfusion has been effective in the treatment of variable fetal decelerations. It is hypothesized that, among those who are at risk for intrapartum morbidity, the optimal time for amnioinfusion is before the occurrence of significant fetal heart rate (FHR) abnormalities or the passage of meconium. In a prospective, randomized trial, 60 women in the latent phase of labor with oligohydramnios (amniotic fluid index ≤ 5 cm) were studied to determine the efficacy of prophylactic intrapartum infusion. Amnioinfusion was performed in 30 women until an amniotic fluid index level at or above 8 cm was reached, and no amnioinfusion was performed in 30 women (controls). All fetuses were at or above 37 weeks' gestation, had normal FHR variability, and had no clinically significant FHR decelerations at the outset.

The infusion group required an average 1.6 infusion sequences to attain an amniotic fluid index level of at least 8 cm, with a mean 379 mL (range, 250–1,000) of normal saline solution infused. The amnioinfusion group had significantly less frequent meconium passage, severe variable decelerations, end-stage bradycardia, and operative delivery for fetal distress, as compared with controls. Mean umbilical arterial blood pH was also significantly higher in the amnioinfusion group. Neonatal outcome, particularly the frequency of nuchal cords, did not differ significantly between groups.

Laboring women at or beyond term with oligohydramnios will benefit from prophylactic amnioinfusion. Prophylactic intrapartum amnioinfusion is a safe, simple, and low-cost procedure that can significantly reduce the incidence of intrapartum morbidity. Further studies are warranted to define the indications, application, and efficacy of this procedure.

▶ Murray Enkin, M.D., Emeritus Professor of Obstetrics and Gynecology, Department of Obstetrics and Gynecology, McMaster University, Hamilton, Ontario, provides the following comment.

▶ Amnioinfusion is a relatively new approach to the treatment of FHR abnormalities, oligohydramnios, and meconium-stained amniotic fluid in labor. Unlike many other new procedures that have been introduced into clinical practice without adequate evaluation, amnioinfusion is being properly studied with randomized controlled clinical trials, albeit so far only with small numbers. The first of these (1) showed a significant reduction in variable decelerations, with a nonsignificant reduction in cesarean section. The Oxford Database of Perinatal Trials (2) lists 10 reports of 7 randomized trials that have been conducted since that time; all of these showed similar results, with improvement in proxy measures of infant well-being but no clear cut effects on more substantive outcomes. Amnioinfusion has a sound theoretical basis, and shows promise of proving to be a useful therapeutic modality. Further trials, with large enough numbers to demonstrate whether the procedure has an effect on clinical outcomes, are required before amnioinfusion can be considered to be therapeutically useful.—M. Enkin, M.D.

References

1. Miyazaki FS, Nevarez F: *Am J Obstet Gynecol* 153:301, 1985.
2. Hofmeyr GJ: Overviews of amnioinfusion. Oxford Database of Perinatal Trials, 1990.

Outcomes of Care in Birth Centers: The National Birth Center Study
Rooks JP, Weatherby NL, Ernst EKM, Stapleton S, Rosen D, Rosenfield A (Columbia Univ, New York; Natl Assoc of Childbearing Centers, Perkiomenville, Penn)
N Engl J Med 321:1804–1811, 1989   5–4

Originally established to serve rural communities, birth centers are now appearing in urban communities. Birth centers are nonhospital facilities designed to provide family-centered maternity care for women at low risk of obstetric complications. Safety is the primary concern. The labor, delivery, follow-up care, and outcomes of a large number of women admitted in labor to birth centers were studied.

Data on 11,814 women admitted to 84 free-standing birth centers from 1985 to 1987 were analyzed. The women were at lower-than-average risk of poor pregnancy outcomes according to many but not all recognized demographic and behavioral factors. Seventy-one percent had minor or no complications, and 7.9% had serious emergency complications during labor and delivery or soon thereafter. Such complications included thick meconium and severe shoulder dystocia. One in 6 women was transferred to a hospital; 2.4% had emergency transfers. Twenty-nine percent of nulliparous women and 7% of parous women were transferred. The frequency of emergency transfers, however, was the same. Cesarean section was needed in 4.4%. None of the mothers died. Overall, the intrapartum and neonatal mortality rate was 1.3 per 1,000 births. Rates of infant mortality and low Apgar scores were comparable to those among low-risk hospital births.

Birth centers are a safe, acceptable alternative to hospital confinement for selected women, especially those who have had children. Such care leads to relatively few cesarean sections.

▶ It is encouraging to inspect the actual data from the 84 U.S. birth centers and note the low infant morbidity and mortality. Though 17,856 mothers enrolled in these free-standing birth centers planning to deliver, far fewer (66.2%) actually did! The main reason not to deliver in the birth center was prenatal complication (2,557 women). Thus, in a select low-risk population, even with this qualification, birth centers compare quite nicely with low-risk deliveries in hospital. In evaluating these results it is important to note that if there was a death in any patient referred to a hospital it was included as a complication of the birth center. The low cesarean section rate of 4.4% is further evidence that present hospital practices may be aversive to many women.—M.H. Klaus, M.D.

Vaginal Birth After Cesarean Delivery: Results of a 5-Year Multicenter Collaborative Study

Flamm BL, Newman LA, Thomas SJ, Fallon D, Yoshida MM (Kaiser Permanente Med Ctr, Northern Calif and Southern Calif Regions; Univ of California, Irvine)

Obstet Gynecol 76:750–754, 1990

5–5

Many physicians remain reluctant to attempt vaginal birth after previous cesarean delivery without large studies conclusively demonstrating the safety of this policy. In this multicenter study that began in 1984, 11 medical centers participated in a collaborative project involving a trial of labor after a previous cesarean delivery.

Of the 15,098 women with previous cesarean sections seen during the 5-year study, 5,733 (38.0%) underwent a trial of labor. Successful vaginal births were achieved in 4,291 (74.8%). The rate of trial of labor ranged from 14% to 63% among the 11 institutions and the vaginal birth rate ranged from 68% to 89%. Among patients with previous cesarean operations for cephalopelvic disproportion or failure to progress, 65% of those who attempted vaginal birth were successful. The overall incidence of uterine rupture was 1.7 per 1,000 (10/5,733), and was not affected by the number of previous cesarean operations or use of oxytocin during labor. No maternal deaths occurred. The perinatal morbidity rate, using the 5-minute Apgar score, was 0.9%. The perinatal mortality rate was 6 per 1,000, a rate slightly less than the overall perinatal mortality rate of 10 per 1,000 in all participating hospitals. One perinatal death related to uterine rupture occurred, but the patient labored at home.

This study presents overwhelming evidence on the safety and efficacy of vaginal birth after previous cesarean operations. The policy of routine repeat cesarean delivery should be abandoned.

▶ Peter Boylan, M.B., Master, National Maternity Hospital, Dublin, Ireland, provides his insight and commentary on this article.

▶ This is a most welcome study that demonstrates, again, the safety of vaginal delivery after cesarean section. The study group achieved an enviable 75% vaginal delivery rate among 5,733 patients. Perhaps 1 of the more significant sentences in the entire publication is the following: "Our medical-legal consultants concluded subsequently that vaginal birth after cesarean is well within the current standard of care and that special consent forms were no longer necessary." It is now apparent that women who are not given trial of labor after a previous cesarean section are not getting the best standard of care. The paper also supports the safe use of oxytocin and epidural analgesia in this group of patients. While the authors are to be congratulated, one might quibble in a minor way with their final conclusion that no other method offers such a profound potential for reducing the overall cesarean delivery rate in the United States. Perhaps efforts should be directed at preventing the original cesarean section by adopting a medical (1) rather than a surgical approach to the treatment of dystocia, the root cause of the current cesarean epidemic.—P. Boylan, M.B., M.R.C.O.G.

Reference

1. Boylan P, et al: *Am J Perinat Med*, in press.

Prognosis for Twins With Birth Weight <1500 gm: The Impact of Cesarean Section in Relation to Fetal Presentation
Rydhström H (Univ Hosp, Lund, Sweden)
Am J Obstet Gynecol 163:528–533, 1990   5–6

The impact of cesarean section on intrapartum and neonatal mortality and long-term morbidity of twins weighing less than 1,500 g was studied using national data at the Medical Birth Registry, Stockholm. A total of 862 twins born between 1973 and 1983 were studied. Of these, 357 were identified with cerebral palsy and/or mental retardation 8 years after birth using questionnaires sent to various agencies caring for disabled children. Groups were stratified based on birth weight and period of delivery.

The cesarean section rate increased from 7.7% in 1973 to 1976 to 68.9% in 1981 to 1983, and intrapartum and neonatal mortality decreased from 51.7% to 29.1% during the same periods. Intrapartum and neonatal mortality decreased in twin II born either vaginally or abdominally, but remained relatively constant in twin I. Overall, the relative risk for intrapartum and neonatal mortality after vaginal/abdominal birth was 1.5, with 95% confidence limits of 1.0 to 2.3. The risk did not differ significantly for twin I or twin II in vertex or breech presentation, even when the only indication for operation was prematurity.

The rate of cerebral palsy and/or mental retardation was 8.8% in 1973 to 1976 and 8.0% in 1977 to 1988; the difference was not significant. For twins born in breech presentation, the rate was similar for the first period (cesarean section rate 6.0%) and the second period (cesarean section rate 59.6%).

Cesarean section appears to have little impact on fetal outcome for low birth weight twins, even after considering fetal presentation.

▶ Providing comment on this article as well is Peter Boylan, M.B., Master, National Maternity Hospital, Dublin, Ireland.

▶ This is an important study that fails to support the liberal use of cesarean section for twins with a birth weight less than 1,500 g. This is particularly interesting in view of the fact that no advantage was found even for twins where the baby was presenting by the breech. The study was a retrospective one based on the prospective collection of data in the Swedish system where very accurate records are kept of all births during the year. The study is also interesting in that there was no decline in incidence of cerebral palsy during the decade examined, despite a 10-fold increase in cesarean delivery. This again is further evidence against the influence of peripartum events as a cause of long-term neurologic deficit. The study provides support for those who wish to continue with a conservative approach toward the care of women and babies around the time of delivery. It is becoming more apparent with the passage of time that cesarean birth rates may be used as an index of the quality of care given to women, and that a low cesarean section rate equates with a high standard of care.—P. Boylan, M.B., M.R.C.O.G.

Neonatal and Maternal Outcome in Low-Pelvic and Midpelvic Operative Deliveries

Robertson PA, Laros RK Jr, Zhao R-L (Univ of California, San Francisco; San Francisco Med Ctr)
Am J Obstet Gynecol 162:1436–1444, 1990

---

pH of Umbilical Cord Artery Blood Gases
of Operative Vaginal Deliveries Versus
Matched Cesarean Sections

Method	pH < 7.10 (%)	Significance
Midforceps	46.8	
Cesarean section	20.3	$p < 0.001$
Midvacuum	28.9	
Cesarean section	15.1	—
Low-forceps	41.7	
Cesarean section	26.3	$p < 0.05$
Low-vacuum	24.1	
Cesarean section	26.1	—

(Courtesy of Robertson PA, Laros RK Jr, Zhao R-L: *Am J Obstet Gynecol* 162:1436–1444, 1990.)

The American College of Obstetrics and Gynecology has redefined the concept of outlet, low-pelvic, and midpelvic operative vaginal delivery using a −5 to +5 scale system of station. Using these new definitions, neonatal and maternal outcomes were compared retrospectively in 95 midforceps and 52 midvacuum vaginal deliveries vs. 290 cesarean sections with a second stage of labor longer than 30 minutes at similar station, and 921 low-forceps and 347 low-vacuum deliveries vs. 64 cesarean sections of similar station and second stage longer than 30 minutes.

Compared with matched cesarean sections, all vaginal operative deliveries, both forceps and vacuum, showed significantly decreased estimated blood loss, maternal hospital stay, and maternal morbidity. In terms of neonatal outcome, both midforceps and midvacuum vaginal deliveries were associated with a significant increase in the frequency of active neonatal resuscitation and an increase in base deficit for the umbilical artery. Furthermore, midforceps delivery was associated with a significantly increased rate of admission to the intensive care nursery and an increased risk of significant birth trauma. Both midforceps and low-forceps delivery were associated with a significant increase of neonates with cord arterial pH below 7.1 and increase of base deficit, even after exclusion of cases of fetal distress (table).

Midpelvic delivery has substantial detrimental effects on the neonate compared with cesarean section at similar station. Thus, when considering a midforceps or midvacuum operative vaginal delivery, the potential risks to the neonatal must be carefully balanced against the maternal benefits.

▶ Life is a series of compromises; however, there can be no compromise when it comes to maternal and fetal safety. As such there is an ever diminishing role for instrumental deliveries. Judicious midforceps deliveries were not necessarily harmful to the fetus according to Dierker (1), and Baerthlein (2) concluded that the vacuum appears to be safe for midpelvic delivery when compared with forceps. There remains a problem in training residents in midpelvic procedures so that cesarean section becomes the preferred route of delivery. The case matched study from Robertson et al. for the first time uses the new definitions from the College, but it does nothing to allay the concerns of those who believe that midforceps deliveries should be abandoned. Midforceps deliveries resulted in beaten up, depressed, acidotic neonates who required more admissions to neonatal intensive care units. The costs, any which way you measure them, are unacceptably high. The debate of vacuum versus cesarean section for delays during the second stage of labor will continue, but forceps, a lost art, should be eliminated from contention (3). (See also Abstract 7–3.)

We are not born to sue, but to command.—William Shakespeare

A.A. Fanaroff, M.B.B.Ch.

References

1. Dierker LJ Jr, et al: 1987 YEAR BOOK OF NEONATAL AND PERINATAL MEDICINE, Abstract 4–1.
2. Baerthlein: 1987 YEAR BOOK OF NEONATAL AND PERINATAL MEDICINE, Abstract 4–2.
3. 1990 YEAR BOOK OF NEONATAL AND PERINATAL MEDICINE, Abstract 5–15.

True Knots in the Umbilical Cord: Clinical Findings and Fetal Consequences

Matorras R, Diez J, Pereira JG, Montoya F, Gutiérrez de Terán G, Aranguren G, Rodríguez-Escudero FJ (Universidad del País Vasco, Hospital de Cruces, Baracaldo, Spain)
J Obstet Gynaecol 10:383–386, 1990

5–8

There are differing opinions on the clinical consequences of a true knot in the umbilical cord. Fetal mortality rates ranging from 4% to 40% have been reported, but there are frequently concomitant pathologic factors. To clarify further, 87 singleton pregnancies with true knots in the umbilical cord were studied and compared with a control group consisting of 87 pregnancies delivered immediately after each case of true knot.

The incidence of umbilical cord knot was 0.68% (89/13,091). Factors associated with true knots were multiparity, long cords, and presence of nuchal cords. True knots were not associated with greater fetal morbidity or mortality. Apgar scores, umbilical cord analysis, and fetal heart rate tracings were similar in both groups. Likewise, perinatal mortality (1.1% vs. 2.3%) and neonatal morbidity (9.2% vs. 6.9%) were similar in both groups.

In general, true knots in the umbilical cord are not associated with greater fetal loss or higher neonatal morbidity.

▶ Though true knots are observed more often with long cords and in multiparous women they were not associated with an increased incidence of fetal or neonatal distress. Benirschke and Driscoll (1) note that to determine that the fetal death is caused by a true knot it is necessary to find a reduction or disappearance of Wharton's jelly, distal venous congestion, and at least partially occlusive vascular thrombi. Though other observers have noted an increased perinatal mortality ranging from 4% to 6% with a true knot, in this report true knots were not associated with any greater fetal morbidity. It is interesting that the 89 cases of true knot occurred in 13,091 deliveries. Seventeen percent of the infants had 2 knots and 1 infant had three. It is impressive in this large series that a true knot was not associated with an increased incidence of neonatal problems.—M.H. Klaus, M.D.

Reference

1. Benirschke K, Driscoll SG: *The Pathology of the Human Placenta.* New York, Springer-Verlag, 1974, pp 159–162.

Clavicular Fractures in Neonates
Joseph PR, Rosenfeld W (Winthrop-Univ Hosp, Mineola, NY; State Univ of New York at Stony Brook)
Am J Dis Child 144:165–167, 1990   5–9

The reported incidence of clavicular fracture in newborns varies widely from .2% to 3.5%. The frequency of such injuries was prospectively determined in 626 consecutive infants who were delivered vaginally in a 32-month period.

There were 18 (2.9%) clavicular fractures. Only 2 infants had signs and symptoms of fracture on initial examination; 9 fractures were diagnosed at the time of discharge when swelling over the clavicle was minimal, and 7 were found at the first office visit. The most reliable sign of clavicular fracture in the hospital was difficulty feeling the clavicular margins. No obstetric complications occurred. Of the 18 infants, 13 were girls, and 13 fractures were on the right side.

Most newborns with a fractured clavicle have no symptoms and no marked physical findings in the first few days of life, emphasizing the need for repeated examinations.

▶ Every now and again it would appear as if the wheel needs to be rediscovered. Such is the case with this prospective study that reaffirms the value of careful neonatal physical examination and follow-up. It represents the clinical experience of a single physician who notes that the majority of neonates with fractures of the clavicle are asymptomatic, and their fractures are only detected by physical examination. Surprisingly, infants with clavicular fractures appear to experience minimal discomfort. Waiting for textbook signs such as crepitus, an asymmetric Moro, or extensive bruising before considering the diagnosis will result in most clavicular fractures remaining undetected.

Most things break including hearts. The lessons of life amount not to wisdom, but to scar tissue and callus.— Wallace Stegner

A.A. Fanaroff, M.B.B.Ch.

Birth Asphyxia and the Intrapartum Cardiotocograph
Murphy KW, Johnson P, Moorcraft J, Pattinson R, Russell V, Turnbull A (John Radcliffe Hosp, Oxford; Univ of Stellenbosch, Tygerberg, South Africa)
Br J Obstet Gynaecol 97:470–479, 1990   5–10

The results of using the intrapartum cardiotocography for predicting low pH at birth have been reported to be poor, possibly because of poor

---

Indications for Intervention in Fetal Interest (Fetal Sampling or Operative Delivery) Agreed Upon by All 3 Investigators	Duration (min)
Fetal heart rate abnormality	
Uncomplicated tachycardia: 160–180 bpm	120
Uncomplicated tachycardia: >180 bpm	60
Bradycardia: <100 bpm	20
Moderate variable decelerations >50 bpm, >30 <60 s	120
Severe variable decelerations >50 bpm, >60 s	40
Late decelerations (lag time >20 s)	40
Reduced baseline variability: <5 bpm	60
Complicated tachycardia: FHR >160 bpm, late or moderate/severe variable decelerations and reduced baseline variability	40

Abbreviation: bpm, beats per minutes.
(Courtesy of Murphy KW, Johnson P, Moorcraft J, et al: *Br J Obstet Gynaecol* 97:470–479, 1990.)

interpretation. To investigate further, the intrapartum cardiotocographs of 38 severely asphyxiated term infants and 120 healthy term infants were reviewed retrospectively and independently but 3 investigators who were unaware of the clinical outcome.

The interobserver agreement was good (Kappa statistic = 0.74). Abnormalities on cardiotocography were present in 87% of infants with asphyxia, compared with 29% of controls. The abnormality was considered severe enough to result in significant fetal metabolic acidosis at delivery in 61% of asphyxiated infants compared to 9% of controls. These differences were highly significant ($P < 0.001$).

By using traditional criteria for fetal distress (table), fetal blood sampling was considered to be indicated in 58% of the asphyxia group and 20% of controls, but it was performed in only 16% and 8%, respectively. Operative deliveries for fetal distress were performed more often on the asphyxia group, but the frequency of operative deliveries among those with an abnormal cardiotocogram did not differ between the asphyxia and control groups. Furthermore, the median response times of the delivery suite staff for abnormal fetal heart rate (FHR) problems were similar in the asphyxia and control groups whether the FHR changes were moderate or severe, based on the Krebs' cardiotocograph scoring system.

Interpretation of the intrapartum cardiotocograph remains a major problem, and a more objective method of interpretation should be found.

▶ Interpretation of FHR patterns remains central to identification of fetal distress. Distressingly, 30 years since its introduction there is scant evidence for its efficacy in low-risk pregnancy. Old-fashioned auscultation is equally effective in low-risk pregnancy and perhaps even for premature infants (1). In high-risk pregnancies poor interpretation, technical failures, and combinations thereof have resulted in poor predictibility of low pH at birth. Murphy et al. have attempted to validate the usefulness of cardiotocography in pregnancies complicated by asphyxia.

Asphyxia was based on a combination of low Apgar scores, umbilical artery metabolic acidosis, the need for assisted ventilation in the delivery room, meconium aspiration, or seizures within 48 hours of birth. Few will quibble with this definition. A methodical search through their database yielded the asphyxiated infants and suitable controls. The perinatal history and the monitoring strips were then presented to the review panel who were blinded as to the outcome of the infants. The panelists agreed on when fetal blood gases should be done but only predicted acidosis accurately about 70% of the time. The overall impression of the panel was that although abnormal FHR patterns occurred with greater frequency and severity in the asphyxiated infants the response time was not shorter than in the control infants. There was not a faster response in the presence of fetal bradycardia or tachycardia, limited oscillations or baseline variability, no accelerations, and late or severe atypical variable decelerations, i.e., low Krebs' scoring system. Although there is a strong association between abnormal FHR monitoring, low pH and Apgar, and poor postnatal outcome the high rate of false positives (low specificity) is a major problem with fetal cardiotocography. The major recommendations of the panel were to improve the interpretation of FHR monitoring and to increase the number of scalp blood gases. Ongoing in-service education, more systematic strategic review of tracings, and central monitoring stations may also contribute to better interpretation. Computer analysis of the tracings is on the horizon (2). I also see interpretation of FHR monitoring becoming the major quality issue on the obstetric service. The net effect is to identify asphyxia earlier and to reduce the need for cesarean sections. Then I rudely awaken from my dream.

And we forget because we must,
and not because we will.— Matthew Arnold

A.A. Fanaroff, M.B.B.Ch.

References

1. Shy KK: *N Engl J Med* 322:588, 1990.
2. Pello LC: *Br J Obstet Gynecol* 95:1128, 1988.

A Device for Domiciliary Neonatal Resuscitation

Milner AD, Upton CJ, Green J, Stokes GM (City Hosp; Univ Hosp, Nottingham, England)
Lancet 335:273–275, 1990

5–11

Basic neonatal resuscitation facilities are lacking in most developing countries, and this may account for more than 1 million infants deaths per year and hypoxic encephalopathy in many more. A simple, inexpensive device was developed to aid in neonatal resuscitation in these countries.

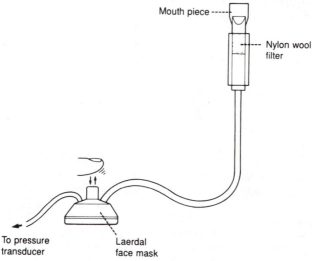

Mouth piece

Nylon wool filter

To pressure transducer

Laerdal face mask

Fig 5–2.—Resuscitation device. (Courtesy of Milner AD, Upton CJ, Green J, et al: *Lancet* 335:273–275, 1990.)

Causes of Death According to Smoking Status

	% of deaths (*no*)	
Cause of death	Non-smokers	Current smokers
All causes	100 *(302)*	100 *(1792)*
All cardiovascular	58 *(174)*	51 *(907)*
CHD	43 *(129)*	38 *(675)*
Stroke	6 *(19)*	5 *(95)*
All cancers	28 *(84)*	33 *(587)*
Lung cancer	3 *(10)*	15 *(265)*
All other causes	15 *(44)*	17 *(298)*

(Courtesy of Milner AD, Upton CJ, Green J, et al: *Lancet* 335:273–275, 1990.)

The resuscitation device is a face-mask T-piece system. It consists of a silicone rubber tube, 1 cm in diameter, mounted into the dome of the round silicone rubber face-mask (Laerdal face mask) and a disposable mouthpiece with an integral filter of nylon wool (Fig 5–2). The total system resistance is 8 cm/H_2O)/L/second.

A total of 68 volunteers with and 82 volunteers without previous experience on neonatal resuscitation were instructed on the use of the mouth-tube/face-mask system. They were told to hold the face-mask over the mouth and face of a neonatal manikin with 1 hand and to produce expiratory flow through the face-mask for 6 to 10 seconds while intermittently occluding the port of the face-mask to produce an inflation pressure.

Median inspiratory pressures achieved by volunteers without neonatal resuscitation experience were similar to those of experienced volunteers (table). The median respiratory rate and median maximum and median mean pressures were similar to those generally recommended for neonatal resuscitation. Most participants found the system to be effortless and easy to use.

The mouth-tube/face-mask is a simple and inexpensive device appropriate for use in neonatal resuscitation in developing countries. It requires only 1 hand and is easier than mouth-to-mouth resuscitation.

▶ There is beauty in its simplicity. This is a simple, easy to learn and easy to teach technique. What's more, it is effective and inexpensive. The ability to quickly instruct a naive provider makes this a wonderful tool for centers with minimal staffing. The resuscitation course established in the United States by the American Academy of Pediatrics and the American Heart Association has been broadly accepted. Although there are local disagreements with some of the specifics, the overall principles have been accepted. There should soon be skilled personnel assigned to resuscitate every baby born in every hospital. The toll of perinatal asphyxia on a worldwide basis is staggering. The risk of AIDS has made mouth-to-mouth ventilation an unacceptable risk. The device reported above therefore represents an excellent technique for neonatal resuscitation in developing countries.—A.A. Fanaroff, M.B.B.Ch.

6 Infectious Diseases and Developmental Immunology

Congenital Syphilis Presenting in Infants After the Newborn Period
Dorfman DH, Glaser JH (Bronx Municipal Hosp Ctr; Albert Einstein Coll of Medicine, Bronx, NY)
N Engl J Med 323:1299–1302, 1990   6–1

Syphilis generally is excluded if both the mother and infant are seronegative, but 7 infants were encountered during a 1-year period with symptomatic congenital syphilis in whom serologic tests were negative. The hospitals where these infants were born used a qualitative rapid-plasma-reagin test as the initial screening measure; at delivery, 4 of the infants and their mothers had negative tests. Three of the mothers were seronegative during pregnancy and were not tested at delivery. Two of their infants were seronegative at birth; 1 was not tested.

All 7 infants were seropositive when tested at age 3 to 14 weeks, when symptoms were present. The 5 mothers tested also were seropositive at this time. Four of the infants had a typical diffuse rash; the other 3 were febrile and had aseptic meningitis. All infants had multisystemic disease, as evidenced by liver enlargement, anemia, monocytosis, and increased alkaline phosphatase and and aminotransferase levels. All infants responded to parenteral penicillin treatment. A Jarisch-Herxheimer reaction consistently followed the first dose of antibiotic.

Probably at least some of these mothers acquired syphilis toward the end of pregnancy, accounting for negative serologic test results at the time of delivery. It is best to test all mothers during pregnancy, and all mothers and infants at the time of delivery. Infants who have fever with aseptic meningitis, hepatomegaly, or hematologic abnormalities should be tested for congenital syphilis even if previous tests have been negative.

► There has been a resurgence of syphilis throughout the United States. Rates of congenital syphilis have increased from 2 to 4 per 100,000 live births in 1980 to 18 per 100,000 in 1988. In New York City approximately 10 cases were reported in 1983 and more than 400 cases in 1988. The newer definition wherein any infant whose mother had untreated or inadequately treated syphilis at delivery, regardless of findings in the infant, account in part for the increased reporting. Other cases to be reported include any infant who has a reactive treponemal test for syphilis in addition to physical or radiologic evidence of congenital syphilis, abnormal spinal fluid, reactive test for FTA-ABS-19S-IgM antibody, or cord blood titer 4-fold higher than the mother's. Guidelines for screening the high-risk patients during pregnancy include testing during the first and third trimesters and again at delivery. Unscreened mothers should not be discharged after delivery until their status with regard to syphilis has been determined. Pediatricians need to rehone their skills in diagnosing congenital syphilis, and a high index of suspicion is mandatory, particularly for neonates who are undergrown and those with unexplained jaundice, hepatomegaly, skin lesions, nasal discharge, bony lesions, or thrombocytopenia. A comprehensive review of bone lesions by Rasool (1) is helpful reading and indicative of the resurgence of syphilis in Southern Africa. Vigorous and complete treatment with follow-up to detect treatment failures manifested by the presence of a positive Venereal Disease Research Laboratory test beyond 1 to 2 years, a 4-fold rise in the nontreponemal tests, and persistence of clinical signs and symptoms must be implemented.

The short words are best and the old words are best of all.—Winston Churchill

A.A. Fanaroff, M.B.B.Ch.

Reference

1. Rasool M: *J Bone Joint Surg* 71B:752, 1989.

Preliminary Study of Breastfeeding and Bacterial Adhesion to Uroepithelial Cells
Coppa GV, Gabrielli O, Giorgi P, Catassi C, Montanari MP, Varaldo PE, Nichols BL (Univ of Ancona, Ancona, Italy; Baylor Univ, Houston)
Lancet 335:569–571, 1990   6–2

Bacterial adhesion to epithelial surfaces is usually established by binding of the bacteria to the specific receptors of the host cell surface. The receptors are mostly oligosaccharide residues of glycoproteins and glycolipids on cell membranes. Human milk contains a substantial amount of oligosaccharides, which have been found to inhibit adhesion of *Streptococcus pneumoniae* to human pharyngeal and buccal epithelial cells. The present study provides preliminary evidence that human milk may help protect against infection of the urinary tract.

Thirty days after delivery 24-hour urine samples were obtained from 10 nursing mothers and their infants. A sample of milk was also taken from each mother. The oligosaccharide content of these specimens was analyzed by thin-layer and high-performance liquid chromatography. The effect of oligosaccharide fractions from a 500-mL pool of colostrum on bacterial adhesion to uroepithelial cells was tested on a strain of *Escherichia coli* isolated from an infant with a urinary tract infection.

The oligosaccharide profile in each woman's breast milk and urine was very similar. The pattern of oligosaccharide excreted in the urine by the infant correlated strongly with that of the mother's milk. Daily oligosaccharide excretion by the infants was 300 to 500 mg, and excretion by the mothers was 500 to 800 mg. When tested on an *E. coli* strain isolated from an infant with a urinary tract infection, the high-molecular-weight sialylated oligosaccharides had no inhibitory effect, but neutral oligosaccharides caused inhibition of bacteral adhesion that increased as the size of the oligosaccharides decreased.

Breastfeeding may have a preventive effect against urinary tract infection in both mother and infant.

► We described in the 1988 YEAR BOOK OF NEONATAL AND PERINATAL MEDICINE (p 11) a report by A. Prentice noting that in breastfed infants the secretory A levels in the urine are 3-fold greater than bottle fed infants. Now we have another possible defense mechanism—oligosaccharides from breast milk that are secreted into the infant's urine and significantly reduce the adhesion of pathogenic *E. coli* from sticking to renal epithelium. Please stay tuned; I am sure we have not heard the complete explanation for why breastfed infants have a reduced number of urinary tract infections.—M.H. Klaus, M.D.

Effect of Breast-Feeding on Antibody Response to Conjugate Vaccine
Pabst HF, Spady DW (Univ of Alberta, Edmonton)
Lancet 336:269–270, 1990   6–3

A previous study of the cell-mediated immune response to vaccination with Bacille Calmette-Guérin (BCG) suggested that breastfeeding may be a useful adjunct to vaccination of infants. Evidence was found for enhancement by breastfeeding of an active humoral immune response.

Fifty-nine breastfed and formula-fed infants were immunized at ages 2, 4, and 6 months with CRM-197 diptheria-toxin/*Hemophilus influenzae* type b polyribose phosphate (PRP) conjugate vaccine. Antibody levels were measured before and at 7 months and again at 12 months after immunization; lymphocyte transformation to different mitogens was also tested. In addition, breastfed infants were changed to formula feeding at a mean age of 4.5 months.

Antibody levels did not differ significantly between groups before immunization; however, they were significantly higher in the breastfed infants at 7 months and 12 months after immunization when compared with formula-fed infants. The antibody levels at 7 months were independent of levels measured before immunization. Lymphocyte transformation results were almost similar in both groups.

Because breastfeeding enhances the active immune response in the first year of life, the feeding method should be considered when evaluating vaccine studies in infants.

► The authors previously have shown that breastfeeding augments the cell-mediated immune response to vaccination with BCG. These observations suggest to the authors that the immune regulatory system of the infant receives maturational signals through breastfeeding. Recent studies in the laboratory suggest that fractions of human colostrum stimulate as well as suppress some functions of lymphocytes (1).—M.H. Klaus, M.D.

Reference

1. Mincheva-Nilsson L, et al: *Clin Exp Immunol* 79:463, 1990.

Evaluation of Coagulase-Negative Staphylococcal Isolates From Serial Nasopharyngeal Cultures of Premature Infants
Hall SL, Riddell SW, Barnes WG, Meng L, Hall RT (Univ of Missouri–Kansas City School of Medicine, Kansas City, Mo)
Diagn Microbiol Infect Dis 13:17–23, 1990   6–4

Cogulase-negative staphylococci (C-S) are the leading cause of nosocomial infections in neonatal intensive care units (NICUs). To assess patterns of colonization with C-S in very low birth weight (<1,750 g) infants over prolonged periods of hospitalization, nasopharyngeal cultures were obtained weekly on 28 very low birth weight infants hospitalized for a mean of 8 weeks (range, 4–15). Isolates were identified with 4 screening parameters: species, biotype, antibiotic susceptibility pattern, and slime production. Isolates from the same infant with highly similar screening parameters then underwent phage typing and plasmid analysis to increase the likelihood of establishing strain identity.

A total of 125 isolates from 96 cultures grew C-S, and 105 were evaluable. Nasopharyngeal colonization with C-S increased from 12% on admission to 75% by week 2 of hospital stay, then gradually declined to 30% by week 6 and remained stable through week 10 (Fig 6–1). There were no significant differences among C-S isolates from week 1 compared with week 10 in terms of distribution of species, slime positivity, or multiply antibiotic resistant strains. Although 1 bioptype of *Staphylococcus epidermidis* was recovered from 46% of infants, only 1 infant was colonized with a predominant type of *S. epidermidis*. There was marked variability in C-S isolates in individual infants from week to week.

Thirteen pairs of isolates recovered from 12 infants on 2 or more weeks were identical by phage typing and plasmid analysis. Of these, 7 had concordant results for all the screening parameters, 6 showed minor changes in the biotype, and 2 showed resistance to an additional antibiotic. There were no instances of identical strains changing slime production from week to week.

Very low birth weight infants are very likely to become colonized with C-S in the first 2 weeks after admission in an NICU, but colonization decreases thereafter. There is marked variability among C-S isolates from individual patients from week to week. Furthermore, individual strains do not appear to acquire virulence characteristics, e.g., those characterized as *S. epidermidis,* slime positive, and/or multiply antibiotic resistant, and neither do these characteristics convey selective advantage to C-S

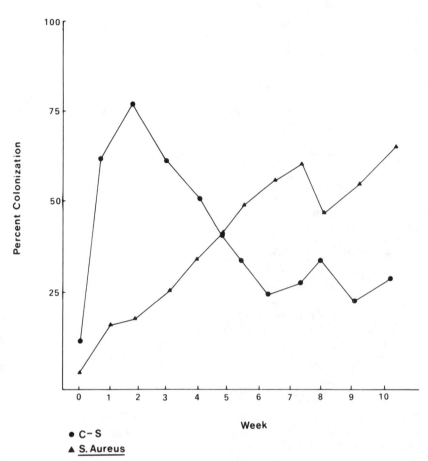

Fig 6–1.—Percent nasopharyngeal colonization with staphylococci among 28 very low birth weight infants by week of NICU stay. *Circles* = C-S, *triangles* = *Staphylococcus aureus*. (Courtesy of Hall SL, Riddell SW, Barnes WG, et al: *Diagn Microbiol Infect Dis* 13:17–23, 1990.)

bacteria colonizing infants in this study. Rather, many different strains of multiply antibiotic resistant C-S are prevalent in the NICU, with approximately 50% producing slime throughout the study period.

▶ Nosocomial infections contribute to the excessive morbidity and mortality that characterize low birth weight and extremely low birth weight infants. Slime producing *S. epidermidis,* the predominant pathogen in the NICU, accounts for many of the nosocomial infections in this subpopulation. Despite this the patterns of colonization and the specific characterization of the organism has received little attention. The interrelationship and perhaps interdependency of *S. epidermidis* and *S. aureus* were an interesting byline in this report. This study therefore addresses an area of need that will contribute ultimately to solving this slimy problem. See also Abstract 6–5.

Slime, in the grains of State,
like smut in the corn,
from the top infected.—*Stanley Kunitz*

A.A. Fanaroff, M.B.B.Ch.

Association of Intravenous Lipid Emulsion and Coagulase-Negative Staphylococcal Bacteremia in Neonatal Intensive Care Units

Freeman J, Goldmann DA, Smith NE, Sidebottom DG, Epstein MF, Platt R (Brigham and Women's Hosp, Boston; Brockton/West Roxbury VA Med Ctr, West Roxbury, Mass; Harvard Univ)
N Engl J Med 323:301–308, 1990   6–5

Coagulase-negative staphylococci (C-S) are the leading cause of bacteremia in neonatal intensive care units (NICUs). A case-control study of 882 infants was conducted in 2 NICUs during 1982 to determine the potential risk factors for this nosocomial infection. Forty-five infants had nosocomial bacteremia with C-S, and 38 were included in the study after excluding neonates with birth weights of less than 700 g. The 76 control infants without bacteremia were matched according to hospital, birth weight, and date of discharge.

The 38 study patients and 76 matched controls were similar with respect to 27 indicators of the severity of the underlying illness. Of the 20 therapeutic measures that were possible risk factors for nosocomial bacteremia, only the administration of intravenous lipid emulsion and the use of nonumbilical central venous catheters were strongly associated with nosocomial bacteremia caused by C-S. The overall relative odds of bacteremia after the intravenous administration of lipid emulsion were 5.8 (95% confidence interval, 4.1–8.3). After exposure to nonumbilical central venous catheters the odds were 3.5 (95% confidence interval, 1.4–8.3).

Because intravenous lipid emulsion was used frequently (68.4% of patients), 56.6% of all cases of nosocomial bacteremia could be attributed to administration of lipids, whereas the attributable risk to exposure to nonumbilical central venous catheters was 14.9%. The induction time for bacteremia after administration of lipids, usually through peripheral catheters, was less than 1 day, compared to 5.5 days with the use of central venous catheters not associated with administration of lipids.

A strong and independent association of C-S bacteremia with intravenous lipid emulsion was also confirmed on a similar analyses of data on another 31 neonates treated in 1988. In this study, the relative odds of bacteremia were 5.3 (95% confidence interval, 3.5–6.7).

The risk of C-S bacteremia in infants in NICUs can be attributed primarily to intravenous administration of lipids. Because lipids are critical for the nutritional support of premature neonates, further studies are warranted to determine the pathogenesis and prevention of lipid-associated bacteremia.

▶ The ubiquitous *Staphylococcus epidermidis* has emerged during the past decade as the dominant pathogen in the NICU. Long considered merely a normal skin commensal that frequently contaminated blood cultures, it is the predominant cause of nosocomial infections in low birth weight infants. The retrospective case-controlled review of patients with staphylococcal bacteremia has tagged intravenous lipid infusions as the prime accomplice. Intravenous lipids provide essential calories and fatty acids for premature infants; however, they also provide an environment conducive for the staphylococci to flourish. The combination of an immature infant with a central venous line receiving intravenous lipid supplementation is the typical scenario for *S. epidermidis* sepsis. The organism secretes slime, which helps to adhere to the catheters and renders it inaccessible to antibiotics. Vancomycin has become the most effective agent for treating the bacteremia, but it is necessary to remove the central lines and perhaps temporarily discontinue intravenous lipid infusions. The only good news from the above analysis is that the organism did not appear to be that virulent and 37 of 38 infected infants survived.

The snotgreen sea. The scrotumtightening sea.—James Joyce

A.A. Fanaroff, M.B.B.Ch.

Extra Hospital Stay and Antibiotic Usage With Nosocomial Coagulase-Negative Staphylococcal Bacteremia in Two Neonatal Intensive Care Unit Populations

Freeman J, Epstein MF, Smith NE, Platt R, Sidebottom DG, Goldmann DA (Brigham and Women's Hosp, Boston; Brockton/West Roxbury VA Med Ctr, West Roxbury, Mass; Harvard Univ)
Am J Dis Child 144:324–329, 1990

6–6

Coagulase-negative staphylococci (C-S) are an important cause of nosocomial bacteremia in neonatal intensive care units (NICUs). Two comparison infants were matched with each of 38 bacteremic infants by hospital, birth weight, and nearest date of discharge. Comparison subjects also remained in the hospital for as long as it took for bacteremia to occur in the bacteremic infant.

The onset of bacteremia occurred an average of 20 days into hospitalization. Despite having comparable birth weights and severity of underlying illness, bacteremic infants remained in the hospital a mean 19.8 days longer than the nonbacteremic comparison subjects. Bacteremic infants received antibiotics an average of 11.2 days longer than nonbacteremic infants. Vancomycin hydrochloride was given to 52.6% of the bacteremic infants, compared with only 5.3% of the comparison infants. All of the nonbacteremic infants and 37 of the 38 bacteremic infants survived.

Nosocomial bacteremia with C-S is a late complication of hospitalization that occurs in infants who have already survived for a relatively long time. This bacteremia seems to be associated with significantly longer hospitalizations and antibiotic treatment but not with significant increases in mortality.

▶ How little difference there is clinically between the bacteremic infants and the comparison groups. The comparison groups even had similar percent of infants with reduced platelets and immature neutrophils. Does this suggest that in some of the bacteremic infants the blood culture may be contaminated? Other than increasing the length of the hospital stay the bacteremia had little effect on morbidity. We continue to require more predictive criteria for the presence of a systemic infection in a young neonate.—M.H. Klaus, M.D.

Pregnancy Outcomes Among Mothers Infected With Human Immunodeficiency Virus and Uninfected Control Subjects

Minkoff HL, Henderson C, Mendez H, Gail MH, Holman S, Willoughby A, Goedett JJ, Rubinstein A, Stratton P, Walsh JH, Landesman SH (State Univ of New York, Brooklyn; Albert Einstein Coll of Medicine, Bronx, NY; Natl Inst of Child Health and Human Development, Bethesda, Md; Natl Cancer Inst, Bethesda, Md; Westat)
Am J Obstet Gynecol 163:1598–1604, 1990   6–7

To compare the health status of HIV-positive and HIV-negative mothers and their infants at birth, a prospective study of 101 seropositive pregnant women and 129 seronegative pregnant women was designed. The HIV-positive women were predominantly asymptomatic. The course of pregnancy and short-term neonatal outcomes of 91 seropositive women and 126 seronegative women were assessed.

Seropositive mothers had a significantly higher incidence of sexually transmitted diseases (17.6% vs. 7.1%) and more medical complications during pregnancy (43% vs. 25%). No other infrequent obstetric complications, i.e., toxemia or endometriosis, were associated with serologic status. When confounding variables such as drug use, tobacco use, or age of mother were controlled, the mother's serologic status was not significantly associated with birth weight, gestational age, head circumference, or Apgar scores of live infants. Average infant birth weight was slightly higher in the seropositive mother group.

More frequent infectious complications and a higher incidence of premature rupture of membranes were noted among seropositive women. Pregnancy outcomes were more affected by drug use and smoking than by detectable viral effects. Birth weight and height, head circumference, and Apgar scores were not related to maternal serologic status.

▶ It is important to note that only 3% of the seropositive women in this study had AIDS. There is evidence from other studies that there is an increased incidence of pregnancy complications for women with AIDS, including reduced birth weight. There is a substantial risk of serious infections during pregnancy among those whose T4 cell counts decreased to less than 300/mm^3. Significantly seropositive women had a higher rate of infectious complications and sexually transmitted diseases were diagnosed twice as often in the seropositive women. In this population the pregnancy outcomes were more influenced by drug use and smoking than by effects of the HIV.—M.H. Klaus, M.D.

Prevalence of Maternal HIV Infection Based on Unlinked Anonymous Testing of Newborn Babies

Peckham CS, Tedder RS, Briggs M, Ades AE, Hjelm M, Wilcox AH, Parra-Mejia N, O'Connor C (Inst of Child Health; Univ College and Middlesex School of Medicine; Hosps for Sick Children, London; St Helier Hosp, Carshalton, Surrey, England)
Lancet 335:516–519, 1990   6–8

Anti-HIV in newborns' serum, which reflects transplacental antibody, is an indirect measure of maternal infection and does not necessarily mean fetal or neonatal infection. A preliminary study was undertaken to establish the laboratory and logistic methods for unlinked anonymous testing of anti-HIV-1 in blood routinely obtained from newborn infants.

Neonatal screening involved the testing of blood samples routinely collected and then dried on filter paper (Guthrie cards). A total of 114,515 dried blood spots obtained from cards collected in 3 Thames regions were tested for HIV-1 antibody. Twenty-eight samples were confirmed to be antibody positive by Western blot (seroprevalence of .24/1,000). This technique was sensitive, specific, and less expensive than more conventional enzyme-linked immunosorbent assays.

Unlinked anonymous screening of newborn infants should be extended to monitor the spread of HIV infection in the heterosexual population. It can also be used to target preventive strategies and to provide better health care.

▶ How strange it will be in years from now when historians try to explain why we kept HIV results anonymous. Even now this makes little sense as various therapeutic regimes are being developed to treat the disease in an early phase. If suddenly syphilis appeared as a new disease would we have the same policy? In addition, the absence of information on the HIV carrier state of patients is a real disservice to the caretakers in case of a needle stick.—M.H. Klaus, M.D.

Neonatal Herpes Simplex Meningoencephalitis: EEG Investigations and Clinical Correlates

Mikati MA, Feraru E, Krishnamoorthy K, Lombroso CT (Harvard Univ; Massachusetts Gen Hosp, Boston)
Neurology 40:1433–1437, 1990   6–9

Neonatal herpes simplex virus meningoencephalitis (NHSV-ME) has a very high morbidity and mortality in all age groups. The use of the elec-

Predominant Background EEG Features at Various Stages
of NHSV-ME*

EEG findings	Days 1-4	Days 5-11	Day 12 and later
Very low voltage background	5	11	9 §
Other background abnormalities	2 †	2 ‡	—
Normal EEG	1	—	1
Total	8	13	10

*Numbers in the table indicate the number of patients manifesting that EEG finding.
†Other background abnormalities consisted of dysmature background in both patients.
‡Other background abnormalities included a dysmature background in 1 patient and a burst suppression EEG in another.
§In 2 of the 9 patients, EEG was consistent with electrocerebral silence.
(Courtesy of Mikati MA, Feraru E, Krishnamoorthy K, et al: *Neurology* 40:1433–1437, 1990.)

troencephalogram (EEG) to recognize a multifocal periodic pattern has been examined. The usefulness of EEGs, CSF tests, and CT was compared in the early diagnosis of NHSV-ME.

Sequential EEGs of 15 patients with NHSV-ME were compared with clinical and laboratory findings (table). Most (88%) of the patients with NHSV-ME showed an abnormal EEG with nonspecific background and paroxysmal abnormalities. In 3 of these patients, CT and ultrasound were normal at the time, pointing to greater sensitivity of the EEG in detecting early cerebral involvement. The multifocal periodic pattern, a nonspecific finding by itself, is highly suggestive of NHSV-ME when associated with clinical findings and inflammatory CSF.

The EEG is a sensitive test that is superior to radiologic procedures in detecting early cerebral involvement in suspected NHSV-ME. Initial normal findings should not preclude diagnosis if NHSV-ME is suspected; sequential EEGs and repeated tests are recommended.

▶ The sexually transmitted infections continue to plague newborns. The reemergence of syphilis (see Abstract 5–1), the continuing toll of cytomegalovirus and herpes, and the appearance of HIV together with *Chlamydia* are all responsible for significant morbidity and even mortality (1). This review of 15 cases of herpes encephalitis pales in the face of the multicenter study just published (2,3). The EEG findings are not pathognomonic, but were earlier indicators than any of the radiologic findings of significant brain involvement. For a long time the EEG in the neonate was not considered to be much importance. Today it is critical to have personnel skilled in reading newborn EEGs in order to make the right decisions in managing neonates with complex multisystem disorders (see Abstracts 7–6, 7–7, and 17–10).

In the multicenter controlled trial no significant difference was found between acyclovir and vidarabine in adjusted morbidity and mortality. There were no deaths among the 85 infants with localized HSV infection; 15% of the 71 infants with encephalitis died, and 57% of the 46 neonates with disseminated infection died.

Neurologic impairment was most frequent in the survivors with encephalitis, seizures, infection with HSV type 2, and those infants with 3 or more recurrences of vesicles in the skin, eye, or mouth.

My heart aches and a drowsy numbness pains
My sense as though of hemlock I had drunk.—John Keats

A.A. Fanaroff, M.B.B.Ch.

References

1. 1990 YEAR BOOK OF NEONATAL AND PERINATAL MEDICINE, Abstracts 6–1 through 6–4; 6–17 through 6–19.
2. Whitley R, et al: *N Engl J Med* 324:444, 1991.
3. Whitley R, et al: *N Engl J Med* 324:450, 1991.

IgA Antibodies for Diagnosis of Acute Congenital and Acquired Toxoplasmosis

Stepick-Biek P, Thulliez P, Araujo FG, Remington JS (Palo Alto Med Found; Stanford Univ; Inst de Puericulture de Paris)
J Infect Dis 162:270–273, 1990   6–10

The search continues for newer methods with greater sensitivity and specificity for early diagnosis of congenital and acquired infection with *Toxoplasma gondii*. The role of an enzyme-linked immunosorbent assay (ELISA) for IgA toxoplasma antibodies in the diagnosis of acute congenital and acquired toxoplasmosis was evaluated in 5 groups of patients.

The IgA ELISA was positive in 12 pregnant women who seroconverted during gestation and in 10 patients with biopsy-proven toxoplasmic lymphadenitis. In the latter patients, the highest titers were noted within the first months after onset of clinical signs. Toxoplasma IgA antibodies were also present in 8 of 9 infants/fetuses with congenital toxoplasma infection, 4 of whom had no demonstrable IgM antibodies. In contrast, only 1 of 20 patients with AIDS and biopsy-proven toxoplasmic encephalitis and none of the 20 adults with chronic *Toxoplasma* infection had demonstrable IgA antibodies.

These data show that demonstration of IgA toxoplasma antibodies can be useful in the diagnosis of acute congenital and recently acquired toxoplasmosis. Determination of IgA antibody should be included in the screening of pregnant women, prenatal diagnosis, and testing of newborn infants suspected of having congenital *Toxoplasma* infection.

▶ We are indebted to Dr. Remington and his colleagues for their many contributions to our understanding of infectious diseases in the newborn in general and, specifically, of congenital toxoplasmosis. Toxoplasmosis is a charter member of the expanding "Torch" syndromes. The need to identify toxoplasmosis infection in the fetus served as the impetus for the refinement of the cordocentesis technique (see the 1990 YEAR BOOK), which has been of enormous diagnostic and therapeutic benefit in many disorders of the fetus.

The above report is part of the continuing search for techniques to identify infection in the adult in the early stages, as well as to distinguish the fetus or newborn who is infected from those who have merely acquired maternal antibodies. previous reports with the use of IgA antibodies had yielded conflicting results, with some investigators considering them to be of little importance for the diagnosis of acute infection; others, useless. The conclusion of this limited investigation was that IgA antibody to toxoplasmosis was of value for diagnosing acute infection and should be included for "screening pregnant women, for prenatal diagnosis and for testing newborns when there is reason to suspect congenital *Toxoplasma* infection." The caution against the possibility of cord blood being contaminated with maternal blood was duly noted and filed.—A.A. Fanaroff, M.B.B.Ch.

Prophylactic or Simultaneous Administration of Recombinant Human Granulocyte Colony Stimulating Factor in the Treatment of Group B Streptococcal Sepsis in Neonatal Rats
Cairo MS, Mauss D, Kommareddy S, Norris K, van de Ven C, Modanlou H (Childrens Hosp of Orange County, Orange, Calif; Miller Children's Hosp, Long Beach, Calif; Univ of California, Irvine)
Pediatr Res 27:612–616, 1990   6–11

The overall mortality rate from group B streptococcus (GBS) sepsis remains significantly high despite newer advances in antibiotic therapy. Experimental GBS in neonatal animals suggests that an altered granulopoiesis characterized by reduced neutrophil proliferative pools, neutrophil storage pools, neutropenia, and polymorphonuclear cell dysfunction may be a major factor in the increased mortality to GBS sepsis. Recombinant human granulocyte colony stimulating factor (rhG-CSF) has been shown to induce neutrophilia and modulate neutrophil proliferative pools and neutrophil storage pools in the newborn rat. Prophylactic or simultaneously administered human rhG-CSF could enhance neonatal host response and subsequently reduce the mortality associated with GBS infection in the newborn.

The adjuvant effect of rhG-CSF was studied in GBS septic Sprague-Dawley newborn (<36 hours) rats treated with and without antibiotic therapy. After inoculating newborn rats with GBS at various concentrations, it was established that an LD_{50} of 3×10^6 organism/g would be used in the studies. After GBS inoculation, the newborn ratrs were randomized into 1 of 4 treatment groups, with rhG-CSF administered simultaneously or 6 hours after GBS inoculation, in 2 separate studies.

In the simultaneous studies, rhG-CSF was administered with GBS inoc-

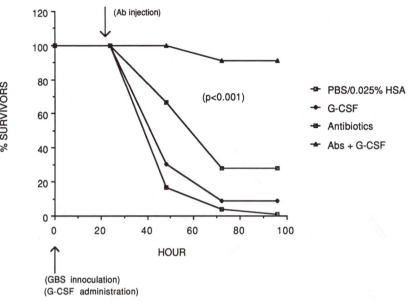

Fig 6–2.—Percent survival for groups of 20 or more neonatal rats from litters of 8–10 animals from 2 to 3 separate experiments after s.c. injection with GBS at 3×10^6 colonies/g body weight and adjuvant therapy. Adjuvant therapy at hour 0 included either i.p. rhG-CSF (5 μg/kg) or PBS/.025% HSA. Additionally, antibiotics (Abs) (gentamicin, 6.5 mg/kg/day, and ampicillin, 150 mg/kg/day) were administered intramuscularly 24 hours after GBS to the last 2 groups. $P < .001$ reflects comparison between 91% survival in G-CSF and Abs vs. Abs alone (72 hours). (Courtesy of Cairo MS, Mauss D, Kommareddy S, et al: *Pediatr Res* 27:612–616, 1990.)

ulation; group 1 received only PBS/.025% human serum albumin, group 2 received rhG-CSF only, group 3 received gentamicin and ampicillin only, and group 4 received rhG-CSF and antibiotics. At 24 hours, there was approximately 100% survival in all treatment groups. By 72 hours, there was a significant difference in survival among treatment groups. The survival rate was 4% in group 1, 9% in group 2, and 28% in group 3. In contrast, the survival rate was significantly increased (91%) in group 4 (Fig 6–2). In the prophylactic studies, rhG-CSF was administered 6 hours before GBS inoculation. Similarly, the survival rate was significantly increased (70%) in animals who received antibiotics plus rhG-CSF compared with the other 3 treatment groups.

Simultaneous or prophylactic pulse administration of rhG-CSF may have a synergistic and protective effect on survival in antibiotic-treated experimental GBS in the neonatal rat.

▶ The art of medical practice is to apply the scientific jewels from the research laboratories to tenable patient diagnostic or therapeutic modalities. It has been most exciting to witness the birth of the recombinant technology. We are already observing its use in the diagnosis of genetic and infectious disorders and starting to glimpse its therapeutic potential. Neutropenia and bone marrow depletion have been associated with high mortality rates in neonates with disseminated streptococcal infections (1–3). Recombinant CSF has the potential to rapidly reconstitute the white cell population that is paramount to the host defense. The rat model discussed above is part of the necessary preliminary bouts before the main event. Granulocyte-macrophage CSF has been used in adults with radiation marrow depression and infections. No doubt its introduction in to the neonatal intensive care unit will be heralded soon. Let's hope that it lives up to our high expectations.— A.A. Fanaroff, M.B.B.Ch.

References

1. Christenson RD, et al: *Pediatrics* 70:1, 1982.
2. Baley JE, et al: *Pediatrics* 80:712, 1987.
3. Cairo MS, et al: *Am J Pediatr Hematol Oncol* 11:227, 1989.

Evaluation of an Intravenous Immunoglobulin Preparation for the Prevention of Viral Infection Among Hospitalized Low Birth Weight Infants
Piedra PA, Kasel JA, Norton HJ, Gruber WC, Garcia-Prats JA, Baker CJ (Baylor Univ, Houston; Vanderbilt Univ, Nashville)
Pediatr Infect Dis J 9:470–475, 1990   6–12

Infectious diseases have been acknowledged as a significant contributing factor to the death of low birth weight infants. In the first year of life infants are at exceptionally high risk of primary infection with respiratory viruses.

In the present study an intravenous immunoglobulin (IVIG) preparation was evaluated prospectively in hospitalized low birth weight infants for the prevention of respiratory virus infection. Premature neonates were studied from October 1987 through July 1988. Weekly cultures were performed on nasopharyngeal secretions and daily clinical data were obtained on each infant.

Ninety-one infants with birth weights of between 500 and 1,750 g were randomized to receive either IVIG, 500 mg/kg (46 infants), or 5% albumin-normal saline (placebo), 10 mL/kg (45 infants), between days 3 and 7 of life, 7 days later, and every 14 days thereafter for a maximum of 5 doses. The demographic and life event data during pregnancy were similar in both groups. Birth weight, gestational age, gender, age at entry in the study, and incidence of respiratory distress syndrome at birth were also comparable in both groups of premature infants.

A total of 26 viruses were isolated from 25 infants. There were 13 viral infections in the IVIG group and 12 in the palcebo group. The severity of disease, as evaluated by clinical factors and the outcomes of virus-infected infants, were not different in the IVIG-treated and placebo groups. Adenoviruses accounted for 57.7% of the viral isolates and cytomegalovirus accounted for 23.1%.

In this study the use of IVIG did not prevent or modify adenovirus and cytomegalovirus infections in premature infants.

▶ The host defense mechanism of the premature infant renders it ill prepared for existence outside the safe confines of the uterus. There are deficiencies in cellular and humoral immunity that are compounded in their exposure to a wide array of pathogens. Attention has focused recently on the transient hypogammaglobulinemia that characterizes the most immature infants. Multicenter studies are addressing the question as to whether intermittent infusions of immunoglobulin can prevent nosocomial infections. The results are eagerly anticipated and should be available in the near future. The above report is discouraging in that immunoglobulin infusions failed to protect against adenovirus, herpes, or cytomegalovirus infections. No conclusions could be drawn regarding respiratory syncytial virus, a major pathogen for hospitalized infants with chronic lung disease, which was not encountered in this series. The $64,000 question is whether nosocomial infections can be reduced by prophylactic immunoglobulin infusions. The key may lie in the antibody profile of the infusate. The presence of functional antibody in adequate quantities probably determines the efficacy. See the 1989 YEAR BOOK OF NEONATAL AND PERINATAL MEDICINE, p 237 and pp 274–275, and the 1990 YEAR BOOK OF NEONATAL AND PERINATAL MEDICINE, pp 132–134.

The brightest flashes in the world of thought are incomplete until they have been proved to have their counterparts in the world of fact.—John Tyndall

A.A. Fanaroff, M.B.B.Ch.

Swaddling and Acute Respiratory Infections
Yurdakok K, Yavuz T, Taylor CE (Ministry of Health, Ankara, Turkey; Gulveren Health Ctr, Ankara, Turkey; Johns Hopkins Univ)
Am J Public Health 80:873–875, 1990   6–13

The ancient practice of swaddling is common in Turkey and China, where infants are tightly bound in cloth from the neck to the feet immediately after birth. Partial swaddling leaves the infant's arms free, whereas complete swaddling does not. Preliminary evidence suggests that swaddling may interfere with normal respiration and predispose to pneumonia. Because pneumonia is the leading cause of death among children in both China and Turkey, particularly in neonates, a cross-sectional study was undertaken to assess the relationship between swaddling and acute respiratory infections or pneumonia in 186 infants aged 3 to 12 months (mean, 6.8). Of these, 92 had been either partially or completely swaddled for at least 3 months.

Radiographically confirmed pneumonia and a history of at least 2 upper respiratory infections were each about 4 times more common among swaddled infants than unswaddled infants (Fig 6–3). The incidence of pneumonia was 24.1% among partially swaddled infants and 11.6% among completely swaddled infants, compared with 3.2% in unswaddled infants; the difference was highly significant. Further studies are attempt-

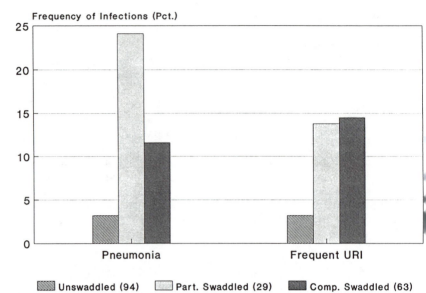

Fig 6–3.—Swaddling and respiratory infections. (Courtesy of Yurdakok K, Yavuz T, Taylor CE: *Am J Public Health* 80:873–875, 1990.)

ing to provide more precise information on time relationships between swaddling and pneumonia.

▶ Since pneumonia is a major cause of mortality in the developing world, it is important to consider why swaddling increases the incidence. Do the swaddled and unswaddled infants come from different populations? Or is it possible that swaddling binds the chest sufficiently to prevent the infant from regular sighing (or deep breath), which is known to prevent alveolar collapse by altering pulmonary surface tension? An atelectatic lung would be more susceptible to infection. Another possibility is that very tight swaddling could reduce the effectiveness of coughing.—M.H. Klaus, M.D.

7 The Nervous System

Qualitative Changes of General Movements in Preterm Infants With Brain Lesions

Ferrari F, Cioni G, Prechtl HFR (Univ of Modena, Italy; Univ of Pisa, Italy; Univ Hosp, Groningen, The Netherlands)

Early Hum Dev 23:193–231, 1990

7–1

Neural dysfunction in preterm infants may manifest itself in changes in the quality of specific movement patterns, such as general movements. Qualitative assessments of general movements were performed in 14 low-risk premature infants and 29 high-risk premature infants with intraventricular-periventricular hemorrhage and/or leukomalacia as seen on ultrasound. Sequential 1-hour video recordings of the unstimulated infants in the incubator were performed during the preterm period and then continued during the postterm period until about 20 weeks. Movement patterns were analyzed based on the classification of Prechtl, and quantification of motility was done in 12 matched pairs of low-risk and high-risk preterm infants. Neurologic follow-up was performed between 1 and 3 years of corrected age.

The rate of distinct movement patterns did not differ significantly between the low-risk and high-risk preterm infants, except for the lower incidence of isolated arm movements in the brain-damaged infants. When the quality of general movements was assessed, all but 1 of the 14 low-risk preterm infants had normal quality of general movements, whereas all 29 infants in the high-risk group had an abnormal quality.

A semiquantitative estimation of various aspects of the abnormal general movements made possible a typology of abnormal patterns. The first type included all trajectories with poor repertoire, i.e., the sequence of successive movement components was monotonous and arm, leg, and trunk movements did not occur in normal sequence. Eight infants had this trajectory, and all had a normal outcome. One additional infant was mentally retarded. The most frequent trajectory was characterized by cramped-synchronized general movements and was present in the remaining 20 infants. The outcome in these patients was 2 monoplegias of the leg, 3 hemiplegias, 5 diplegias, and 9 quadriplegias; 1 infant was blind. These developmental trajectories were more accurate predictors of neurologic outcome than those based on the nature and localization of the lesion; all but 1 of 29 infants were classified correctly, and the only misclassification was the infant who was blind.

Qualitative assessment of general movements from video-recordings is a reliable, quick, cheap, and totally nonintrusive method for the early detection of functional impairment of the nervous system in the neonatal period.

▶ From a master of fetal and infant development and his group comes a completely novel and original method for assessing the normality of development in an immature neonate. This is one of the most creative papers reviewed during the past year! The procedures are the result of at least 10 years of work in Groningen and evaluate the qualitative changes of spontaneous movement. The process is nonintrusive and the same criteria can be used for the fetus and preterm infant. One hour of behavior is videotaped and the sections containing movement can be viewed over a short period of time if the tape is first viewed at high speed. The analysis uses a type of gestalt perception that allows for high interobserver reliability. By viewing spontaneous motor development at various ages the evolution to normality or abnormality can be viewed. This approach is a distinct departure from the traditional neurologic technique of looking for whether abnormal reflexes or signs are present. Interestingly, this work comes nearly 40 years after Prechtl first described the normal states of consciousness in full-term infants. His long and continuing interest as a baby watcher continues to be unusually rewarding. I recommend beginning this work by reading an editorial by Prechtl (1).—M.H. Klaus, M.D.

Reference

1. Prechtl HFR: *Early Hum Dev* 23:151, 1990.

Gross Motor Milestones in Preterm Infants: Correction for Degree of Prematurity
Allen MC, Alexander GR (Johns Hopkins Hosp; Kennedy Inst for Handicapped Children; Johns Hopkins Univ, Baltimore)
J Pediatr 116:955–959, 1990   7–2

The emphasis on early intervention in the first 3 years of life of infants with developmental delay, as generated by Public Law 99-457, has brought attention to the importance of identifying very preterm infants who would benefit from intervention services. The effect of the degree of prematurity on the age of acquisition of gross motor milestone attainment was studied in 100 high-risk, very preterm (<32 weeks) infants with normal neurologic examination results at 12 and 24 months. Age at acquisition for 12 motor milestones were determined based on chronologic age from the date of delivery and term age equivalent, correcting for degree of prematurity. The results were compared with those of normal term infants. For very preterm infants, the mean gestational age was 27.8 weeks (range, 23–32 weeks) and mean birth weight was 1,034 g (range, 490–1,770 g). Half of the infants were boys and 70% were black. The mean duration of follow-up was 38 months.

For each gross milestone, the mean chronologic age of milestone acquisition was 2 to 3 months later for very preterm infants, compared with

Mean Ages at Gross Motor Milestone Attainment

Milestone	Term Infants* (mean)	Age (mo) at milestone attainment Premature infants		n
		Term age equivalent (mean ± SD)	Chronologic age (mean ± SD)	
Roll over P to S	3.6	3.5 ± 1.7	6.3 ± 1.8	97
Roll over S to P	4.8	4.4 ± 1.5	7.2 ± 1.6	97
Sit with support	5.3	5.5 ± 1.4	8.3 ± 1.5†	100
Sit without support	6.3	6.6 ± 1.4	9.4 ± 1.6‡	97
Creep	6.7	5.6 ± 1.6	8.4 ± 1.7	82
Come to sit	7.5	8.1 ± 1.9	11.0 ± 2.1	97
Crawl	7.8	7.5 ± 1.6	10.4 ± 1.8	93
Pull to stand	8.1	8.2 ± 1.6	11.0 ± 1.7	96
Cruise	8.8	8.9 ± 1.5	11.7 ± 1.7	96
Walk	11.7	11.9 ± 2.0	14.7 ± 2.2	99
Walk backward	14.3	14.0 ± 2.3	16.6 ± 2.7	69
Run	14.8	14.4 ± 2.7	17.0 ± 3.1	79

Abbreviations: P, prone; S, supine.
*Data from Capute AJ, Shapiro BK, Palmer FB, et al: *Dev Med Child Neurol* 27:635–643, 1985.)
†Student t test: P = .05 compared with term infants.
‡Student t test: P = .05 compared with term infants.
(Courtesy of Allen MC, Alexander GR: *J Pediatr* 116:955–959, 1990.)

normal term infants. In contrast, after correction for degree of prematurity, the mean term age equivalent of milestone attainment for very preterm infants was nearly equivalent to that of term infants (table). There were no consistent sex differences, but black infants attained the milestone earlier than white infants.

Very preterm infants attain motor milestones sequentially at a rate expected for degree of prematurity. Chronologic age is not a valid measure of determining motor delay in very preterm infants.

▶ This is a simple but important study. The data generated can be used to save families and caretakers of premature infants much grief. The measure of continuing to correct for prematurity through the first 2 years of life will help distinguish those infants with true delays in their gross motor milestones from those who are merely developmentally appropriately immature. It should be routine, when counseling families of immature babies, to repeatedly, whenever the opportunity presents itself, to point out the need to correct for prematurity. The importance of correcting for prematurity is greater for cognitive than motor development. Black infants achieve motor milestones earlier than white, with the exception of rolling from prone to supine. Assessment based on chronologic age, with failure to correct for prematurity, results in overdiagnosis of motor delay, unnecessary referral, and unnecessary grief and anxiety for the family.

Come forth into the light of things, let nature be your teacher.—Wordsworth

A.A. Fanaroff, M.B.B.Ch.

Facial Nerve Palsy in the Newborn: Incidence and Outcome
Falco NA, Eriksson E (Brigham and Women's Hosp; Children's Hosp Med Ctr, Boston)
Plast Reconstr Surg 85:1–4, 1990   7–3

Congenital facial nerve palsy is the expression of any of several disease processes, broadly classified as developmental and acquired. Acquired palsies are caused by birth trauma, and the use of obstetric forceps has been implicated in most patients. Patients with facial palsy related to birth trauma were retrospectively identified and characterized.

The records of infants born with facial weakness or paralysis in a 5-year period at 1 hospital were reviewed. Of 44,292 infants delivered between 1982 and 1987, 92 had congenital 7th nerve palsy; 81 of these were acquired, yielding an incidence of 1.8 per 1000. Of these 81 patients, 74 (91%) were associated with forceps delivery. Obstetric forceps were used in only 19% of all deliveries during the period studied. The average weight of the infants with acquired palsies was 3.55 kg, compared with an overall mean of 3.23 kg; 59% of the mothers of the affected infants and 37% of controls were primigravidas (Fig 7–1). The incidence of additional birth injuries was also much greater among infants with acquired palsies than among the general newborn population. A complete recovery occurred in 89% of the affected infants.

Congenital traumatic facial palsy has definable risk factors and a favorable outcome. Significant risk factors for acquired facial palsy were forceps delivery, birth weight of 3,500 g or greater, and primiparity.

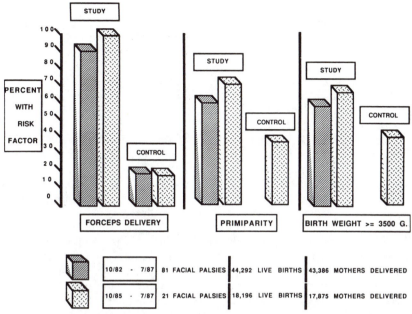

Fig 7–1.—Risk factors for acquiring facial palsy at birth. Control groups are the general population of newborns and of women delivered at the Brigham and Women's Hospital. Among the control groups, parity and birth weight were not consistently documented until October of 1985; the last 22 months of the study (October 1985 to July 1987) and the study as a whole (October 1982 to July 1987) are graphed separately. (Courtesy of Falco NA, Eriksson E: *Plast Reconstr Surg* 85:1–4, 1990.)

▶ An asymmetric crying face in a newborn is a disturbing feature for the family and physicians alike. This is a comprehensive review of facial nerve palsy in the newborn. Facial nerve palsy is predominantly an acquired lesion, with forceps intervention accounting for 91% of the acquired lesions. Notably, 79% of these had signs of external trauma to the head or face, including lacerations, ecchymosis, molding, and cephalohematomata. It was reassuring to note that 59 of 66 infants followed had complete recovery, the majority within 2 weeks of delivery. The primary causes of facial palsy included Mobius syndrome, hemifacial macrosomia, and hypoplasia of the depressor anguli oris muscle. My impression was that the latter was underreported, probably a reflection of the fact that the cases were identified from retrospective chart reviews. The conservative approach to management by a surgical subspecialist was refreshing to observe. Radiologic, electrodiagnostic, and brain stem studies were recommended for developmental palsies. Surgery was not necessary during the first year of life for obstetric palsy.—A.A. Fanaroff, M.B.B.Ch.

Posthypoxic Glucose Supplement Reduces Hypoxic-Ischemic Brain Damage in the Neonatal Rat
Hattori H, Wasterlain CG (VA Med Ctr, Sepulveda, Calif; Univ of California, Los Angeles)
Ann Neurol 28:122–128, 1990   7–4

Glucose load during hypoxia appears beneficial for the recovery of brain slices from hypoxia. However, adverse effects have also been reported, such as worsening of the hypoxic brain injury and increased mortality. The effect of posthypoxic glucose supplement was studied in a neonatal hypoxic-ischemic rat model. After bilateral ligation of the carotid arteries, the rats were exposed to an 8% oxygen atmosphere for 1 hour. The animals received glucose or saline either immediately or 1 hour after hypoxia, and the extent of hypoxic-ischemic damage was assessed histologically 72 hours later.

Glucose supplement given immediately after the insult provided significant protection against the hypoxic-ischemic infarction both in the neocortex and striatum. Immediate supplement reduced the volume of neocortical infarction to 37% of the unsupplemented value and attenuated the ischemic damage in the striatum and the dentate gyrus. In the saline-treated pups, brain glucose levels after the insult were low (0.3 mmol/kg). In contrast, glucose supplement produced a rapid rise in brain glucose level to 3 to 5 mmol/kg over the next 2 years. Plasma and brain lactate levels behaved similarly in saline-treated pups, gradually falling down to baseline level during the first hour of recovery. Glucose supplement slightly retarded the fall in lactate levels. At any period of this neonatal model, the brain lactate levels (9 mmol/kg) did not exceed the toxic level, suggesting that full cortical infarction can develop even if brain lactate levels are low.

Posthypoxic glucose supplement immediately after the insult can be beneficial in neonatal hypoxic-ischemic encephalopathy. In addition, cerebral infarction can develop independently of lactate accumulation in the neonatal model of incomplete ischemia.

▶ The pathogenesis and therapy of hypoxic-ischemic encephalopathy has become the focus of intense investigation. The disruption of the protective mechanism of the neurone is occurring at multiple sites within the cell. Each avenue is being explored to determine whether prophylactic or rescue therapy is feasible. There has been a considerable shift of opinion with regard to the role of glucose in asphyxiated animals. Pretreating immature animals with glucose prolongs survival during hypoxia, but in mature animals elevated blood glucose during ischemia aggravates brain damage. This latter information served as the basis for clinically contraindicating high glucose levels in the presence of asphyxia. More recent in vitro studies reveal that high glucose levels aid the recovery of brain slices from hypoxia. The benefits appear to accrue from maintenance of ATP levels. Hattori evaluated the effect of posthypoxic glucose supplementation in a neonatal hypoxic-ischemic model and concluded that it was beneficial. Siesjo (1) postulated that "the low intracellular glucose is involved in the mechanism of damage and that glucose by refueling the recovering brain tissue restores membrane potentials, increases uptake of released glutamate, pumps out cations, and sequesters intracellular calcium ions." Neuroprotection from glucose could also be through a number of mechanisms other than as an energy source.

Vannuci (2) was able to demonstrate increased glucose transport into the brain during hypoxic ischemia without significantly changing glucose consumption or lactate accumulation. He proposed clinical trials of glucose supplementation to mothers at risk for delivering infants with hypoxia-ischemia. At that time we advocated caution until more data were available. Additional information does now support his contention and clinical trials appear warranted.—

A.A. Fanaroff, M.B.B.Ch.

References

1. Siesjo BK: *J Cereb Blood Flow Metab* 1:155, 1981.
2. 1988 YEAR BOOK OF NEONATAL AND PERINATAL MEDICINE, Abstract 6–3.

Reduction of Perinatal Hypoxic-Ischemic Brain Damage With Allopurinol
Palmer C, Vannucci RC, Towfighi J (The Milton S Hershey Med Ctr of the Pennsylvania State Univ, Hershey, Penn)
Pediatr Res 27:332–336, 1990

7–5

Cytotoxic free radicals are generated during cerebral hypoxia-ischemia and reperfusion. Allopurinol is both a xanthine oxidase inhibitor and free radical scavenger, and may reduce hypoxic-ischemic damage. The potential neuroprotective effect of allopurinol on the developing brain of the 7-day-old rat pup was evaluated. Hypoxic-ischemic injury to the right cerebral hemisphere was produced by ligation of the right common carotid artery, followed by 3 hours of hypoxia with 8% oxygen. At random, the rats received either allopurinol, 130-138 mg/kg, or an equal volume of saline 30 to 45 minutes before the hypoxia. Some animals were sacrificed at 42 hours of recovery to evaluate brain water content and others were killed at 30 or more days for neuropathologic examination.

There were 18 allopurinol-treated and 23 saline-treated pups that survived. Allopurinol significantly reduced brain water content in the cerebral hemisphere ipsilateral to the carotid artery ligation, compared to the saline-treated pups. Allopurinol had no effect on the hemisphere contralateral to the ligation. Furthermore, neuropathologic damage was significantly less in allopurinol-trated pups than in the saline-treated pups. Infarction occurred in only 2 of 13 allopurinol-treated pups, compared to 10 of 14 saline-treated pups.

High-dose allopurinol substantially reduces hypoxic-ischemic brain damage in 7-day-old rats by reducing both cerebral edema and extent of perinatal hypoxic-ischemic brain damage.

▶ Cells that have died cannot be resurrected. It is the adjacent cells that have sustained injury that are most vulnerable to reperfusion injury. A host of agents are being investigated as the pathogenesis of reperfusion injury is clarified. During cerebral hypoxia-ischemia there is depletion of tissue stores of ATP, which is degraded to hypoxanthine. With reperfusion this is converted to xanthine by xanthine oxidase and superoxide, and hydoxyl free radicals are generated. Allopurinol inhibits xanthine oxidase and scavenges free radicals and has been successfully used to reduce ischemic injury in the rat brain and other organs. The group from Hershey that has riveted its attention on hypoxic-ischemic brain damage report here the benefits of allopurinol in a rat pup model.

It is a far cry from the controlled asphyxia of a rat pup to the human situation; nonetheless, progress is being registered and it will not be long before many of these agents, affectionately referred to as lazaroids, are subjected to extensive clinical testing in human neonates. Neonatologists eagerly await the addition of this new group of agents to their therapeutic arsenal.

I am going to give my psychoanalyst one more year, then I'm going to Lourdes.—Woody Allen

A.A. Fanaroff, M.B.B.Ch.

Power Spectral Analysis of the EEG of Term Infants Following Birth Asphyxia

Bell AH, McClure BG, Hicks EM (Royal Maternity Hosp; Royal Belfast Hosp for Sick Children, Belfast)
Dev Med Child Neurol 32:990–998, 1990   7–6

Despite fetal monitoring advances, birth asphyxia is still a major problem. Assessment of the newborn's brain in cases of hypoxic-ischemic encephalopathy has been done through clinical examination, imaging techniques, and biochemical methods. The electroencephalogram (EEG) has been used for assessment to facilitate management in the critical first few hours of an infant with hypoxic-ischemic encephalopathy.

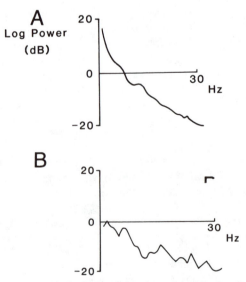

Fig 7–2.—Power spectrum EEG after birth asphyxia: **A,** good outcome; **B,** poor outcome. (Courtesy of Bell AH, McClure BG, Hicks EM: *Dev Med Child Neurol* 32:990–998, 1990.)

Power spectral analysis was performed on the EEGs of 16 term infants with hypoxic-ischemic encephalopathy (Fig 7–2). Analysis was performed at regular intervals during the first 5 days of life, and infants were followed for a total of 18 months. Neurodevelopment of the infants was assessed at a mean age of 24.5 months. Comparison of absolute power on day 1 between infants with different neurodevelopmental outcomes showed significant differences between the 2 groups in all frequency bands. Absolute power was significantly reduced, particularly in the slow frequency bands, in infants with poor outcome. The difference was most marked on day 1, with most information gained on days 1 to 3. Other forms of neurologic assessment are of most value after 1 week of age.

Consistent with work done on raw EEGs, power spectral analysis of EEGs of infants with hypoxic-ischemic encephalopathy relates to infants' outcome. The absolute power on the delta and theta ranges and total EEG power are most useful. Electroencephalograms and power spectral analysis can provide objective results in the critical first few days.

▶ Max Wiznitzer, M.D., Assistant Professor of Pediatrics, Rainbow Babies and Children's Hospital, Cleveland, offers these words of wisdom regarding the EEG interpretations.

▶ The early identification of neonates with irreversible brain injury due to hypoxic-ischemic encephalopathy has always been difficult. Severe background abnormalities on early EEG are related to poor neurologic outcome. However, mild and moderate abnormalities on initial EEG are less useful and require analysis of any change in serial EEG over 1 to 2 weeks to predict outcome. The development of any method to shorten this interval is important for short-term and long-term therapeutic intervention. One use could be differentiation of high-risk and low-risk groups for pharmacologic "brain rescue" after a hypoxic-ischemic event. This study suggests that a processed EEG method (power spectral array) might provide such a method. Processed EEG allows for presentation of the large amount of data within conventional EEG in a more organized and understandable way. It is important to match physiologic EEG states in a study population. In the normal newborn, power is dependent, in part, on level of alertness and the type of sleep state. In this study, most children were in an indeterminate state, allowing for better comparison. Training in EEG interpretation appears necessary to identify state and avoid artifact. The presence of reduced absolute pattern in the poor outcome group is not surprising because this decrease in amplitude usually accompanies significant neonatal brain dysfunction. Verification of these pilot data by a prospective study of a larger cohort would provide a valuable tool for the early establishment of neurologic prognosis.—M. Wiznitzer, M.D.

EEG Monitoring of Therapy for Neonatal Seizures

Hakeem VF, Wallace SJ (Univ Hosp of Wales, Cardiff)
Dev Med Child Neurol 32:858–864, 1990   7–7

The effectiveness of anticonvulsant therapy of neonatal seizures is usually assessed clinically. However, continuous electroencephalography (EEG) monitoring indicates that seizures in the neonate are often subclinical. The effectiveness of anticonvulsant therapy in 11 healthy full-term and preterm infants with seizures was assessed using continuous EEG recording with an immediate cot-side print-out. After 32 weeks' gestation, the EEG showed periods of quiet and active sleep, whereas seizures are evident as episodes of greatly increased power output.

Seven infants were given phenobarbitone. Six infants responded clinically, but 4 showed EEG subclinical seizure bursts that persisted or recurred within 2 hours of treatment. One patient responded clinically to chloral hydrate but seizure discharges recurred briefly within 40 minutes. Another patient treated with chloral hydrate showed persistent subclinical EEG bursts. Three babies were given benzodiazepines. Bolus doses of diazepam appeared to be rapidly effective, but EEG seizure discharges recurred immediately after treatment. However, infusions of diazepam or clonazepam were eventually associated with persistent control of clinical and EEG seizures.

Clinical observation is a poor predictor of the effectiveness of anticonvulsant therapy in neonatal seizures, and conventional anticonvulsants are rarely completely effective. Continuous EEG monitoring is essential for optimal therapeutic intervention.

▶ Max Wiznitzer, M.D., Assistant Professor of Pediatrics, Rainbow Babies and Children's Hospital, Clevelend, offers these words of wisdom regarding the EEG interpretations.

▶ Many studies, including this one, have demonstrated that the majority of neonatal seizures have no discernable clinical features, but only EEG correlates. Electrical seizures may cause further brain tissue injury and need to be controlled. Until recently, the diagnosis of electrical seizures has been difficult because the use of conventional EEG at the bedside requires training in interpretation and equipment use. Continuous monitoring methods such as compressed spectral array (CSA), which process the raw EEG data into a more comprehensible format, provide a technique for rapid identification of electrical seizures that can be learned quickly by physicians and nurses involved in the child's daily care. In our experience, these personnel rapidly learn the CSA patterns associated with the individual child's seizures. The equipment is smaller than a conventional EEG machine, and, in some models, can store EEG data for up to 24 hours, allowing later review of abnormal events. The use of 4 channels allows for coverage of most neonatal electrode sites. It should be used in conjunction with conventional EEG, which provides information about background activity and location of seizure foci. This technology, similar to continuous ECG monitoring used in intensive care units, should allow us to rapidly treat subclinical seizures and avoid their potential long-term effects.—M. Wiznitzer, M.D.

Antenatal and Intrapartum Factors Associated With the Occurrence of Seizures in the Term Infant

Patterson CA, Graves WL, Bugg G, Sasso SC, Brann AW Jr (Emory Univ)
Obstet Gynecol 74:361–365, 1989   7–8

In previous investigations an association between early neonatal seizures and perinatal events, particularly asphyxia, has been defined. To identify antenatal and intrapartum factors associated with seizures in term newborns, 40 term infants who had seizures within 72 hours of birth were compared with 400 controls by using logistic regression analysis.

The risk of early neonatal seizures in these term infants was 1.05 per 1,000 live term births. Factors associated with increased risk of seizures in term infants were antenatal anemia, antenatal bleeding, asthma, meconium-stained amniotic fluid, presentation other than occiput anterior, fetal distress, and shoulder dystocia. The individual predictive value of these factors was low (table), but the combination of these factors in a logistic regression model identified a group of infants for whom the odds of having a seizure were approximately 1 in 100.

This analysis confirmed a strong association between seizures and factors that increase the risk of fetal asphyxia.

▶ Seizures during the neonatal period are indicators of the quality of perinatal care. This analysis is an academic exercise that because of low sensitivity yields little practical information. If the criteria whereby 90% of the infants who will seize are used, then at the same time 35% of the patients who will not have seizures will erroneously be identified as being at risk. On the other hand, manipulating the risk factors so that all the patients who will not have seizures are eliminated, i.e., 100% specificity, only 38% of those who will seize are identified, i.e., low sensitivity. We are forced to conclude that although the underlying risk factors for perinatal seizures are known, that knowledge is useful only for grouped data and is not applicable to individuals.

Sensitivity, Specificity, and Predictive Value for Variables Included in Logistic Regression Model

Variable	Sensitivity	Specificity	Predictive value
Antenatal anemia	15.0	93.8	0.25
Antenatal bleeding	7.5	99.3	1.04
Asthma	7.5	99.0	0.78
Meconium in amniotic fluid	62.5	75.6	0.27
Presentation other than OA	27.5	92.3	0.37
Fetal distress	45.0	93.5	0.72
Shoulder dystocia	7.5	99.3	1.04
Logistic regression model*	58.0	94.0	0.99

Note: Data are presented as percentages.
Abbreviation: OA, occiput anterior.
*Cutoff point = .3.
(Courtesy of Patterson CA, Graves WL, Bugg G, et al: *Obstet Gynecol* 74:361–365, 1989.)

The stars have not dealt me the worse they could do
My pleasures are plenty, my troubles are two.
But oh, my two troubles they reave me of rest,
The brains in my head and the heart in my breast.—A.E. Housman

A.A. Fanaroff, M.B.B.Ch.

Neonatal Cocaine-Related Seizures
Kramer LD, Locke GE, Ogunyemi A, Nelson L (King/Drew Med Ctr, Los Angeles)
J Child Neurol 5:60–64, 1990   7–9

Cocaine abuse is associated with a variety of severe acute neurologic complications, including ischemic stroke, subarachnoid and intraparenchymal hemorrhage, headaches, syncope, seizures, and death. Sixteen children with presumed cocaine-related seizures caused by maternal consumption were examined at age 16 hours to 8 years. All were assessed only because of requests for neurologic consultation. The mothers' pregnancy histories were similar.

The children uniformly had postdelivery tremulousness, irritability, and excessive startle responses. Shortly after birth each child started to have stereotypic episodes with ictal electroencephalographic confirmation in 7 cases. Eight neonates continued to have seizures after the first month of life.

Several mechanisms may be involved in a child with cocaine-related seizures. Transient changes in neurochemistry in the neonatal period may be precursors of long-term changes and epilepsy. Case-control studies are needed to determine the degree of long-term potential for the induction of epilepsy by cocaine.

▶ Cocaine has assumed center court as the noxious drug of the decade. The epidemic continues unabated and the lexicon of adverse effects continues to expand. Neonatal cocaine-related seizures is the theme of this report. Focal seizures are attributed to cerebral infarction or ischemia without infarction. The authors are, however, forced to speculate on the etiology of the seizures in the 15 patients without focal CT lesions. This they are not shy to do and changes in catecholamines, cholinesterase degradation system, amines, or direct toxicity of cocaine are all implicated. The concept of "kindling," in which repeated high-dose cocaine administration results in seizures at much lower doses, is also raised. In summary, "transient changes in neurochemistry during the neonatal period may be precursors to long-term alterations and subsequent epilepsy." It remains to be established that the seizures are directly related to cocaine exposure.

It is so soon that I am done for I wonder what I was begun for.—
Anonymous

A.A. Fanaroff, M.B.B.Ch.

Value of Sonography in the Diagnosis of Intracranial Hemorrhage and Periventricular Leukomalacia: A Postmortem Study of 35 Cases

Carson SC, Hertzberg BS, Bowie JD, Burger PC (Duke Univ Med Ctr)
AJNR 11:595–601, 1990   7–10

Cerebral sonography is widely used to detect germinal matrix hemorrhage and periventricular leukomalacia, but investigators have had difficulty determining the accuracy of the method because, to do so, it is necesary to compare sonographic images with histologic findings after death and periventricular leukomalacia is often not fatal. An autopsy study was performed on brain specimens from 35 infants who died at less than 1 year of age during a 10-month period. Twenty-two infants were born prematurely and died of cardiorespiratory insufficiency within the first week of life. Sonographic images of formalin-fixed brain specimens were compared with histologic findings in whole-brain sections to determine the sensitivity and specificity of sonography for detection of germinal matrix hemorrhage and periventricular leukomalacia.

Twenty-one of 35 brains had abnormalities on pathologic examination; 11 brains had germinal matrix hemorrhage. Sonography identified germinal matrix hemorrhage in 6 cases, but only 3 of these were hemorrhages seen pathologically, so the sensitivity and specificity of sonography were 27% and 88%, respectively. Both hemorrhages larger than 5 mm were identified by sonography, but all but 1 of 11 lesions 5 mm or smaller were overlooked (Fig 7–3), as were 2 resolving bilateral hemorrhages. If only those hemorrhages larger than 5 mm are considered, the sensitivity of sonography was 100% and the specificity was 91%. On pathologic examination 3 brains had choroid plexus hemorrhages, none of which were predicted by postmortem sonography. However, sonography made 5 false positive predictions of choroid plexus hemorrhage, for an overall sensitivity of 0% and specificity of 85%. Of 5 hemorrhages in the cerebral parenchyma and cerebellum, sonography identified 3 as ab-

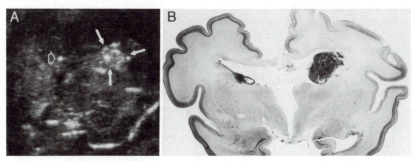

Fig 7–3.—**A**, coronal sonogram obtained post mortem illustrates sensitivity of sonography for large germinal matrix hemorrhages, but its insensitivity for smaller lesions. Area of increased echogenicity on right *(long arrows)* corresponds to germinal matrix hemorrhage, but there is no corresponding abnormality in echogenicity on the left, where a 5-mm hemorrhage was found on pathologic examination. Highly echogenic focus *(short arrow)* is an air bubble in lateral ventricle. **B**, histologic coronal section of specimen imaged in **A** reveals large germinal matrix on right that was visualized by sonography. Darkly staining smaller contralateral hemorrhage was not seen by sonography. Hematoxylin-eosin. (Courtesy of Carson SC, Hertzberg BS, Bowie JD, et al: *AJNR* 11:595–601, 1990.)

normalities, but 2 of these were identified as representing periventricular leukomalacia rather than hemorrhage. Therefore, sonography had a sensitivity of 40% and a specificity of 100% for intraparenchymal hemorrhage.

Four of 7 examples of periventricular leukomalacia/infarction were identified by postmortem sonography, but sonography also identified 4 false positive cases of periventricular leukomalacia/infarction, 2 of which showed an adult pattern of ischemia that could not be classified by sonography because other categories of ischemic injury were not included in the sonographic evaluation. For periventricular leukomalacia/infarction, sonography had sensitivity and specificity of 57% and 86%, respectively. True periventricular leukomalacia was found in only 4 cases, all in infants less than 34 weeks' gestational age. If true periventricular leukomalacia was considered separately, sonographic sensitivity and specificity decreased to 50% and 87%, respectively.

Sonography is useful for detecting larger germinal matrix hemorrhages, but it has limited sensitivity in the early diagnosis of periventricular leukomalacia. The technique appears insensitive for the detection of choroid plexus hemorrhages.

▶ Ron A. Cohen, M.D., Pediatric Radiologist, Children's Hospital Oakland, California, offers his thoughts on this selection.

▶ The accuracy and specificity of ultrasound in diagnosing periventricular leukomalacia and hemorrhage was limited. Classic histologic periventricular leukomalacia overlaps sonographically in this study with hemorrhage, infarction, and white matter gliosis.

In practice, increased periventricular echogenicity represents ischemic-hypoxic injury that may or may not be hemorrhagic. Follow-up ultrasound several weeks later may demonstrate areas of cystic encephalomalacia. To more accurately assess areas of parenchymal injury, MRI is being increasingly used for follow-up of affected infants.

Premature infants normally have areas of increased echogenicity adjacent to portions of the lateral ventricles. They are usually symmetrical, less echogenic than periventricular leukomalacia, and are most prominent near the trigone region. Histologic examination demonstrates layers of migrating glial cells. Follow-up examinations reveal normal deep white matter.

Other patterns of focal and diffuse ischemic-hypoxic injury also occur in newborns. Small ventricles may be present in normal newborns and are therefore not specific for cerebral edema. Infarcted areas demonstrate increased echogenicity of cortex and/or white matter. However, the findings are often subtle even when severe injury is present. Clinical suspicion and follow-up studies are required to make an accurate diagnosis and provide useful information regarding prognosis.—R.A. Cohen, M.D.

Neurosonographic Features of Periventricular Echodensities Associated With Cerebral Palsy in Preterm Infants

Pidcock FS, Graziani LJ, Stanley C, Mitchell DG, Merton D (Thomas Jefferson Univ Hosp, Philadelphia)
J Pediatr 116:417–422, 1990   7–11

Because periventricular leukomalacia probably represents the results of ischemic injury to subcortical white matter, the risk of cerebral palsy was determined in 127 preterm infants whose neonatal neurosonograms demonstrate periventricular echogenic abnormalities. The infants had sonographic evidence of increased periventricular echodensity and were followed up to ages 18 to 24 months.

Spastic cerebral palsy was diagnosed in 26 infants, all of whom had moderate to severe periventricular echodensities superior and lateral to the caudothalamic notch. Similar changes were present in 36 infants without cerebral palsy, 19 of whom had cyst formation. Intracranial hemorrhage was more frequent in infants in whom cerebral palsy developed, but did not increase the predictive value of neurosonography. All 24 infants with diparesis or quadriparesis had cysts and periventricular echodensities.

Sonographic abnormalities in the anterior parietal region are helpful in predicting the development of cerebral palsy (table). Although sensitive, periventricular echodensity is not very specific for cerebral palsy. Spastic cerebral palsy is unlikely to develop in the absence of periventricular echodensities and cyst formation, if grade IV intracranial hemorrhage also is absent.

▶ Cranial ultrasonography is of immense value in monitoring the course of preterm infants as well as determining features indicative of neurodevelopmental outcome (1–3). Surviving infants born at less than 33 weeks' gestation with echodensities and cysts larger than 2 mm comprise the group under scrutiny. The echodense lesions were classified as mild, moderate, or severe, and cysts larger than 3 mm were classified as large, those below 3 mm as small. Cystic changes were paramount to the development of cerebral palsy and once again

Diagnostic Accuracy of Neurosonographic Findings for Predicting Cerebral Palsy in Study Population

Test result	Sensitivity (%)	Specificity (%)	Predictive value Positive (%)	Negative (%)	Efficiency (%)
Mild PVE, no cysts	0	58	0	69	46
Mild PVE, ≤2 mm cysts	0	80	0	76	64
Mild PVE, ≥3 mm cysts	0	97	0	79	77
Mod/sev, no cysts	0	83	0	76	66
Mod/sev, ≤2 mm cysts	31	83	32	82	72
Mod/sev, ≥3 mm cysts	69	98	90	93	92

Abbreviations: Mod/sev, moderate severe.
(Courtesy of Pidcock FS, Graziani LJ, Stanley C, et al: *J Pediatr* 116:417–422, 1990.)

had the best positive (90%) and negative predictive values (93%), and were the most sensitive and specific neurosonographic findings for predicting cerebral palsy. All 26 infants with spastic cerebral palsy had lesions, including cystic changes, superior or lateral to the caudothalamic notch. The location and cystic changes are indicative of damage to the corticospinal tract. Serial ultrasound examinations diminish the chances for misreads and incorrect interpretation. Careful characterization is critical as the prognosis is dependent on the situation and size of the lesions, with cystic lesions larger than 3 mm spelling out great risk for spastic cerebral palsy. Periventricular leukomalacia probably results from ischemic injury and may be established in utero (see Abstract 7–1). Although these data are of great prognostic value the natural history and prognosis for echodense lesions without cystic changes remain to be elucidated. See also Abstracts 7–13 and 10–3.—A.A. Fanaroff, M.B.B.Ch.

References

1. Graziani LJ, et al: *Pediatrics* 78:88, 1986.
2. Graham M, et al: *Lancet* 2:593, 1987.
3. Boyzinski MEA, et al: *Dev Med Child Neurol* 30:342, 1988.

Thalamic Hemorrhage With Intraventricular Hemorrhage in the Full-Term Newborn
Roland EH, Flodmark O, Hill A (Univ of British Columbia; British Columbia Children's Hosp, Vancouver)
Pediatrics 85:737–742, 1990   7–12

Intraventricular hemorrhage, although common in premature infants, is uncommon in full-term newborns. The clinical appearance, associations, and radiologic features and sequelae at 18 months in a group of

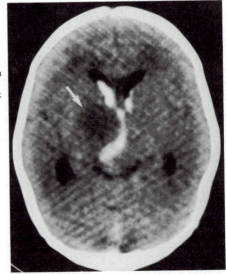

Fig 7–4.—Noncontrast CT scan of brain of full-term newborn with thalamic hemorrhage/intraventricular hemorrhage. Decreased tissue attenuation *(arrow)* is shown in thalamus adjacent to hemorrhage in thalamus. (Courtesy of Roland EH, Flodmark O, Hill A: *Pediatrics* 85:737–742, 1990.)

Neurologic Outcome at 18 Months of Age

Neurologic Outcome	Infants With Germinal Matrix/ Intraventricular Hemorrhage and Choroid Plexus/ Intraventricular Hemorrhage (n = 7)	Infants With Thalamic Hemorrhage/ Intraventricular Hemorrhage (n = 12)	*P* Values
Normal	0	2	.51
Developmental delay			
Mild/moderate	5	9	.99
Severe	1	1	.99
Hydrocephalus	2	7	.35
Seizures (after 1 mo of age)	4	8	.99
Cerebral palsy†	2	10	.05†
Death	1	0	.37

Note: Germinal matrix/intraventricular hemorrhage + choroid plexus/intraventricular hemorrhage and thalamic hemorrhage/intraventricular hemorrhage were compared using the 2-tailed version of Fisher's exact test.
*P < .05 denotes statistically significant difference between groups.
(Courtesy of Roland EH, Flodmark O, Hill A: *Pediatrics* 85:737–742, 1990.)

full-term newborns with an unusually high incidence of thalamic hemorrhage associated with intraventricular hemorrhage were described.

Of 19 full-term infants with intraventricular hemorrhage diagnosed by CT before 1 month of age, thalamic hemorrhage was documented in 12. Most of the infants had predisposing factors for cerebral venous infarction, including sepsis, cyanotic congenital heart disease, and coagulopathy. The clinical appearance and outcomes for the infants with thalamic hemorrhage associated with intraventricular hemorrhage were similar to those of infants with intraventricular hemorrhage originating from other sites. However, there was an increased incidence of cerebral palsy in infants with thalamic hemorrhage associated with intraventricular hemorrhage. A definitive diagnosis could be established on the basis of characteristic radiologic anomalies (Fig 7–4, table).

Thalamic hemorrhage seems to be the most common source of intraventricular hemorrhage in full-term infants, especially in those with uneventful birth histories and those in whom clinical abnormalities developed after the first week of life. Definitive diagnosis relies on the observance of radiologic abnormalities on CT scans, cranial ultrasonography, or cerebral angiography. Neurologic sequelae occur commonly, and only a minority of the infants appeared neurologically and developmentally normal at 18 months of age.

▶ Commenting on this article is Majeed Al-Mateen, M.D., Director, Neurology, Children's Hospital Oakland, California.

▶ The authors' conclusion that thalamic hemorrhage appears to be the most common source of intraventricular hemorrhage in full-term infants is a departure from the largely held view that in the full-term infant intraventricular hemorrhage arises primarily from bleeding in the choroid plexus. Two major pathogenic mechanisms thought to play a role in intraventricular hemorrhage in the term neonate, i.e., trauma and perinatal hypoxic-ischemic events, were not applicable to the cases in this series. The data suggest that coagulopathy and sepsis rank highest among the possible predisposing factors to thalamic hemorrhage. Venous occlusion involving the internal cerebral vein, leading to hemorrhagic infarction, seems a plausible mechanism in the neonate who after an uneventful first week of life, having survived the trauma of birth and escaping hypoxic injury, succumbs to rheological turmoil caused by infection of a hematological defect. The clinical presentation with signs of increased intracranial pressure was due, at least in part, to the development of hydrocephalus that contributed to neurologic morbidity. It would therefore be interesting to compare the neurologic outcome of a group of full-term infants with thalamic hemorrhage and intraventricular hemorrhage to that of full-term infants with thalamic and/or basal ganglia hemorrhage without intraventricular hemorrhage. Nevertheless, the significantly higher incidence of cerebral palsy in infants with thalamic hemorrhage and intraventricular hemorrhage in this study allows us to refine our prognostic statement.—M. Al-Mateen, M.D.

Frequent Handling in the Neonatal Intensive Care Unit and Intraventricular Hemorrhage

Bada HS, Korones SB, Perry EH, Arheart KL, Pourcyrous M, Runyan JW III, Anderson GD, Magill HL, Fitch CW, Somes GW (Univ of Tennessee, Memphis; Memphis State Univ)
J Pediatr 117:126–131, 1990   7–13

A decrease in the handling of ill premature babies has been recommended for the prevention of periventricular-intraventricular hemorrhage (PV-IVH). Neonatal intensive care unit procedures and normal physical or spontaneous activity cause arterial hypertension, which may result in rupture of the germinal matrix capillaries and PV-IVH. Also associated with increases in blood pressure during handling are reductions in transcutaneous oxygen pressure, at times to hypoxic levels, which may also predispose infants to PV-IVH.

A prospective, clinical study was carried out in 156 premature infants with a birth weight of no more than 1,500 g, but without major congenital malformations. Sixty-two infants who did not have PV-IVH or who had grade 1 PV-IVH within 1 hour after birth were randomly assigned to the reduced manipulation protocol; the other 94 infants were assigned to standard care. A bedside microcomputer-based data acquisition system was used to monitor the duration of rest or the number of interventions per day.

On the first day of life the study group spent 72.3% of the day (17.4 hours) at rest, compared with 64% of the day (15 hours) for the control group. The differences between the groups were apparent only during the first 48 hours after which the duration of rest increased and the number

Comparison of Mortality and Morbidity Rates

	Reduced manipulation (n = 62)	Standard manipulation (n = 94)
Discharge*		
Age (days)	61 ± 48	52 ± 27
Weight (gm)	1749 ± 545	1834 ± 562
Days with supplemental O_2*		
FIO_2 <40	13 ± 31	10 ± 18
FIO_2 ≥40	11 ± 52	2 ± 6
Days with ventilator support*	10 ± 16	12 ± 15
Age at death†		
≤7 Days	9 (14)	7 (07)
>7 Days	4 (06)	10 (09)
Bronchopulmonary dysplasia†	10 (17)	19 (21)
Patent ductus arteriosus†		
No treatment	12 (20)	14 (16)
Medically treated	9 (15)	10 (11)
Necrotizing enterocolitis†,‡	4 (05)	9 (10)

Abbreviation: FIO_2, fraction of inspired oxygen.
*Values are expressed as mean ± standard deviation.
†Values are expressed as number (%).
‡Stages 2 and 3.
(Courtesy of Bada HS, Korones SB, Perry EH, et al: *J Pediatr* 117:126–131, 1990.)

of interventions decreased in both groups. By the fifth day of life, 76% of the study group's day was spent at rest, compared with 73% of the control group's day.

The incidence of grades 2 to 4 or severe PV-IVH did not differ significantly between the study and control groups. At age 24 hours grades 2 to 4 PV-IVH were noted in 13% of the study group and 18% of the control group. Daily cumulative incidence did not differ between groups nor did the mean age at the time of extension of the PV-IVH. Severe PV-IVH occurred in 10% of the study group and in 13% of the control group. The clinical course of the infants assigned to the study and control groups was similar. The mortality and morbidity of the 2 groups in the neonatal period are compared in the table.

Low birth weight and low 5-minute Apgar scores were significant predictive variables for the development of severe PV-IVH. These findings also underscored the role of prematurity and asphyxia in the pathogenesis of PV-IVH.

No relationship between frequent handling and PV-IVH was demonstrated, even when other perinatal risk factors were taken into account. The overall risk of PV-IVH is significantly affected by low birth weight and factors indicative of perinatal asphyxia.

▶ Efforts at prevention of PV-IVH have featured prominently in the brief history of the YEAR BOOK OF NEONATAL AND PERINATAL MEDICINE (1–5). Nurseries across the land have already proclaimed that minimal handling reduces the incidence of PV-IVH. However, under the critical glare of the prospective study, no relationship between frequent handling and hemorrhage was established. I am convinced that strong proponents of minimal handling will not abandon their stations. Nor should they. The concept makes sense and the interventions for the infants should be planned and coordinated so that the infant is minimally disturbed. Periventricular-intraventricular hemorrhage may be too crude an end point to demonstrate the benefits of minimal handling. Minimal handling does no harm, which is more than can be said for many other interventions in the intensive care arena.

If we believe a thing to be bad, and we have a right to prevent it, it is our duty to try and prevent it, and damn the consequences.—Lord Milner

A.A. Fanaroff, M.B.B.Ch.

References

1. 1987 YEAR BOOK OF NEONATAL AND PERINATAL MEDICINE, Abstract 16–2.
2. 1988 YEAR BOOK OF NEONATAL AND PERINATAL MEDICINE, Abstract 12–2.
3. 1989 YEAR BOOK OF NEONATAL AND PERINATAL MEDICINE, Abstracts 6–8 and 6–9.
4. 1990 YEAR BOOK OF NEONATAL AND PERINATAL MEDICINE, Abstract 16–4.
5. 1991 YEAR BOOK OF NEONATAL AND PERINATAL MEDICINE, Abstracts 7–11, 10–3, and 15–9.

Measurement of Progressive Cerebral Ventriculomegaly in Infants After Grades III and IV Intraventricular Hemorrhages
Brann BS IV, Qualls C, Papile L, Wells L, Werner S (Univ of New Mexico, Albuquerque)
J Pediatr 117:615–621, 1990   7–14

The clinical management of posthemorrhagic ventricular dilation after intraventricular hemorrhage in preterm infants is problematic. Physicians must ascertain whether the ventricle size is static or is increasing and requires intervention. Guidelines were created that may help predict which infants with severe IVH will require intervention.

Serial cranial sonograms were obtained to measure the rate of growth of cerebral ventricular volumes in 48 preterm infants with and without intraventricular hemorrhage. There were 3 groups of infants: 22 with no intraventricular hemorrhage, 13 with hemorrhage and acute ventricular dilation, and 13 with hemorrhage and progressive ventricular dilation that required intervention. Clinical criteria and the subjective assessment of increasing ventricular size on weekly cranial sonograms were the basis of the decision to intervene. The rate of cerebral ventricular volume growth in infants with intraventricular hemorrhage who needed intervention was greater than that in infants without intraventricular hemorrhage and those with intraventricular hemorrhage and acute ventricular dilation. Guidelines were generated and confirmed in 10 infants.

The simplest guideline for predicting the need for intervention is to obtain a single volume measure. At some point, the ventricular volume will be so large that there is little doubt about whether hydrocephalus will develop. If the total lateral cerebral ventricular volume (TVV) reaches 30 mL by age 21 days, there is almost a 90% certainty that the infant will need intervention. If the volume is 30 mL by age 28 days, there is a greater than 90% chance. Using the frontooccipital circumference (FOC) as an indirect measure of intracranial volume and dividing TVV by FOC improves predictive power. A TVV/FOC ratio of .9 mL/cm by age 17 days gives a 90% certainty that an infant needs intervention. A stricter guideline with better predictive capability involves determining the rate at which the lateral cerebral ventricles are enlarging.

▶ The pliability of the CNS is sorely tested in infants with intraventricular hemorrhage. The natural history of ventricular dilatation was well-described by Dykes et al. (1). A critical clinical decision is to know when to intervene for progressive cerebral ventriculomegaly. The first order of business is to prove that the ventricles are continuing to dilate. Sequential ultrasonography provides direct visualization of the status of the ventricles but the concurrent evaluation of ventricular size is largely subjective; hence, the determination of ventricular volume represents a step forward. The ratio of ventricular volume to head circumference accurately predicted the need for intervention in 90% of infants by age 17 days. This is a small series; progressive hydrocephalus was noted in up to 50% of the subjects and the optimal time for intervention has yet to be determined. (Not all infants requiring intervention can be expected to be identified.)

There is little doubt this is a high-tech study. We are forced to have faith in both the mathematical and statistical modeling and the computer must remain on its best behavior. Verification of the mathematical model has been published by this group (2).

This report does add a further dimension to the evaluation and treatment of infants with intraventricular hemorrhage and ventriculomegaly. The primary objective of this study was to establish consistent predictive criteria for intervention. This was accomplished. We will closely follow its impact on the long-term outcome of these infants.

Healing is a matter of time, but it is sometimes also a matter of opportunity.—Hippocrates

A.A. Fanaroff, M.B.B.Ch.

References

1. 1990 Year Book of Neonatal and Perinatal Medicine, Abstract 18–4.
2. Brann BS IV, et al: *J Ultrasound Med* 9:1, 1989.

Randomised Trial of Early Tapping in Neonatal Posthaemorrhagic Ventricular Dilatation

Ventriculomegaly Trial Group (Whitelaw A, Radcliffe Infirmary, Oxford)
Arch Dis Child 65:3–10, 1990

In a large, multicenter trial conducted over a 3-year period 157 infants with posthemorrhagic ventricular dilatation were randomized to receive either early repeated CSF taps or conservative management. Outcome was assessed in terms of neurodevelopmental condition at age 12 months.

Thirty infants died and 6 were not available for follow-up. During the first 14 days after randomization the early treatment group had 5 times more taps and 12 times more CSF removed than the group managed conservatively. Infection of the CSF occurred in 7 infants in the early treatment group and 4 of the conservatively managed infants. Sixty-two percent of the survivors in both groups ultimately had ventricular shunts inserted.

When neurodevelopmental assessment was performed in 121 survivors at age 12 months, 103 (85%) had abnormal neuromotor signs and 88 (73%) had disabilities. The distribution and severity of abnormal neuromotor signs were similar in both treatment groups, regardless of whether parenchymal lesions were present at the time of entry into the study. Nearly all infants with parenchymal lesions had neuromotor impairment, but early treatment was associated with a significant reduction in other impairments.

These findings provide no evidence that early tapping in neonatal posthemorrhagic ventricular dilatation prevents impairment in children who have no parenchymal lesions at the start of treatment. However, early and repeated tapping should be considered in infants with parenchymal lesions.

▶ The observations described in this report emphasize the usefulness of collaborative randomized trials when a specific patient problem is infrequently observed in any 1 unit. In this study 15 different units in 3 countries cooperated to study 121 surviving patients. The high rate of abnormal neuromotor signs (85%) and disability (75%) in this group of infants continues to be discouraging. The 95% follow-up at 1 year is impressive. A further study of these children at 2½ years will be of special interest, especially when it includes assessment of language and perception.—M.H. Klaus, M.D.

Brain Damage in Monozygous Twins

Larroche JC, Droullé P, Delezoide AL, Narcy F, Nessmann C (INSERM U29; Hôpital de Port-Royal, Paris; Maternité Pinard, Nancy; Hôpital Necker, Enfants Malades; Hôpital Cochin; Hôpital Robert-Debré, Paris)
Biol Neonate 57:261–278, 1990   7–16

Twin pregnancies have higher mortality and morbidity rates than singleton pregnancies. In monochorionic twins, hemodynamic interdependency may lead to "transfusion syndrome" involving lesions in the brain and/or viscera. Fifteen monochorionic-diamniotic fetuses and neonates with a great variety of cerebral lesions were reviewed.

In 7 classical cases, the recipient twin was affected and the donor was macerated. In 5 cases, the lesions were described in the donor twin as well. In 10 of 11 cases, fetal ultrasonography indicated a diagnosis of intrauterine growth retardation, death of a fetus, or brain lesions, which was proved by ultrasonography or CT in fetuses born alive and who survived.

Lesions in the recipient twin may result from emboli or necrotic tissue from the macerated co-twin. Blood pressure instability or episodes of severe hypotension might lead to lesions in the recipient twin. In the donor, the lesions result from hypotension or anemia.

Outcome may be summarized in 4 ways. In the classical form, the donor dies in utero and at delivery may be macerated; the recipient, born alive with cerebral or visceral lesions, dies soon after birth or survives with lesions or survives and develops normally. Both fetuses may die in utero. Both fetuses may be born alive and 1 may die soon after birth with cerebral damage. In other cases, both infants may be born alive and survive with or without lesions.

▶ Although the precise incidence of twin-twin transfusion is unknown, perhaps 8% to 16% of monozygous twins, it is well recognized that the impact on both fetuses may be devastating. In the classic form the donor twin is affected first and dies in utero. Necrotic tissue from the dead fetus subsequently results in ischemic infarcts in the brain and/or viscera of the surviving twin. Given the many combinations of outcomes, as designated in the above abstract, Murphy's law prevails, so that the win-win situation, both twins surviving intact, occurs relatively infrequently. Larroche et al. are to be complimented on providing a new perspective of the phenomenon of feto-fetal transfusion. The focus, as might be anticipated from a neuropathologist, is on identification of brain lesions in utero, with confirmation after delivery. The small series is reported in exquisite detail and accompanied by high quality illustrations. Strikingly, leukomalacia was evident, beyond any doubt, in a macerated stillbirth. (This reinforces the need for comprehensive autopsies on all perinatal losses.)—A.A. Fanaroff, M.B.B.Ch.

Prenatal and Perinatal Factors in the Etiology of Cerebral Palsy
Torfs CP, van den Berg BJ, Oechsli FW, Cummins S (Univ of California, Berkeley)
J Pediatr 116:615–619, 1990   7–17

The best way to keep one's word is not to give it.—Napoleon

Cerebral palsy occurred in 41 of 19,044 children born between 1959 and 1966 to mothers whose pregnancies were monitored, for an incidence of 0.2%. In these cases cerebral palsy did not reflect progressive disease or a neural tube defect. All the children without cerebral palsy served as a control group.

Significant prenatal and gestational predictors of cerebral palsy included another birth defect, low birth weight, low placental weight, abnormal fetal position, and premature separation of the placenta (Table 1). Maternal antecedents included an unusually long or unusually short

Table 1—Fetal Prenatal Risk Factors: Distribution (%) in Children With CP and Control Subjects and Risk Ratios

Condition	CP cases		Control subjects (%)	RR	95% CI
	%	(No.)			
Birth weight <2500 gm*	17.1	(7)	6.8	2.8	0.8-6.3
Birth weight <2000 gm*	14.6	(6)	3.8	4.2	1.8-10.2
Abnormal fetal presentation*,†	14.6	(6)	4.3	3.8	1.6-9.1
Low placental weight*	24.0	(7)	8.7	3.6	1.5-8.4
Gestation <37 wk	17.1	(7)	8.8	2.1	1.0-4.8
Severe birth defect other than CP and sequelae*,	41.5	(17)	2.9	15.6	8.1-30.0
Nonsevere birth defect in addition to CP	41.5	(17)	10.4	6.1	3.1-11.8

Abbreviations: RR, risk ratios; CI, confidence interval.
*Associated with CP in Nelson and Ellenberg study.
†Breech, face, transverse.
(Courtesy of Torfs CP, van den Berg BJ, Oechsli FW, et al: J Pediatr 116:615–619, 1990.)

interval between pregnancies and unusually long menstrual cycles. Delayed crying, reflecting birth asphyxia, and abnormal delivery were also associated with occurrence of cerebral palsy (Table 2). Children who had seizures within 48 hours of birth were at high risk of cerebral palsy. Birth asphyxia was present in 22% of infants with cerebral palsy, and these

Table 2—Delivery and Perinatal Factors: Distribution (%)
in Children With CP and Control Subjects and Risk Ratios

Condition	CP cases %	(No.)	Control subjects (%)	RR	95% CI
Abnormal delivery*,†	14.6	(6)	4.3	3.8	1.6-9.0
Instrument delivery‡	58.5	(24)	52.5	1.3	0.69-2.4
Time to cry >5 minutes*	22.0	(9)	2.9	9.0	4.3-18.8

*Associated with CP in Nelson and Ellenberg study.
†Breech, face, transverse.
‡Forceps or cesarean section.
(Courtesy of Torfs CP, van den Berg BJ, Oechsli FW, et al: *J Pediatr* 116:615–619, 1990.)

infants had other prenatal risk factors that might have compromised their recovery.

Future etiologic studies of cerebral palsy should focus on prenatal, gestational, and neonatal risk factors, including genetic and environmental aspects that have not yet been investigated.

▶ Improvements in obstetric management have reduced the perinatal mortality rate but have not decreased the prevalence of cerebral palsy. The contribution of asphyxia to cerebral palsy has been challenged by Nelson and Ellenberg from their analyses of the Collaborative Perinatal Project (1,2). Torfs subjects the California Child Health and Development data, from a smaller, racially different cohort, to similar analysis and draws similar conclusions. Seventy-eight percent of children with cerebral palsy did not have birth asphyxia, whereas 2.9% of control subjects had birth asphyxia but recovered without neurologic damage. The majority of variables associated with cerebral palsy were gestational or maternal risk factors that were present before labor and delivery. This important message must be transmitted throughout the nation so that obstetricians will not be held accountable for that over which they have not had the resources to thwart. See also References 3–5.—A.A. Fanaroff, M.B.B.Ch.

References

1. Nelson KB, Ellenberg JH: *Am J Dis Child* 139:1031, 1985.
2. Nelson KB, Ellenberg JH: *N Engl J Med* 315:81, 1986.
3. 1987 YEAR BOOK OF NEONATAL AND PERINATAL MEDICINE, Abstract 6–9.
4. 1989 YEAR BOOK OF NEONATAL AND PERINATAL MEDICINE, Abstract 19–5.
5. 1990 YEAR BOOK OF NEONATAL AND PERINATAL MEDICINE, Abstracts 9–7 and 9–8.

8 Behavior

Effects of Prenatal Methadone Exposure on Sex-Dimorphic Behavior in Early School-Age Children
Sandberg DE, Meyer-Bahlburg HFL, Rosen TS, Johnson HL (North Shore Univ Hosp–Cornell Univ Med Coll, Manhasset, NY; New York State Psychiatric Inst, New York; Columbia Univ, New York)
Psychoneuroendocrinology 15:7–82, 1990   8–1

Animal studies have shown that prenatal exposure to morphine can alter the pattern of sex-dimorphic behavior in children, possibly through opiate-induced suppression of testosterone synthesis by the fetal testis in males; the mechanism is less clear in females. Whether in utero opiate exposure in humans is associated with changes in nonreproductive sex-dimorphic behaviors in children of women maintained on methadone during pregnancy was assessed. Thirty children of methadone-exposed women and 16 children of drug-free mothers were followed until they were at least 6 to 8 years old. Standard questionnaires completed by the primary caretakers served as assessment instruments.

Methadone-exposed boys showed significantly more stereotypically feminine behavior than nonexposed male control subjects, even after exclusion of maternal polydrug abuse. For girls, there were no significant differences between methadone-exposed and control groups.

Prenatal methadone exposure may be associated with gender-atypical behavior in boys. Long-term assessment of prenatal drug exposure in humans should include assessment of gender role behavior.

▶ This report is presented not as a major finding but to describe some of the studies presently underway. The stimulus for this work arose from studies in rats that demonstrated that prenatal exposure to morphine interfered with the development of normal adult sexual behavior. Unfortunately, the authors faced many difficulties in trying to obtain more definitive data. Sample sizes were small and became even smaller when separating out the polydrug users, and the results are anything but clear-cut. The finding that exposure in utero may be associated with altered sexual behavior suggests only that further explorations are indicated.—M.H. Klaus, M.D.

Behavioral States in Normal Mature Human Fetuses
Pillai M, James D (Bristol Maternity Hosp, England)
Arch Dis Child 65:39–43, 1990   8–2

Distinct behavioral states have been described in fetuses corresponding to the first 4 of 5 behavioral states in infants (quiet sleep, S1; active/rapid eye movement sleep, S2; quiet awake, S3; active awake without crying, S4; and with crying, S5). In fetuses, these states are designated 1F to 4F. To evaluate variations in behavior in healthy mature fetuses, 80 low-risk fetuses were studied by real-time ultrasound between 36 and 42 weeks' gestation. Fetal eye, head, trunk, and upper limb movements were observed, and fetal heart rate was recorded for a mean duration of 103.7 minutes per recording.

Three different behavioral patterns were observed: 1 quiescent pattern, 1F, and 2 active patterns, 2F and 4F. The latter 2 active patterns accounted for 67% of the total recording time (table). The most common behavioral pattern was state 2F, which occurred 58% of the time. State 1F was seen 30% of the time, and 4F occurred 9% of the time. In the remaining 3% of observation time, fetal behavior was indeterminate. Cy-

Number and Duration of Each Behavioral State in 80 Fetuses of 36 to 42 Weeks' Gestation

	Behavioural State				
	1F	2F	4F	Indeterminate	Total
No of episodes	121	150	21	25	317
Mean Duration (mins)	20.8	31.6	37.8	9.2	26.1
SD	8.6	19.5	30.4	5.6	18.1
Range (mins)	3-38	3-94	4-137	3-20	3-137
Total mins in each state	2516	4785	794	231	8326
% time in each state	30.2	57.5	9.5	2.8	

State 1F = no eye movements, no somatic movement except for the occasional startle, and narrow variability of the baseline heart rate. State 2F = continuous eye movements, frequent bursts of somatic movements, heart rate accelerations with movement, and wide baseline variability. State 4F = continuous eye movements, almost continuous somatic movements, and a sustained tachycardia.
(Courtesy of Pillai M, James D: *Arch Dis Child* 65:39–43, 1990.)

cling of quiescent and active states occurred in 96% of the fetuses within 100 minutes of starting the recording.

State 1F was characterized by absence of eye movements and somatic movements, except for the occasional startle, and a fetal heart rate pattern with little baseline variability. State 2F was characterized by continuous eye movements, frequent bursts of somatic movements, and a fetal heart rate with wide baseline variability and accelerations with movement. In State 4F, continuous eye movements with almost continuous somatic movements and sustained tachycardia were observed. Indeterminate behavior had no distinct pattern and occurred at transition between different states.

The existence of 3 of 4 behavioral states previously described in human fetuses is confirmed. The third state, 3F, may occur infrequently, if at all, in the fetus. These behavioral cycles may indicate integrity and maturity of neurologic development. Although its clinical application may be limited, there is a need to redefine the normal limits for the current biophysical fetal tests.

▶ Maureen Hack, M.B., Ch.B., Professor of Pediatrics, Director of the Follow-Up Program, Rainbow Babies and Childrens Hospital, Case Western Reserve University School of Medicine, Cleveland, comments as follows:

▶ Documentation of fetal states is arduous and time consuming and therefore has very little clinical application; however, the state of the fetus needs to be considered when evaluating the biophysical profile. This study of behavioral states in term fetuses replicates that of Nijhuis et al. in Groningen (1). Apparently not much has changed with fetal states over the past decade. If fetal states are considered to be equivalent to the postnatal states of normal newborns, then it is puzzling to me why state 3F, which is equivalent to the quiet-awake newborn state, was not documented. This quiet-awake state is considered to be important for learning, whereas in human newborns the active-awakeness is considered to be related to external needs. If there is no quiet-awake state in utero, can it mean that the fetus in utero cannot learn? Although only a small percentage of time (6%–11%) was spent actively awake, it would be interesting to understand what determines these periods.—M. Hack, M.B., Ch.B.

Reference

1. Nijhuis JG, et al: *Early Hum Dev* 6:177, 1982.

Circadian Rhythms in Preterm Infants: A Preliminary Study
Mirmiran M, Kok JH, de Kleine MJK, Koppe JG, Overdijk J, Witting W (Netherlands Inst for Brain Research; Univ of Amsterdam)
Early Hum Dev 23:139–146, 1990   8–3

Circadian rhythms have been found in humans from midgestation. These rhythms were studied in 9 preterm infants under fairly constant environmental conditions in a nursery unit. The method used to record the rhythmicity of body temperature and rest-activity in these infants had been developed for long-term continuous recordings of several physiologic variables in humans. In 5 of 9 infants circadian rhythms (recorded at 28 to 34 weeks' conceptual age) were found in body temperature; however, rhythmicity was not detectable in other physiologic variables.

An active biologic clock is already functional in preterm infants. In these infants, circadian rhythmicity is present in certain physiologic variables (body temperature) but not in others. The method used for studying circadian rhythms is simple and reliable enough to record and analyze circadian rhythms in several physiologic variables even in very young infants.

▶ Circadian rhythms have been well documented in the fetus but have been elusive in the newborn. It is strange that a biologic clock, turned on in utero, would stop ticking during the neonatal period. The fetal heart rate shows a circadian rhythm from as early as 22 weeks' gestation (1), and wouldn't you know it but the fetus is most active during maternal sleep (2). The central neuronal oscillators underlying the generation of circadian rhythms in mammals are located in the anterior hypothalamus (suprachiasmatic nucleus) (3). One can only wonder if these neurons are reset with the major hormonal and physical changes accompanying the birth process. Mirmiran's investigation should be regarded as preliminary, merely establishing the validity of the technology. Finding evidence of circadian rhythmicity with temperature is a bonus. Further exploration will reveal the inner workings of the biologic clock in the newborn. See also Abstract 4–3.

Time is the school in which we learn
Time is the fire in which we burn.—*Delmore Schwartz*

A.A. Fanaroff, M.B.B.Ch.

References

1. de Vries JIP, et al: *Early Hum Dev* 15:33, 1987.
2. Patrick J, et al: *Am J Obstet Gynecol* 142:363, 1982.
3. Moore RY: *Fed Proc* 42:2783, 1983.

Short-Term Effects of Early Suckling and Touch of the Nipple on Maternal Behaviour
Widström A-M, Wahlberg V, Matthiesen A-S, Eneroth P, Uvnäs-Moberg K, Werner S, Winberg J (Karolinska Hosp; Univ of Stockholm)
Early Hum Dev 21:153–163, 1990   8–4

The effects of early suckling, if any, when skin-to-skin contact was held constant were investigated within 30 minutes after birth in 57 primiparous mothers and their healthy full-term infants. Infants of 32 mothers were helped to suckle during the first hour of life. The control infants

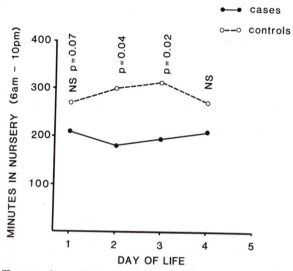

Fig 8–1.—The case and control infants' median time spent in the nursery from 0600 hours to 2200 hours, day 1 to day 4. (Courtesy of Widström A-M, Wahlberg V, Matthiesen A-S, et al: *Early Hum Dev* 21:153–163, 1990.)

were first suckled during the 8th hour of life. Skin-to-skin body contact was held constant in both case and control groups. Mother-infant interaction during breast-feeding, infants' time in the nursery, and different aspects of breast-feeding were assessed. Prolactin and gastrin in maternal serum were determined before and after breast-feeding 4 days post partum.

Only 6 of the 32 case infants sucked during the first hour. However, there were significant differences between cases and controls. In the case group, in which all infants had touched or licked the areola and nipple, mothers left their infants in the nursery a significantly shorter time (Fig 8–1). Also, significantly more case mothers talked to their infants during breast-feeding. Median gastrin concentrations were significantly lower in cases than controls before and after breast-feeding.

Infants' early touch of their mothers' areola and nipple appears to positively influence the mother-infant relationship in the first 4 days of life. It was also associated with lower maternal gastrin levels, suggesting that it influences maternal neuroendocrine functions. Ten months after birth, there were no differences between cases and controls.

▶ It is surprising that just touching the mother's nipple in the first hour of life would so affect her behavior. The acute sensitivity of the nipple is in line with 7 of 9 studies that reveal suckling of the nipple in the first hour of life markedly increases both the initial success and overall length of breast-feeding. It is, however, at variance with anthropologic observations that in nearly 50% of societies in which breast-feeding is successful, nursing begins after the first 24 hours of life. In any case it is another reason to allow parents private time with their infants in the first hours of life and encourage early suckling. In my experience when the infant is first taken to the breast initial licking of the mother's nipple is more common than vigorous sucking. Is the infant learning the scent of the mother during this early period?—M.H. Klaus, M.D.

Neonatal Facial and Cry Responses to Invasive and Noninvasive Procedures
Grunau RVE, Johnston CC, Craig KD (BC Children's Hosp; Univ of British Columbia, Vancouver; McGill Univ, Montreal)
Pain 42:295–305, 1990   8–5

It is difficult to assess pain in neonates. Whether the crying and facial activity induced by an invasive procedure, intramuscular vitamin K injection, could be distinguished from responses to noninvasive tactile events such as applying disinfectant solution to the umbilical cord stump and rubbing the thigh with an alcohol swab was studied in 36 healthy infants weighing more than 2,500 g at birth. Crying was analyzed by computer, and facial activity was analyzed by the Neonatal Facial Coding System. The infants were about 2 hours old when observed.

Significant procedure effects were found for total facial activity and latency to facial movement. The invasive procedure tended to produce brow bulging, squeezing shut of the eyes, deepening of the nasolabial furrow, and mouth opening. Crying, when it occurred, tended to be higher-pitched and more intense after the injection than after the noninvasive procedures.

Acute invasive procedures on newborns tend to alter facial expression and to produce earlier, longer-lasting crying. The facial display may reflect the infant's reaction to pain as predominantly affective and sensory-discriminative, with little or none of the cognitive meaning that allows older persons to cope with the experience.

▶ Linda Franck, M.S., R.N., Director of Critical Care Nursing at Children's Hospital Oakland, California, contributed this commentary:

▶ In this current study, the authors continue their rigorous scientific exploration of the expression of pain in newborns. The study paradigm addresses the relevant question of whether the neonatal response to noninvasive stimuli can be differentiated from the response to invasive (and presumably more painful) stimulation. In addition, the descriptive elements of the neonatal pain response are further delineated. The authors' discussion of the theoretical, methodological, and statistical concerns is most thoughtful and should be required reading. Further understanding of the pain responses of healthy full-term infants will lead to better methods for assessing and treating neonatal pain. However, we are a long way from direct application of such work to those who need it most: critically ill or premature infants who experience prolonged and invasive procedures (and whose faces are covered with tape and tubes). It's a crying shame that more research of the caliber of this study is not currently underway.— L. Franck, M.S., R.N.

Preference for Infant-Directed Speech in the First Month After Birth
Cooper RP, Aslin RN (Virginia Polytechnic Inst and State Univ, Blacksburg; Univ of Rochester)
Child Dev 61:1584–1595, 1990   8–6

Adults modify certain linguistic and paralinguistic aspects of their speech when talking to young children. Infant-directed (ID) speech may serve important social, attentional, and language-related functions in early development. Infants may be perceptually predisposed to attend to certain acoustic features of ID speech. Two experiments were done to determine whether infants much younger than those previously studied prefer ID speech.

Both experiments used a modification of the visual-fixation-based auditory-preference procedure. Experiment 1 involved 12 infants who were 1 month old, and experiment 2 involved 16 infants who were 2 days old. The experiments assessed whether the infants looked longer at a visual stimulus when looking produced ID as opposed to adult-directed (AD) speech. Both groups of infants preferred ID to AD speech. Although the absolute magnitude of the ID speech preference was significantly greater, with the older infants looking for longer durations than the younger infants, subsequent analysis revealed no significant difference in the relative magnitude of this effect. Differences in the overall looking times between the groups seemed to reflect task variables instead of speech processing differences (Fig 8–2).

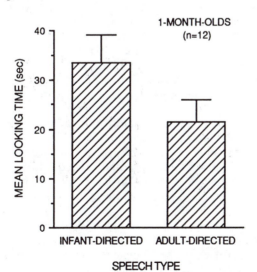

Fig 8–2.—Mean looking times (in seconds) of 1-month-old subjects from experiment 1 (including standard errors). (Courtesy of Cooper RP, Aslin RN: *Child Dev* 61:1584–1595, 1990.)

Infants' preferences for the exaggerated prosodic features of ID speech is present from birth and may not be related to specific postnatal experiences. However, prenatal auditory experiences with speech may also play a role.

▶ Not only do newborns appear to be more interested in ID speech, which has a higher overall pitch, slower tempo, longer pauses, and increased emphatic stress, but normal mothers use ID speech 70% of the time in the first hours of life when they talk to their infants. There is apparently a beautiful matching between the way the mother talks to her infant and what the neonate likes to hear. All this occurs even though mothers don't take classes in how to talk to their infants.—M.H. Klaus, M.D.

Does Infant Carrying Promote Attachment? An Experimental Study of the Effects of Increased Physical Contact on the Development of Attachment
Anisfeld E, Casper V, Nozyce M, Cunningham N (Columbia Univ, New York)
Child Dev 61:1617–1627, 1990   8–7

Previous studies suggest that close physical contact in the early months of life is an antecedent to the development of attachment between mother and infant. Forty-nine women, aged 18 to 37 years, from a low-income clinic population who delivered at a large inner-city hospital were randomly assigned to an experimental group or a control group. Mothers in the experimental group carried their infants in soft baby carriers (more physical contact), and mothers in the control group received infant seats (less physical contact). It was hypothesized that increased physical contact would promote greater maternal responsiveness and more secure attachment between infant and mother.

When the infants were 3½ months old, analysis of a video recording of a play session between mother and infant showed that mothers in the experimental group were more contingently responsive to their infants' vocalizations. When the infants were 13 months old, they were administered the Ainsworth Strange Situation, a procedure that activates the infant's attachment systems by putting him or her through a series of separations and reunions with his or her mother and a stranger. Analysis of the videotape indicated that significantly more infants in the experimental group were securely attached to their mothers.

For low-income, inner-city mothers, there may be a causal relationship between increased physical contact and subsequent security of attachment between infant and mother. Further confirmation in other low-income populations and larger population samples is warranted.

▶ This beautifully designed and executed study demonstrates that giving a newly delivered mother a soft infant carrier shortly after delivery significantly alters her infant's behavior some 13 months later when they were studied in a structured observation known as the Ainsworth Strange Situation. In this standardized test the infant and mother at the beginning are alone together in a room. They are observed during a sequence where a stranger enters the room, and after a short time the mother leaves the room and then returns. In addition, in a play session at 3½ months the experimental mothers were more responsive to their infants. It is surprising that it is possible to so easily alter by a simple intervention the behavior of a woman who has been molded by 18 to 30 years of previous experiences. During a time where caregivers are overwhelmed by the high incidence of child abuse it is refreshing to consider that we may be able to alter some maternal behaviors with such a low-cost intervention. A much larger trial is certainly now in order.—A.A. Fanaroff, M.B.B.Ch.

Persistent Perceptions of Vulnerability Following Neonatal Jaundice
Kemper KJ, Forsyth BW, McCarthy PL (Univ of Washington; Yale Univ)
Am J Dis Child 144:238–241, 1990   8–8

Although treatments for neonatal jaundice are considered both safe and effective, these treatments may later be associated with symptoms of the vulnerable child syndrome that may persist. Mothers of otherwise healthy infants with jaundice and demographically similar infants without jaundice were surveyed and compared 6 months after discharge from the hospital. Sixty-three mothers of infants with jaundice and 69 mothers of infants without jaundice participated in the study.

At 6 months 17% of mothers of infants with jaundice were still primarily breastfeeding, compared with 32% of mothers in the comparison group. Mothers of jaundiced infants were more likely to have tried a number of different formulas than mothers in the comparison group. There were no significant differences in responses between the groups on the Bates Infant Characteristics Questionnaire. The 2 groups also had similar scores on the Forsyth Child Vulnerability Scale at 6 months.

Mothers of children with jaundice did not report being more worried than mothers in the comparison group that their infants "might not make it." A similar percentage of mothers in both groups reported anxiety about leaving infants with other caretakers. Surprisingly, by 6 months, mothers of infants with jaundice were willing to separate from their infants for much longer periods than were mothers in the comparison group.

Both groups reported some health problems other than jaundice during the first 6 months, but mothers of infants with jaundice were more likely to consider these problems serious. Mothers of infants with jaundice also had higher use of health care facilities. Mothers of infants who had been treated with phototherapy had the highest rate of health care use.

Jaundice was strongly associated with the number of formulas a mother had tried, use of special formulas, and high use of health care facilities. The questionable benefits of treating moderate jaundice should be weighed against these risks.

▶ The findings reported here were also noted 30 years ago by Kennell (1). Parents are especially sensitive to what caretakers tell them about their infants.

Winnicott (2) noted, "At the beginning no mother fully believes in her baby, she cannot believe she has produced a normal baby." Too often we present material without ever asking how parents understand what we have told them. We should always ask parents what they understood about what we have told them. Over 50% of the time they are confused about what we discuss with them. To prevent the perception of vulnerability long after a neonatal pertubation it is important to be optimistic with parents unless we are absolutely sure the infant will die.—M.H. Klaus, M.D.

References

1. Kennell, JH, Rolnick A: *Pediatrics* 26:832, 1960.
2. Winnicott DW: *The Child, the Family and the Outside World*. Reading, Mass, Addison-Wesley, 1987.

9 Gastroenterology and Nutrition

Effect of Dietary Omega-3 Fatty Acids on Retinal Function of Very-Low-Birth-Weight Neonates
Uauy RD, Birch DG, Birch EE, Tyson JE, Hoffman DR (Univ of Texas Southwestern Med Ctr, Dallas)
Pediatr Res 28:485–492, 1990   9–1

Essential fatty acid accretion during late gestation and postnatally is essential for the developing retina in humans. Thirty-two neonates with very low birth weight (1,000-1,500 g) were randomly assigned to diets of formula with different ω-3 fatty acid content or normative human milk. The diets were designed to test whether the 18:3 ω-3 fatty acid was essential for optimal retinal development or whether ω-3 long-chain polyunsaturated fatty acids (LCPUFA) from marine sources were also required. Previous studies in chicks support the specific need for long-chain ω-3 fatty acids in early life.

The group fed formula enhanced with the long-chain derivatives eicosapentaenoic acid and docosahepaenoic acid in fish oil was closest to the human-milk fed group in both retinal function and biochemical markers of ω-3 fatty acid status. Formulas based on corn oil as an essential fatty acid supply have low 18:3 ω-3, and no commercial formulas presently contain long-chain ω-3 derivatives. Cone function was not affected by dietary essential fatty acids. The electroretinographic data showed a selective effect of ω-3 fatty acid on rod function.

Omega-3 FA is apparently an essential nutrient for optimal retinal development. Altered retinal function and fatty acid composition of blood lipids was found in low birth weight neonates fed an ω-3-deficient diet. Patients receiving enteral or parenteral nutrition with low or absent ω-3 supply have reported nonspecific visual changes and peripheral neuropathy. Long-chain ω-3 PUFAs are necessary to sustain rod function similar to that in a normative human-milk fed group.

▶ Offering commentary on this selection is William B. Pittard, III, M.D., Professor of Pediatrics, Director, Division of Neonatology, Medical University of South Carolina, Charleston:

▶ This article potentially describes yet another of numerous components in mothers' milk that makes it uniquely tailored to the needs of the newborn. Unlike the immunoprotective components of mothers' milk that play a passive host defense role, the ω-3 fatty acids may play an active role in brain and retinal function. Altered neonatal electroretinogram responses are reported in this study in infants with a deficiency in the essential dietary fatty acid, linolenic acid. Since linolenic acid is not produced in the human body, is not contained in commercial formulas, and is present in human milk, this study clearly generates interest. Further, since the conversion of linolenic acid to LCPUFAs is limited in premature infants, the LCPUFAs may also represent (at least for premature infants) essential fatty acids. This potential dietary requirement is similar to that for the amino acids taurine and cystine. These two amino acids are biochemically derived from the essential amino acid methionine. In premature infants, the conversion to taurine and cystine from methionine is limited, potentially making both of them, at least transiently, essential dietary amino acids. In the kitten an exogenous supply of taurine seems to be required for the development of a normal retina. Further, cystine and taurine, just like the ω-3 LCPUFAs, are both found in ample concentrations in mother's milk. Despite the fact that there is little tangible data indicating that adverse clinical symptomatology accompanies neonatal cystine or taurine deficiency, commercial formulas now contain these amino acids in concentrations similar to those found in human milk. Perhaps the ω-3 fatty acids should also be in commercial formulas. Although Dr. Uauy has successfully demonstrated a difference in the rod electroretinogram responses of premature infants with a plasma and red blood cell membrane deficiency of ω-3 fatty acids as compared to those who were sufficient, the clinical relevance of these observations is not clear. Further, based on ANOVA, less than half of the variance in electroretinogram findings between very low birth weight neonates with sufficient and deficient ω-3 fatty acids was explained by red blood cell and plasma ω-3 LCPUFA content. Thus, one wonders what additional factors other than ω-3 fatty acids contributed to these differences in electroretinogram responses. Do these changes predict long-term deficiencies in visual status or are they transient phenomena? Do these electroretinogram changes represent permanent retinal dysfunction or will these retinal responses return to normal when the infants are placed on an ω-3 fatty acid sufficient diet? Dr. Uauy's paper and the background data provided in its introduction offer genuine food for thought. It leaves the reader with the anxiety that although we do not have an adequate yardstick to assess the clinical relevance of the electroretinogram alterations measured, such a yardstick may soon be found with disquieting results. Yes, once again another uniqueness of mothers milk is postulated!—W.B. Pittard, III, M.D.

Taurine Depletion in Very Low Birth Weight Infants Receiving Prolonged Total Parenteral Nutrition: Role of Renal Immaturity
Zelikovic I, Chesney RW, Friedman AL, Ahlfors CE (Univ of Tennessee; Univ of Wisconsin; Univ of California, Davis)
J Pediatr 116:301–306, 1990   9–2

Depletion of the β-amino acid taurine in early life could potentially have deleterious effects on the developing brain and retina. Although it is abundant in human milk and supplemented infant formulas, taurine is not always found in total parenteral nutrition (TPN) solutions. In a prospective, controlled study, plasma and urinary taurine concentrations were determined in 7 very low birth weight (gestational age < 28 weeks, birth weight ≤ 1,000 g) sick infants who received a taurine-free TPN solution from day 3 or 4 of life for a period of 32 to 49 days and thereafter were formula-fed (group P). The values were compared with those of 8 sick infants matched by gestational age and birth weight who received formula or human milk from day 3 or 4 of life (group E), and 10 healthy, full-term, formula-fed infants, aged 1 to 18 weeks (group C). Blood samples were obtained weekly between postnatal weeks 3 and 18.

Between postnatal weeks 3 and 7, mean plasma taurine values were significantly lower in group P compared with group E and group C. After initiation of feeding, mean plasma taurine levels increased to normal in group P. Between weeks 3 and 5, the mean values of fractional excretion of taurine were markedly increased in groups P and E compared with group C. In contrast, during the same period, low urinary taurine values were present in 2 larger, older infants receiving TPN whose plasma taurine values were in the normal range. After week 5, urinary taurine values were in the control range in all groups.

Taurine levels in the body are regulated at the luminal membrane of the renal tubular epithelium. The marked hypertaurinuria in very low birth weight infants during the first weeks of life, despite extremely low plasma taurine values, suggests the limited ability of the immature kidney to adapt to low taurine intake by up-regulation of tubular urine reabsorption. The combination of renal immaturity and the absence of taurine in TPN solutions given to very low birth weight infants may result in depleted taurine body pools during early life. These findings strongly suggest the need for taurine supplementation of TPN solution administered to very low birth weight infants.

▶ Taurine resides predominantly in the cells and plays a vital role in the developing brain and retina. Deficiency has been manifested by abnormal electroretinograms or brain stem evoked responses. Taurine accumulates in the fetus late in the third trimester, rendering the pool size smaller in preterm infants. Also, the biosynthesis of taurine from methionine and cysteine is limited by low levels of the converting enzymes in these infants. Renal tubular immaturity prevents premature infants from conserving taurine even in the face of depleted stores and falling plasma levels. This report effectively documents the development of taurine depletion during TPN without added taurine, implicating all the above factors. No specific deleterious features are attributed to the low taurine levels, but the authors speculate on the benefits of taurine supplementation of TPN solutions. I was surprised by the selection of the so-called control group. My contention is that normal plasma levels should be established from breastfed term infants rather than those fed formula. See also references 1 and 2.—A.A. Fanaroff, M.B.B.Ch.

References

1. Sturman JA: *Ann NY Acad Sci* 477:196, 1986.
2. Tyson JE, et al: *Pediatrics* 83:406, 1989.

Chronological Development of the Fetal Stomach Assessed Using Real-Time Ultrasound

Nagata S, Koyanagi T, Horimoto N, Satoh S, Nakano H (Kyushu Univ, Fukuoka, Japan)
Early Hum Dev 22:15–22, 1990   9–3

Growth of the fetal stomach has been shown to be linear across gestation. It is hypothesized that this is not so, but rather, there exist some different time periods underlying the chronologic development of gastrointestinal functions. To test this hypothesis, chronologic changes in the maximum longitudinal and anteroposterior gastric dimensions were measured in 618 fetuses from 14 to 41 weeks' gestation using real-time ultrasound (Fig 9–1).

Piecewise linear regression analysis showed 3 significant critical points for both longitudinal and anteroposterior dimensions at exactly the same gestational age at 26–27, 32–33, and 36–37 weeks' gestation (Fig 9–2). Both dimensions increased from 16–17 weeks to 26–27 weeks of gestation, remained fairly constant between 26–27 and 32–33 weeks, increased again from 32–33 weeks to 36–37 weeks, and then decreased from 36–37 to 40–41 weeks.

There are 4 biologically different periods underlying the development of gastric function in the human fetus that correspond to the time periods divided by the 3 critical points of gestational age. The increase in gastric dimensions from 16–17 to 26–27 weeks complements fetal growth, and the fairly constant dimensions between 26–33 weeks suggest the initiation of fetal gastric functions. The fetal stomach dimensions begin to in-

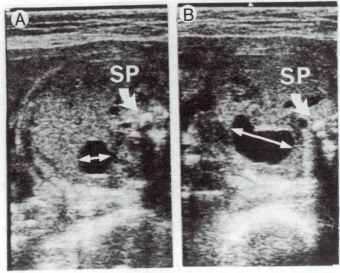

Fig 9–1.—Ultrasound image of the fetal stomach at 29 weeks of gestation. *Arrows* indicate longitudinal (**B**) and anteroposterior (**A**) dimensions. SP = spine. (Courtesy of Nagata S, Koyanagi T, Horimoto N, et al: *Early Hum Dev* 22:15–22, 1990.)

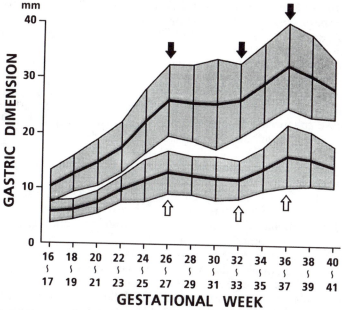

Fig 9–2.—Shown are chronological changes in the gastric dimensions with advance in gestation obtained from 618 fetuses from 16 to 41 weeks of gestation. The mean values are within the range of ±1 SD of longitudinal (top) and anteroposterior (bottom) dimensions. *Filled arrows* indicate critical points in the longitudinal dimension, and *open arrows* indicate critical points in the anteroposterior dimension. (Courtesy of Nagata S, Koyanagi T, Horimoto N, et al: *Early Hum Dev* 22:15–22, 1990.)

crease again at 32–33 weeks, relating to the initiation of lower esophageal sphincter activity in utero and swallowed amniotic fluid, until it reaches maturity by 36–37 weeks. The decrease in fetal stomach size between 36–37 and 40–41 weeks' gestation possibly corresponds to the decrease in turnover of amniotic fluid volume in the fetus.

▶ In utero real-time ultrasound permits a bird's-eye view of the growth of the stomach, and with a little imagination this can be correlated with function. This is a fascinating time motion study of the fetal stomach that results in a plausible thesis wherein physiologic changes account for the various pertubations in gastric dimensions. Knowing the capacity of the stomach is essential in planning feeding strategies. In utero the capacity is evidently determined by gastrointestinal motility and swallowing and production of amniotic fluid, together with lower esophageal sphincteric tone. The rapid increase in dimensions at the "critical time" of 33–34 weeks' correlates with onset of the gag reflex and the ability to coordinate sucking and swallowing. The stomach is thus prepared for the onslaught of enteric feeding from this point in time and forever more.

Life is thirst.—Leonard Michaels

A.A. Fanaroff, M.B.B.Ch.

Early Diet of Preterm Infants and Development of Allergic or Atopic Disease: Randomised Prospective Study

Lucas A, Brooke OG, Morley R, Cole TJ, Bamford MF (Med Res Council Dunn Nutrition Unit, Cambridge; Ipswich Hosp, Suffolk, England)
Br Med J 300:837–840, 1990   9–4

The possible effect of early diet on the development of atopic disease in infancy has provoked much attention and controversy. Premature infants may have enhanced exposure to antigens and consequently may be expected to be at high risk of sensitization and the development of allergic disease.

Two randomized prospective trials were undertaken in 777 infants. All were without any major congenital abnormality and weighed less than 1,850 g at birth. The infants were born between 1982 and 1984.

In trial A, the infants were randomly given banked donor breast milk or preterm formula as their sole diet or (separately randomized) as a supplement to their mother's expressed breast milk. In trial B, infants were given a term formula or preterm formula as the sole diet or as a supplement to their mother's milk. A blind follow-up examination was carried out 18 months after the expected date of birth.

The infants in trial A were first seen for follow-up at 9 months; those in both trials were seen at 18 months. At follow-up, information was obtained on eczema, wheezing (asthma), and sensitivities to food and drugs, and a detailed clinical and neurodevelopmental evaluation was made. Details of atopic or allergic disease in the family were procured during the infants' stay in the neonatal unit.

At 18 months after term there was no difference in the incidence of allergic reactions between dietary groups in either trial. However, in the subgroup of infants with a family history of atopy, those in trial A who were allocated preterm formula rather than human milk had a significantly higher risk of experiencing 1 or more allergic reactions (notably eczema) by the end of the 18 months. Neonates fed formulas based on cows' milk, including those with a high protein content, did not have an increased risk of allergy.

▶ Significantly, only a subgroup of infants whose close family relatives had a history of atopy benefited from breast-feeding. The authors suggested as an explanation that the premature infants immature immunological system permitted a gradual tolerance to develop for cows' milk. Clinically, the study supports the value of taking a family history. This report also demonstrates how much valuable data can be collected in a well-designed study.—M.H. Klaus, M.D.

Effect of Lactose on Mineral Absorption in Preterm Infants

Wirth FH Jr, Numerof B, Pleban P, Neylan MJ (Eastern Virginia Med School, Norfolk; Old Dominion Univ, Norfolk; Ross Labs, Columbus, Ohio)
J Pediatr 117:283–287, 1990   9–5

Preterm infants, especially very low birth weight infants, are given premature-infant formulas that contain only 50% lactose because of their low intestinal lactase activity. However, lactose enhances calcium absorption in term infants, and reduced lactose content in premature-infant formulas may limit calcium absorption in preterm infants at a time when their calcium requirement is very high.

In a controlled, randomized 72-hour balance study, 18 very low birth weight infants (birth weight < 1,400 g) were fed Similac Special Care formula with a 50:50 carbohydrate blend of glucose polymers and lactose (LGP group, no. = 8) or a nearly identical formula with 100% carbohydrate as lactose (lactose group, no. = 10) to determine the effects of dietary reduction of lactose on mineral absorption in preterm infants. The studies were conducted after at least 3 consecutive days of full oral feeds in infants with a mean age of approximately 23 days.

There were no significant differences between the LGP and lactose groups in percentage of calcium, phosphorus, magnesium, zinc, copper, or manganese absorption. These minerals were retained at rates similar to or greater than those in utero. Calcium absorption was 75% of intake, despite an intake of vitamin D that was less than half of the recommended intake for preterm infants.

Reducing the lactose content of premature-infant formulas to 50% apparently does not significantly impair mineral absorption, particularly calcium absorption.

▶ The fundamental question is whether the lactose content of the formula is critical for calcium and other mineral absorption. The background is that lactase activity is reduced before 34 weeks' gestation, lactose enhances calcium absorption in term infants, and the bulk of calcium accretion takes place during the third trimester. Carefully controlled balance studies comparing formulas with 50% lactose and 100% lactose revealed not the semblance of a difference in calcium and mineral absorption or accretion. A simple question therefore yielded the uncomplicated answer that 50% lactose as the source of carbohydrate does not compromise calcium absorption. The study did raise questions about the vitamin D requirements but that is a story for another day.

I eat merely to put food out of my mind.—N.F. Simpson

A.A. Fanaroff, M.B.B.Ch.

Effect of Delivery Room Routines on Success of First Breast-Feed
Righard L, Alade MO (Univ of Lund, Sweden; Obafemi Awolowo Univ, Ile-Ife, Nigeria)
Lancet 336:1105–1107, 1990   9–6

Human infants apparently share the newborn mammal's instinctual response of crawling to the mother's nipple for breast-feeding in the first hour after birth. When this routine is disrupted by separating the infant from the mother for weighing and measuring, the process is disturbed and the infant may not suckle. Sedation of the infant by drugs (e.g., pethidine administered to the mother during labor) may also disrupt the routine.

Seventy-two healthy infants were observed for 2 hours after birth. Decisions by the midwife and mother naturally divided the 72 mothers and infants into a separation group and a contact group. In a group of 34 mothers, the infant was removed from the mother after about 20 minutes. A group of 38 mothers requested at least 1 hour's uninterrupted contact with the newborn.

Of 34 infants in the separation group, 7 sucked correctly, 11 sucked incorrectly, and 16 refused to suck. In the 38 infants in the contact group, 24 sucked correctly, 4 sucked in a faulty manner, and 10 did not suck at all. Of the 26 infants in both groups who did not suck, all but 1 were affected by pethidine.

The difference between the groups showed a significant impact of separation or contact on the success or failure of initial sucking. The recommended course of action is that the naked infant be left on the mother's abdomen undisturbed until the first breastfeeding is accomplished. The infant's efforts to reach the breast should be promoted. Using analgesics during labor that may affect the infant is discouraged.

▶ Though we carefully repress evidence of our animal heritage, it is fascinating that shortly after birth human infants have the ability when they are not disturbed or sedated with residual pethidine received during labor to actually crawl to their mother's nipple and suckle. What is the neonate sensing that stimulates their movement to the nipple? Is it a temperature gradient, odor, or reflexive? It should be emphasized that this activity frequently occurred 20 to 45 minutes after delivery just when we in the United States take the infant away from the mother for a short period for cleaning. This report is additional evidence that maternal analgesia significantly alters neonatal behavior. It may be time to review the hospital care of mothers and infants during the first hour of life. For further evidence on how suckling in the first hour of life alters a mother's behavior see Abstract 8–4.—M.H. Klaus, M.D.

Do Changes in Pattern of Breast Usage Alter the Baby's Nutrient Intake?
Woolridge MW, Ingram JC, Baum JD (Univ of Bristol, England)
Lancet 336:395–397, 1990   9–7

Because the fat concentration in the milk at the end of breast-feeding appears to be directly related to feed length and feed volume, it was hypothesized that the fat concentration in breast milk is lower with incomplete breast emptying. To test this hypothesis, a within-subject, repeated measures, randomized, crossover study was undertaken. The effect of 2 patterns of breast-feeding (either feeding at 1 breast or at 2 breasts during a feed) was studied in 12 mother/infant pairs. The mother was randomly assigned to either breast-feeding pattern at 4 weeks post partum and adopted the alternate pattern at 5 weeks post partum.

The 1-breast per feed policy resulted in a longer feed time and increased volume extraction per breast, higher postfeed fat concetrations, longer interval between use of the same breast, and lower prefeed fat levels, compared with the 2-breast policy. However, the infant's net fat intake per 24 hours did not differ significantly between the 2 patterns.

Breast-fed infants can quickly achieve stable fat intake despite changes in patterns of breast-feeding. Hence, mothers should be encouraged to exercise flexibility and be led by infants during feeding.

▶ It is fascinating how an infant is able to consume a similar fat intake on very different patterns of feeding. There must be a well-integrated system regulating the fat intake. This report supports the data of Dewey and Lonnderdal (1), who suggested that babies regulate their caloric intake by volume and concluded that "the wide range of breast milk volume . . . is due to more variation in infant 'demand' than to inadequacy in milk production." This report is further evidence that the infant should decide the timing and length of the feedings. How do human infants regulate their net fat intake to be so similar to different feeding schedules?—M.H. Klaus, M.D.

References

1. Dewey KG, Lonnerdal B: *Acta Paediatr Scand* 75:893, 1986.

Breast-Feeding Frequency During the First 24 Hours After Birth in Full-Term Neonates
Yamauchi Y, Yamanouchi I (Okayama Natl Hosp, Okayama, Japan)
Pediatris 86:171–175, 1990

9–8

There is no finer investment for any community than putting milk into babies.—Winston Churchill

During the first week of life, breast-fed neonates lose more weight, gain weight more slowly, receive fewer calories, and have higher serum bilirubin levels than do formula-fed neonates. These problems might be ameliorated by increasing the frequency of suckling, which would also have a positive effect on maternal nipple pain and duration of lactation.

Investigators studied 140 healthy, full-term, breast-fed, vaginally delivered neonates to determine the factors that contribute to frequency of breast-feeding during the first 24 hours after birth and the neonatal response to breast-feeding frequency. The infants were kept with their mothers from the time of delivery, and mothers were encouraged to nurse them whenever they appeared hungry. Mothers were told not to limit frequency or length of nursing. Investigators also noted factors that affected the frequency of nursing.

Frequency of breast-feeding ranged from 0 to 11, with a mean of 4.3, during the first 24 hours. Frequency increased significantly to a mean of 7.4 during the next 24 hours. Feeding frequency during the first 24 hours correlated significantly with frequency during the next 24 hours, frequency of meconium passage, age at maximum weight loss, maximum weight loss, weight loss from birth to hospital discharge, breast milk intake on days 3 and 5, and transcutaneous bilirubin readings on day 6. Newborns born between midnight and 6:00 AM were nursed more frequently than neonates born between 1:00 PM and midnight.

Frequent nursing during the first days of life is beneficial to the neonate. Many neonatal clinical problems related to breast-feeding are iatrogenic. These problems could be reduced by educating mothers and nurses and by changing in-hospital practices related to breast-feeding.

▶ Once again the question of breast-feeding frequency and neonatal problems has forged to the forefront. This politely convincing manuscript brought back pleasant memories of the valiant effort by Manoel de Carvalho from Brazil to complete similar studies during his sojourn in Cleveland (1–3). It took considerable charm and patience to persuade the nursing staff to permit unrestricted feeding and grit and perseverance to measure stool bilirubin excretion in newborn babies. Nonetheless he documented that frequent feeding, defined as 8 or more times per 24 hours, was associated with lower peak bilirubin levels, greater breast milk intake, and no increase in maternal discomfort. (We shall say nothing of the discomfort of the nursing staff initially participating in this project.) Breast-fed infants excreted less bilirubin in their stools, supporting the concept of enhanced enterohepatic circulation of bilirubin. The above report from Japan has similar findings, clearly enunciated in the abstract above. Regrettably, the groups are selected after the fact rather than assigning patients to the various feeding groups, i.e., nonrandom selection. The select group who nursed more frequently during the first 24 hours of life appeared to be a hardier breed. They ate more vigorously, lost less weight, and had significantly lower bilirubin levels on day 6. Once again this is a relatively small study. In view of the large number of women who breast-feed and given the noninvasive painless nature of the study it appears prudent to repeat this study, assigning matched groups to frequent or standard feeding regimens. It appears to be a low budget study just waiting to happen. It was interesting to note the civilized practice of keeping the mothers and their healthy full-term infants hospitalized until the 7th day of life, a practice long and no doubt forever banished in the United States.—A.A. Fanaroff, M.B.B.Ch.

References

1. deCarvalho M, et al: *Am J Dis Child* 136:737, 1982.
2. deCarvalho M, et al: *J Pediatr* 107:786, 1985.
3. deCarvalho M, et al: *Pediatrics* 72:307, 1983.

Breast-Milk Amylase Activity in English and Gambian Mothers: Effects of Prolonged Lactation, Maternal Parity, and Individual Variations
Dewit O, Dibbas B, Prentice A (Med Research Council Dunn Nutrition Unit, Cambridge, England; Keneba, The Gambia)
Pediatr Res 28:502–506, 1990

9–9

Breast milk contains an amylase that may contribute to the digestion of carbohydrates during complementary feeding. To assess the quantity and variability of amylase activity in breast milk, 63 English mothers of parity 1–5 and 107 Gambian mothers of parity 1–12 who were at various stages of lactation (0.5–27 months) were studied. Breast-milk amylase activity was measured by hydrolysis of maltotetraose.

Amylase activity was measurable in all breast milk samples. Amylase activity ranged from 0.08 to 3.53 IU/mL, and did not vary during a feed or over 24 hours. Each mother exhibited a characteristic level of activity in her milk. Amylase activity decreased with the progress of lactation (Fig 9–3); it was higher in the first trimester of lactation and decreased significantly by 35% to a plateau at 6 to 27 months. After adjustment for stage of lactation, Gambian mothers of parity 11 or 12 had only half as much of the amylase activity in primiparous mothers. Parity had no effect on activity in English mothers, probably because of the low parity in this group. Using community data on milk volume, the estimated breast-milk amylase intake by breast fed infants ranged from 800 to 1,000 IU/24 hours in the first trimester and 400 IU/24 hours in the second year of lactation.

Breast milk is an important source of amylase in both developed and developing countries. Amylase is secreted into breast milk throughout 2 years of lactation in quantities of potentially valuable digestive capacity. The intake of breast-milk amylase varies widely among children because

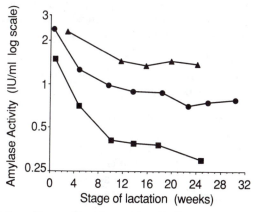

Fig 9–3.—Variations of breast-milk amylase activity with the stage of lactation in 3 mothers who were exclusively breast-feeding. Each mother is represented with a symbol and samples from the same mother are linked by a *solid line*. (Courtesy of Dewit O, Dibbas B, Prentice A: *Pediatr Res* 28:502–506, 1990.)

of differences in breast-milk amylase activity in mothers as well as breast-milk intake.

▶ Note that the amylase level in Figure 9–3 is on a log scale and during the first 8 weeks of life there is a remarkable drop in activity. The high levels in early lactation may be especially useful for the infant since it is at this time that amylase secretion into the saliva and pancreatic juices of the baby are negligible. Importantly, breast-milk amylase survives gastric digestion and remains active in the small intestine. This may be another example of how neatly breast milk matches the needs of the young neonate.—M.H. Klaus, M.D.

Partition of Nitrogen Intake and Excretion in Low-Birth-Weight Infants
Donovan SM, Atkinson SA, Whyte RK, Lönnerdal B (Univ of California, Davis; McMaster Univ, Hamilton, Ontario)
Am J Dis Child 143:1485–1491, 1989   9–10

Because milk from mothers who deliver prematurely ("preterm milk" [PTM]) has higher concentrations of nitrogen, protein, macrominerals, energy, and electrolytes than term milk, it has been speculated that the optimum food for the premature infant may be the mother's milk. To determine the adequacy of feeding solely PTM, compared with a combination of PTM and infant formula, on overall nitrogen retention and to quantitate and partition total nitrogen intake and excretion in low birth weight infants, 24 infants with a mean gestational age of 30.7 weeks and a mean birth weight of 1.36 kg received either PTM only or 50% PTM plus 50% standard infant formula (PTM + F). After 1 week of feeding 72-hour balance studies were conducted, and total nitrogen, nonprotein nitrogen, and whey protein intake and excretion were measured.

Total mean nitrogen intake was 452 mg/kg/day for the PTM group, and 406 mg/kg/day for the PTM + F group; the difference was not significant. There were no significant differences in nitrogen absorption (85%), excretion, and retention (71%) between groups. The contribution

---

Intake and Fecal Excretion of Human Whey Proteins

	PTM Group (n = 23)		PTM + Formula Group (n = 10)	
	Intake	**Excretion (%*)**	**Intake**	**Excretion (%*)**
α-Lactalbumin	425 ± 104	0 (0)	171 ± 32[b]	0 (0)
Serum albumin	102 ± 67	0.56 ± 0.13 (0.5)	57.21	0.34 ± 0.6 (0.6)
Lactoferrin †	492 ± 217[a]	24 ± 26 (5)	262 ± 80[b]	33 ± 22 (13[b])
Lysozyme†	34 ± 10[a]	1.1 ± 1.2 (3[a])	11 ± 8[b]	2.0 ± 1.5 (18[b])
Secretory IgA†	460 ± 383[a]	110 ± 150 (24)	138 ± 83[b]	38 ± 58 (27)

Note: Values represent mean ± standard deviation in milligrams per kilogram per day.
*Calculated as percentage of intake.
†For each protein different superscript letters denote significantly different values between groups (P < .05).
(Courtesy of Donovan SM, Atkinson SA, Whyte RK, et al: *Am J Dis Child* 143:1485–1491, 1989.)

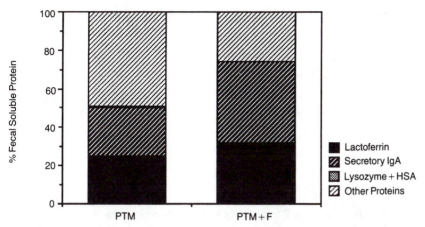

Fig 9–4.—Components of fecal soluble protein (soluble nitrogen minus nonprotein nitrogen) fraction of infants receiving PTM or PTM + F. *Abbreviation: HSA, human serum albumin.* (Courtesy of Donovan SM, Atkinson SA, Whyte RK, et al: *Am J Dis Child* 143:1485–1491, 1989.)

of human milk whey proteins to overall nitrogen intake reflected the composition of the infants' diet. Although the levels of intake of serum albumin, lactoferrin, and lysozyme were higher in the PTM group, excretion of the proteins was similar between groups (table). Combined lactoferrin and secretory IgA (sIgA) accounted for an average 52% and 72% of the soluble protein in feces of infants fed PTM and infants fed PTM + F respectively (Fig 9–4). The mean level of excretion of sIgA was 3-fold higher in the PTM-fed group, reflecting the 3.3-fold higher intake of sIgA.

Premature infants who receive their own mother's milk attain nitrogen balance with nitrogen excretion rates similar to intrauterine growth rates for the first 5 weeks postnatally. Preterm milk provides potentially functional proteins for the low birth weight infants.

▶ The adequacy of PTM for nourishing and nurturing preterm infants is constantly being questioned. On theoretical grounds it should not be sufficient to sustain growth and provide all the prerequisite macro- and micronutrients. However, theories are swept aside and when PTM is fed to preterm infants they will thrive. The composition of the breast milk, including the unique whey proteins such as secretory IgA, lactoferrin, lipase, and lysozyme, and the bioavailability of various factors render breast milk in many ways advantageous. Concerns about the adequacy of the protein are laid to rest in this careful comparative study that uses state-of-the-art technology, which demonstrated that PTM resulted in nitrogen accretion similar to intrauterine growth rates for 5 weeks postnatally. Also, identification of immunologically intact secretory IgA and lactoferrin infers better protection against infection in the gastrointestinal tract. This is confirmed by a multicenter study in Britain where breast milk reduced the incidence of necrotizing enterocolitis, the major gastrointestinal disorder in the intensive care nursery (1). This should serve as a powerful impetus to feed to sick preterm infants their own mother's milk. See also the 1990 YEAR BOOK OF NEONATAL AND PERINATAL MEDICINE, Abstracts 9–6, 9–7, and 9–11.

Things are seldom what they seem
Skim milk masquerades as cream.—*Sir William S. Gilbert*

A.A. Fanaroff, M.B.B.Ch.

Reference

1. Lucas A, et al: *Lancet* 336:1519, 1990.

Metabolic and Clinical Consequences of Changing From High-Glucose to High-Fat Regimens in Parenterally Fed Newborn Infants
Chessex P, Gagne G, Pineault M, Vaucher J, Bisaillon S, Brisson G (Univ of Montreal; Hôpital Sainte-Justine, Montreal)
J Pediatr 115:992–997, 1989

9–11

The mountain sheep are sweeter,
But the valley sheep are fatter;
We therefore deemed it meeter
To carry off the latter.—*Thomas Love Peacock*

Initially, neonates receiving intravenous alimentation are temporarily restricted to preparations in which glucose is the main source of energy. To investigate the metabolic and clinical consequences of changing from high-glucose to high-fat regimens during initiation of parenteral nutrition, 11 newborn infants receiving total parenteral nutrition were studied during 2 consecutive days while given 2 isocaloric (70 kcal/kg/day) and isoproteinic (2.5 g/kg/day) regimens differing only in the source of energy. The infants received a high-dose glucose regimen (12–17 g/kg/day) on the first day, and a high-lipid regimen (2.5–3 g/kg/day) on the second day. The infants, with a mean birth weight of 2.54 kg and mean gestational age of 37 weeks, were studied at a mean postnatal age of 8 days. Both studies were performed under steady-state conditions of incubator and infant temperatures.

The rectal and interscapular temperatures rose significantly from the high-glucose to the high-lipid regimen, despite constant environmental temperature (table). There were no significant changes in the urinary excretion of C peptide or catecholamines associated with the dietary changeover. However, there was a significant decrease in nitrogen retention during the high-lipid regimen from 63.9% to 56%.

Energy source can influence body temperature in infants, and the increase in body temperature may reflect a metabolic adaptation to the rapid change in energy substrates. The specific locations of the changes in body temperature, the rectal and interscapular areas, suggest brown fat activation that results in this diet-induced thermogenesis.

Thermic Response to Parenteral Regimens Differing
by Source of Energy

	High-glucose regimen	High-lipid regimen	Difference
Operative incubator temperature (°C)	31.6 ± 0.7	31.6 ± 0.8	0.01 ± 0.14
Infant temperature (°C)			
Rectal	36.6 ± 0.3	37.0 ± 0.3	−0.36 ± 0.34*
Average skin	35.6 ± 0.3	35.7 ± 0.3	−0.1 ± 0.24
Interscapular (n = 7)	35.6 ± 0.3	36.0 ± 0.3	−0.36 ± 0.15*

Data are expressed as mean ± SD and obtained from 11 patients except when stated otherwise.
*Significant difference between high-glucose and high-lipid regimens, $P < .05$.
(Courtesy of Chessex P, Gagne G, Pineault M, et al: *J Pediatr* 115:992–997, 1989.)

▶ Nutritional and metabolic aficionados will delight in this report. Others will merely nod their heads, acknowledge the quality of the research, and ponder on its significance. The metabolic consequences of shifting energy intake are easy enough to follow. The clinically relevant component of the investigation is that the switch to the lipid regimen is accompanied by an increase in body temperature. The investigators fall far short of satisfactorily explaining this increased temperature that will no doubt provoke future experiments and communications. They do suggest stepwise increases in lipid infusions, which is sound advice.—A.A. Fanaroff, M.B.B.Ch.

Pancreatic Function in Infants Identified as Having Cystic Fibrosis in a Neonatal Screening Program

Waters DL, Dorney SFA, Gaskin KJ, Gruca MA, O'Halloran M, Wilcken B (Royal Alexandra Hosp for Children, Sydney; New South Wales Dept of Health, Sydney, Australia)
N Engl J Med 322:303–308, 1990   9–12

Many centers use the immunoreactive-trypsin assay on dried blood samples from newborns to screen for cystic fibrosis. However, screening is not universally accepted because improved outcomes with screening have yet to be demonstrated. The use of the dried-blood immunoreactive-trypsin assay has been questioned because it has not been validated for the estimated 10% of patients with cystic fibrosis who have sufficient pancreatic function to prevent malabsorption.

To determine whether screening with the immunoreactive-trypsin assay can identify patients with pancreatic sufficiency, pancreatic function was assessed in 78 infants who received a diagnosis of cystic fibrosis based on immunoreactive-trypsin screening. Each evaluation included measurement of fecal excretion of fat, estimation of serum level of pancreatic isoamylase, pancreatic stimulation tests, and sweat chloride test. The mean age at evaluation of the 34 patients who received a diagnosis of cystic fibrosis before 1984 was 2.3 years, and the mean age of the 44 patients who received such a diagnosis after 1984 was 2 months.

The diagnosis of cystic fibrosis was confirmed by the sweat chloride test in 74 of the 78 patients; the other 4 had borderline results on the sweat test. Two patients later had repeat sweat tests that were diagnostic. Twenty-nine infants (37%) with a median age of 4 years had substantial preservation of pancreatic function. These children had growth close to normal and comparable to growth in children with severe pancreatic insufficiency who were receiving oral enzyme therapy. Six of these 29 patients subsequently had pancreatic insufficiency at 3 to 36 months of age.

The serum immunoreactive-trypsin assay used in neonatal screening programs can identify infants with cystic fibrosis who have sufficient pancreatic function to have normal fat absorption. Pancreatic function should therefore be assessed in all infants with cystic fibrosis because not all children who receive a diagnosis of this disease will require enzyme therapy.

▶ This report gives useful data on several issues. First, not all infants with cystic fibrosis require enzyme therapy initially. Second, though fat absorption is normal, pancreatic function may be significantly reduced. Last, it may be time to begin screening all newborn infants for cystic fibrosis.—M.H. Klaus, M.D.

Nutrient Intake and Growth Performance of Older Infants Fed Human Milk
Stuff JE, Nichols BL (Baylor College of Medicine, Houston; Texas Children's Hosp, Houston)
J Pediatr 115:959–968, 1989   9–13

Energy and protein intake of exclusively human milk-fed infants are below recommended levels after the second month of life, and weight-for-age percentiles of these infants fall progressively as well. Whether the ad libitum addition of solid foods to the diet of exclusively human milk-fed infants increases energy intake and reverses the decline in percentiles observed during exclusive feeding with human milk was studied. Forty-five mother-infant pairs from middle and upper income groups who planned to breastfeed exclusively for at least 16 weeks were entered in this longitudinal study. Solid foods were introduced at a time determined by the mother and pediatrician. Weekly or biweekly measures of growth were made from birth to 36 weeks of age, and monthly measures of nutrient intake were made from 16 weeks of age until 10 weeks after solid foods were introduced into the diet.

Solid foods were introduced between 18 and 24 weeks of life. After solid foods were added, daily milk intake declined significantly at a rate of 77 g of milk per day per month. There were no changes in the milk composition during the observation period.

Total daily energy intake increased significantly at a mean rate of 29 kcal/month, but no changes were seen in energy intake after adjustments for body weight were considered. Weight (National Center for Health Statistics percentiles) at 28 weeks were 13 percentiles lower than at birth, whereas length at 28 weeks was 1 percentile lower than at week 1. When compared with peak values at 8 weeks, weight percentiles at 28 weeks had dropped 19 percentiles and length percentiles at 28 weeks had dropped 14 percentiles.

Energy intake levels of human milk-fed infants do not increase after solid foods are added to the diet. In fact, energy levels remain approximately 20% below the recommended levels. Recommendations for the energy requirements of infancy should be reevaluated. The dissimilarities in growth patterns of exclusively breast-fed infants and the reference population raise questions about the adaptive response of human milk-fed infants to different levels of energy intake and the estimation of energy requirements based on the sum of basal metabolism, activity, growth, and diet-induced thermogenesis.

▶ The major argument in this report is based on the weight gain without reference to any of the complex growth processes in the infant, especially the brain. The authors' data and discussion are similar to those of Whitehead and Paul (1) who suggest that, because the rate of weight gain of infants on breast milk decreased after 5 to 6 months, it is not adequate nutrition. Within limits we should be interested in the quality of growth, not its quantity. Breast milk has evolved over centuries to meet the multiple needs of the growing infant in a hostile environment. It does not seem rational to describe it as inadequate if it produces a few less ounces of weight gain. So many other parameters are far more important but difficult to assess such as school performance, length of survival, incidence of cancer etc.—M.H. Klaus, M.D.

Reference

1. Whitehead RG, Paul AA: *Lancet* 2:161, 1981.

Role of Platelet Activating Factor and Tumor Necrosis Factor-Alpha in Neonatal Necrotizing Enterocolitis

Caplan MS, Sun X-M, Hsueh W, Hageman JR (Children's Mem Hosp; Northwestern Univ, Chicago; Evanston Hosp, Evanston, Ill)
J Pediatr 116:960–964, 1990   9–14

Results of previous studies show that platelet activating factor (PAF) and tumor necrosis factor-α (TNF-α) act synergistically to induce necrotizing enterocolitis in the rat. To determine if these mediators may play a role in human necrotizing enterocolitis, PAF, the PAF-degrading enzyme acetylhydrolase, and TNF-α were measured in the plasma of 12 neonates with necrotizing enterocolitis and 8 age-matched controls with similar gestational and postnatal ages and weights.

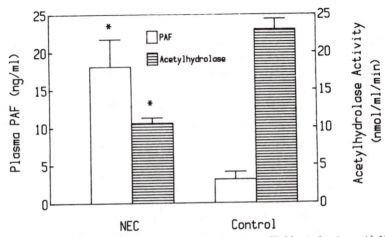

Fig 9–5.—Plasma PAF *(open bars)* and acetylhydrolase activity *(filled bars)* of patients with NEC and controls. Data are expressed as mean ± SEM. *Asterisk* indicates *P* < .01 compared with control values with 2-tailed, unpaired Student *t* test. (Courtesy of Caplan MS, Sun X-M, Hsueh W, et al: *J Pediatr* 116:960–964, 1990.)

Plasma PAF levels were significantly greater in the patients with necrotizing enterocolitis compared with controls (Fig 9–5). Most patients with necrotizing enterocolitis had abnormally high plasma PAF levels (>10 ng/mL), whereas none of the controls did. Plasma TNF-α values were also significantly higher in patients with necrotizing enterocolitis, but individual variations were much greater than for the PAF values. There was no correlation between PAF and TNF-α levels, as well as between severity of the disease and PAF and TNF-α levels. Plasma acetylhydrolase activity was significantly lower in the patients with necrotizing enterocolitis.

Plasma PAF and TNF-α levels are significantly increased in patients with necrotizing enterocolitis and suppressed PAF degradation may contribute to the increased circulating PAF levels in these patients. These findings suggest that PAF and TNF-α may contribute to the pathophysiology of human necrotizing enterocolitis.

▶ Necrotizing enterocolitis remains the preeminent gastrointestinal problem in the intensive care nursery. Asphyxiated low birth weight infants remain the prime candidates for this disorder, which may be prevented by antenatal steroids, the use of breast milk (1), and oral IgA supplementation (2). The pathogenesis of necrotizing enterocolitis remains unclear, with a blurred interrelationship between ischemia, infection, immaturity, immunity, and nutrition. There is marked curiosity now as to the role of cytokines in tissue and organ injury and repair, thus it was timely that their role in necrotizing enterocolitis be investigated. Both PAF and TNF are regarded as potent mediators of bowel necrosis in the rat. Platelet activating factor produces a picture like necrotizing enterocolitis and TNF-α causes intestinal PAF production. In this limited human experience elevated levels of both these mediators suggests that they may indeed play a role in necrotizing enterocolitis. Perhaps a new and fruitful line of investigation has emerged that will clarify the pathogenesis of this puzzling disorder. Until then, cautiously advance feedings with maternal breast milk and await new developments.

We live by our genius for hope;
We survive by our talent for dispensing with it— *V.S. Pritchett*

A.A. Fanaroff, M.B.B.Ch.

References

1. Lucas A, et al: *Lancet* 336:1519, 1990.
2. 1989 YEAR BOOK OF NEONATAL AND PERINATAL MEDICINE, Abstract 8–9.

A Randomized, Controlled Application of the Wallaby Phototherapy System Compared With Standard Phototherapy
Gale R, Dranitzki Z, Dollberg S, Stevenson DK (Bikur Cholim Hosp, Jerusalem; Stanford Univ)
J Perinatol 10:239–242, 1990

9–15

The Wallaby Phototherapy System, a fiberoptic blanket, was compared with conventional phototherapy in 42 full-term infants having nonhemolytic jaundice. Both treatments delivered an average irradiance of 7 μw/cm^2/nm.

Changes in plasma bilirubin did not differ in the study and control groups for up to 48 hours after the start of treatment. Comparable numbers of infants in the 2 groups were taken off treatment at any given interval. Bilirubin levels changed significantly in both the fiberoptic and bililight groups when the initial level exceeded 200 μmol/L.

Use of a fiberoptic blanket is an effective approach to phototherapy for physiologic jaundice. It is as safe as conventional bililight treatment in healthy term infants. Eye patches are unnecessary, and maternal handling of the infant is facilitated.

▶ M. Jeffrey Maisels, M.B., B.Ch., Professor of Pediatrics, Wayne State University School of Medicine, Detroit, University of Michigan Medical School, Ann Arbor, and Chairman, Department of Pediatrics, William Beaumont Hospital, Royal Oak, Michigan, our resident bilirubin commentator, offers the following insightful comments on this paper:

▶ In the early days phototherapy units were constructed in hospital workshops. We progressed to commercially made units, and then from fluorescent light bulbs to halide spot lamps and now, inevitably, fiberoptics. There are already 2 fiberoptic units on the market: the Wallaby Phototherapy System (Fiberoptic Medical Products Inc., Allentown, Penn) and the BiliBlanket (Ohmeda, Columbia, Md). Both systems use a high intensity halogen lamp to generate the light. In the Wallaby device the light is transmitted via a bundle of fiberoptic fibers that fan out on a cummerbund. This can be wrapped around the infant's torso or the baby may simply lie on the mat. The BiliBlanket uses a woven fiberoptic mat to transmit the light. The baby either lies on this or it can be tucked under the infant's shirt. No published data are available to date on the BiliBlanket.

These techniques offer obvious advantages. Mothers can hold their infants and eye patching is probably unnecessary. The data from this and Rosenfeld's studies (1) as well as those of Holtrop et al. (2) show that fiberoptic phototherapy works about as well as conventional phototherapy. It is also a useful adjunct to conventional phototherapy. The efficacy of phototherapy is related to the irradiance (the dose of light delivered) in the blue spectrum and the surface area exposed. Phototherapy is more effective when delivered to both sides of the baby simultaneously, but double light systems are difficult to construct. Fiberoptic blankets offer a simple way to deliver double phototherapy. We studied low birth weight infants in our neonatal intensive care unit and used the Wallaby system to compare double with single phototherapy. The double phototherapy infants received the same irradiance (9.2 μw/cm^2/nm at 400–800 nm) but laid on the Wallaby blanket while they received standard phototherapy. The mean percent decline in bilirubin after 18 hours of treatment was 29% for the double phototherapy group compared with 17% for the single phototherapy group ($P = .002$). This technique should be helpful when we need to reduce the bilirubin level rapidly or prevent a rapid rise in a hemolyzing or badly bruised infant.—M.J. Maisels, M.B.B.Ch.

References

1. Rosenfeld W, et al: *J Perinatol* 10:243, 1990.
2. Holtrop, et al: *Pediatr Res* 209A:27, 1990.

Does Breast-Feeding Protect the Hypothyroid Infant Whose Condition Is Diagnosed by Newborn Screening?
Rovet JF (Hosp for Sick Children, Toronto)
Am J Dis Child 144:319–323, 1990   9–16

Although screening for congenital hypothyroidism permits earlier hormone replacement, there still is some delay before euthyroidism is achieved. Breast milk contains a small amount of thyroid hormone and therefore might protect the infant to some extent.

In this study, thyroid function was monitored in 107 children positively identified as having congenital hypothyroidism at neonatal screening. Ectopic thyroid, dyshormonogenesis, and athyrosis were the causes of the disease in this population. Fifty-eight infants were breast-fed and 49 were formula-fed.

Breast-fed children had significantly higher thyroxine levels than those who were fed formula at ages 1 and 2 months, but not later in the first year of life. When controlling for parental IQ, socioeconomic status, and dose level, there were no significant differences in neuropsychologic functioning. Nevertheless, the children with ectopic thyroids did better on several tasks at age 3 when they were breast-fed as infants.

There is minimal support from these findings that breast-feeding protects infants with congenital hypothyroidism despite higher thyroxine levels in early infancy. Even children with ectopic thyroid glands have not benefited past age 3. Mothers who choose to breast-feed their hypothyroid infants should continue doing so for as long as possible.

▶ Frank J. Gareis, M.D., Endocrinologist, Children's Hospital Oakland, California, provides the commentary for this selection:

▶ The clinical observation that breast-feeding may ameliorate congenital hypothyroidism is coupled with laboratory evidence of small amounts of thyroxine (mainly T_3) in breast milk. The extent to which this is of importance in protecting the developing brain against the adverse effects of untreated hypothyroidism remains open to question, however, and is difficult to assess for a variety of reasons. In the above study, children with congenital hypothyroidism secondary to ectopic thyroids seemed to fare better when breastfed as contrasted with children with congenital hypothyroidism due to thyroid ectopia who were formula fed in infancy. Breast-feeding, however, conferred only a small advantage in terms of T_4 levels and speed at which euthyroidism was achieved once treatment was started. Most importantly, there did not seem to be any long-term advantage when children with congenital hypothyroidism were psychologically tested in later years. What is intriguing about all of this is that breast milk does in fact contain enough thyroxine to be of any significance in infants with hypothyroidism. Incidentally, should we be concerned that breast milk thyroxine might "mask" neonatal thyroid screening studies? Fortunately no, since breast milk thyroxine does not reach peak levels until well after 1 month of age and most thyroid serum studies are done within a few weeks of age.—F.J. Gareis, M.D.

10 The Respiratory Tract

Congenital Bronchopulmonary Malformations: Diagnostic and Therapeutic Considerations

Bailey PV, Tracy T Jr, Connors RH, deMello D, Lewis JE, Weber TR (St Louis Univ)

J Thorac Cardiovasc Surg 99:597–603, 1990

10–1

Forty-five children, aged 13 and younger, who were evaluated and treated for bronchopulmonary malformations between 1970 and 1988 were studied. No sex predominance was evident. Thirty-seven children had solitary lesions, the most frequent being bronchogenic cyst and cystic adenomatoid malformation. Eight patients had 2 abnormalities simultaneously, most often sequestration plus cystic adenomatoid malformation.

Twenty-one of the 45 patients had respiratory symptoms, which in 7 cases were marked. Twelve patients had pulmonary infection. Ultrasonography was helpful in diagnosing cystic adenomatoid malformation and pulmonary sequestration. Forty-two patients survived after excision of the lesion by lobectomy or pneumonectomy. Three neonates died of pulmonary hypoplasia and hypertension; 2 had a concomitant diaphragmatic hernia.

Combinations of different types of bronchopulmonary malformation are not infrequent. All these lesions can be managed operatively shortly after diagnosis. Surgery is well tolerated if significant pulmonary hypoplasia and hypertension are absent.

▶ This manuscript reads like an audit, which is essentially what it is. As with all retrospective chart reviews it is of necessity descriptive rather than mechanistic, yet it contains a few clinical pearls. Bronchopulmonary malformations occur infrequently, as evidenced by a series of 45 patients accumulated at a single center over a 19-year time period. The classification of lesions is based on their temporal relationship with fetal lung growth. The prognosis is excellent unless there is associated pulmonary hypoplasia or hypertension. The lesions may occur in combination and usually are found during the neonatal period. Bronchogenic cysts are the most common lesions encountered. They arise early in development from abnormal budding of the fetal tracheobronchial tree and may cause atelectasis or air trapping. The hallmark of pulmonary sequestration is a lobe that fails to communicate with the tracheobronchial tree and a systemic blood vessel that can be traced below the diaphragm (by ultrasound). Most bronchopulmonary malformations can be pinpointed by a combination of plain x-ray studies and ultrasound. Although CT is highly specific it is rarely necessary, and there are few indications for angiography. Congenital lobar emphysema is part of the spectrum of disturbed lung growth, with abnormalities in airway or alveolar number or alveolar size. Congenital lobar emphysema may

199

produce hydrops fetalis, and it has been successfully operated on in utero (1). Clinicians should be alerted to bronchopulmonary malformations in neonates with respiratory distress and cystic or solid masses on x-ray studies.—A.A. Fanaroff, M.B.B.Ch.

Reference

1. Harrison : *Lancet*, 1990.

Effect of Extracorporeal Membrane Oxygenation on Survival of Infants With Congenital Diaphragmatic Hernia
Van Meurs KP, Newman KD, Anderson KD, Short BL (Children's Natl Med Ctr; George Washington Univ, Washington, DC)
J Pediatr 117:954–960, 1990   10–2

Infants with congenital diaphragmatic hernia symptomatic in the first few hours of life have a high mortality rate. The standard approach has

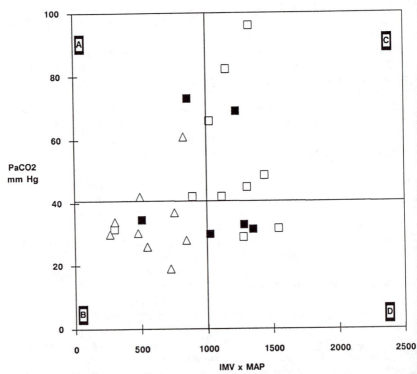

Fig 10–1.—Preoperative ventilation index (intermittent mandatory ventilation × mean arterial pressure) correlated with PaCO₂. Survival rate was 86% in quadrant C compared with 100% mortality rate in study by Bohn D, Tamura M, Perrin D, et al: *J Pediatr* 111:423–431, 1987. Survival rate in quadrants **A**, **B**, and **D** was similar to that reported by Bohn et al. *Open squares* = alive after ECMO therapy; *open triangles* = alive without ECMO therapy; *filled squares* = died after ECMO therapy. (Courtesy of Van Meurs KP, Newman KD, Anderson KD, et al: *J Pediatr* 117:954–960, 1990.)

been emergency surgery with the expectation that hernia reduction would lead to improved respiratory status. To determine the effect of extracorporeal membrane oxygenation (ECMO) on the survival of infants with congenital diaphragmatic hernia, a retrospective study of 31 infants was conducted. Three infants were immediately excluded because of lethal associated anomalies.

Using the Bonn ventilation index, infants assigned to the 100% mortality quadrant were treated with ECMO. The survival rate in this group was 86% when assessed preoperatively and 67% when assessed postoperatively. Comparison of changes that occurred in the ventilation index and arterial carbon dioxide pressure indicated that after repair, 48% of infants deteriorated, 40% improved, and 12% remained unchanged. Of the 12 infants who deteriorated after surgery, 11 were eventually treated with ECMO (Fig 10– 1).

Of 28 infants in the review, 11 were treated by conventional therapy and 10 survived (91%). Of 17 infants treated with ECMO after conventional treatment failed, 10 survived (59%). The overall survival rate was 71%. Extracorporeal membrane oxygenation significantly improved survival in infants with congenital diaphragmatic hernia who had rated a "poor prognosis" on Bohn's ventilation index. Extracorporeal membrane oxygenation is recommended for all infants with congenital diaphragmatic hernia when maximal medical treatment fails.

▶ Contributing this commentary is Eileen K. Stork, M.D., Assistant Professor of Pediatrics, Rainbow Babies and Childrens Hospital, Case Western Reserve University School of Medicine, Cleveland:

▶ Ever since Desmond Bohn published his paper on predictors of mortality in congenital diaphragmatic hernia, ECMO doctors have been busy proving that they can save the unsalvageable, i.e., infants with arterial carbon dioxide pressure greater than 40 plus a ventilation index (MAP × RR) greater than 1,000. Indeed, in this series 6 of 7 infants with congenital diaphragmatic hernia treated with ECMO postoperatively survived despite falling into Bohn's 100% mortality quadrant. Eleven of 12 infants whose carbon dioxide and ventilation index deteriorated postoperatively required ECMO. The overall survival of ECMO-treated patients was 59%, which when combined with the excellent survival rate (91%) in patients with congenital diaphragmatic hernia managed conventionally, brings the overall survival to 71%. The authors contend that, contrary to Bohn's predictions, many patients with congenital diaphragmatic hernia do have adequate lung volume to survive if they can be supported until the pulmonary hypertension abates. Interestingly, 3 of 7 deaths in the ECMO-treated group were attributed to recurrent persistent pulmonary hypertension of the neonate (PPHN) after ECMO therapy. This serves to emphasize the malignant nature of PPHN in this special group of infants, which is likely related to their anatomically truncated pulmonary vascular bed.— E.K. Stork, M.D.

Surfactant Replacement Therapy With a Single Postventilatory Dose of a Reconstituted Bovine Surfactant in Preterm Neonates With Respiratory Distress Syndrome: Final Analysis of a Multicenter, Double-Blind, Randomized Trial and Comparison With Similar Trials
Fujiwara T, Konishi M, Chida S, Okuyama K, Ogawa Y, Takeuchi Y, Nishida H, Kito H, Fujimura M, Nakamura H, Hashimoto T, Surfactant-TA Study Group (Iwate Med Univ; Showa Univ; Saitama Med Coll Med Ctr, Matsudo City Hosp; Tokyo Med Coll; et al)
Pediatrics 86:753–764, 1990   10–3

A double-blind study of modified bovine surfactant (surfactant TA) enrolled neonates weighing 750 to 1,749 g at birth but were appropriate for gestational age and had clinical and radiologic findings of respiratory distress syndrome (RDS) and surfactant deficiency. All required an inspired oxygen fraction of 0.4 or greater after initial stabilization. The dose of surfactant was 100 mg phospholipid per kilogram.

Fifty-four infants received surfactant and 46 received an air placebo in the first 8 hours of life. Active treatment significantly reduced the severity of RDS. Pulmonary interstitial emphysema and pneumothorax were significantly less frequent in surfactant recipients, as was intracranial hemorrhage. Among the smallest neonates, 58% of those given surfactant and 4% of controls survived without intracranial bleeding or bronchopulmonary dysplasia.

A single postventilatory dose of surfactant TA substantially reduced the severity of RDS in this study and decreased both major pulmonary problems and intracranial hemorrhage. It remains to be seen whether earlier treatment or multiple doses would be of further benefit.

▶ Alan Jobe, M.D., Professor of Pediatrics, UCLA Medical Center, and longtime investigator in the surfactant arena, comments as follows:

▶ This multicenter trial from Japan focuses on the effects of a bovine lung extract surfactant on pulmonary complications of RDS and intraventricular hemorrhage. The entry criteria for the trial are unique in that infants had to demonstrate surfactant immaturity based on a bubble test of gastric aspirates, and the infants could not have intraventricular hemorrhage above grade II at entry, permitting the authors to focus more specifically on RDS and intraventricular hemorrhage. On the other hand, the trial included 20 centers to enlist 100 patients and 74% of the infants were outborn, both factors that could influence outcome variables. My general impression is that the trials from Japan have consistently reported more striking effects of surfactant TA on ventilation (mean airway pressures, ventilation indices) than similar trials using the same or similar surfactants in this country. The excellent effects on oxygenation and ventilation are particularly surprising given the high percent of outborn infants and the relatively late treatment at 5.5 hours of age. This general observation, together with large center differences in clinical responses to surfactant noted in the multicenter trials in this country, suggests to me that subtle differences in ventilatory techniques may significantly impact treatment responses and could also influence the incidence of intraventricular hemorrhage. Fujiwara et al. carefully describe a treatment technique that emphasizes rapid surfactant delivery to the distal lung together with stabilization of oxygenation in the infant. Surfactant is administered in aliquots with positioning in a manner similar to the procedures used in this country. However, the surfactant is delivered to the lung by hand bagging with 100% oxygen, followed by an increase in peak inspiratory pressures of 4 cm H_2O using 0.5 second inspiratory times for 15 minutes following treatment. Instillation without increases in pressures, oxygen, or hand bagging can cause transient desaturation, elevated Pco_2 values, and bradycardia, presumably resulting from the acute fluid load to the lung, transient airway obstruction, and air trapping. This potential cardiopulmonary destabilization is generally mild and may be an acceptable tradeoff against uncontrolled bagging and possible hyperoxia from 100% oxygen resulting from treatments by the unexperienced. However, the technique describd in this paper could well result in a more rapid and better surfactant distribution, which may explain the generally better clinical responses noted in Japan. Treatment techniques have not been compared. The techniques used in this country were developed to optimize ease of administration and safety rather than to optimize treatment responses.

The nonpulmonary complications of prematurity (intraventricular hemorrhage, necrotizing enterocolitis, retinopathy of prematurity, and patent ductus arteriosus) have not been altered by surfactant treatment when all the published trials are viewed in aggregate. Individual trials have reported decreased or increased incidences of patent ductus arteriosus or intraventricular hemorrhage, for example. Since trials vary as to patient selection, surfactant, dosing strategy, and other factors, the isolated observations may be real effects applicable only to the unique situations present at the time and place of that trial or just statistical aberrations. In that light, the decreased incidence of intraventricular hemorrhage in this trial could be discounted. However, grades III and IV intraventricular hemorrhage were decreased in the 750 to 1,250 g infants from 36% to 8%, an important difference in terms of long-term outcome. The difference is worth discussion primarily because this trial preselected infants without severe intraventricular hemorrhage to test specifically if intraventricular hemorrhage was impacted by surfactant treatments. The authors suggest that the decrease in intraventricular hemorrhage following surfactant treatment could have resulted from the combination of improved respiratory function and decreased air leaks in the surfactant-treated infants. However, these same effects on air leaks and qualitatively similar effects on lung function are common to all the surfactant trials. My hunch is that the impact on intraventricular hemorrhage may be explained by different treatment and/or ventilation strategies that indirectly impact cardiopulmonary performance in infants with RDS. The issue of treatment techniques was discussed above, and cerebral blood flow can change during and following surfactant treatment. Management strategies for RDS vary widely with the 2 extremes being high tidal volume ventilation using long inspiratory times and slow rates versus low tidal volume ventilation with short inspiratory times at high rates. While most clinicians no doubt generally use some compromise between the 2, the compromises vary—rate versus PEEP versus inspiratory time, etc. The only thing that I am sure of is that there is no best technique for all babies all of the time. There are no studies of how to optimize ventilation strategies following surfactant treatments. The major effect of a surfactant treatment is to increase lung volumes. Acute increases in lung volumes can impact cardiopulmonary performance both positively and negatively. The effect of increased lung volumes will be improved oxygenation; however, overinflation can have very negative effects that could impact intraventricular hemorrhage incidence. The decrease in intraventricular hemorrhage noted by Fujiwara et al. should stimulate us to design studies to try to reproduce and to seek physiologic explanations for the observation. Trials cannot include untreated control groups in the era of licensed surfactants, but trials comparing standard care strategies with logical variations in care procedures are essential.—A. Jobe, M.D.

Single- Versus Multiple-Dose Surfactant Replacement Therapy in Neonates of 30 to 36 Weeks' Gestation With Respiratory Distress Syndrome
Dunn MS, Shennan AT, Possmayer F (Univ of Toronto; Women's Coll Hosp, Toronto; Univ of Western Ontario)
Pediatrics 86:564–571, 1990   10–4

The effectiveness of bovine surfactant replacement therapy, with emphasis on multiple-dose protocol, in neonates of 30 to 36 weeks' gestation with respiratory distress syndrome (RDS) was evaluated in a randomized, controlled trial. Seventy-five neonates of less than 6 hours of age with a diagnosis of RDS were randomly assigned to control, single-dose surfactant, or multiple-dose surfactant groups. Subjects received either 100 mg/kg of bovine surfactant or air placebo, and those in the multiple-dose group received up to 3 additional doses as indicated.

Neonates in both surfactant groups showed a positive response to treatment, with marked improvement in oxygenation by 10 minutes postinstillation. Neonates receiving surfactant could be successfully weaned after the first does of surfactant and had significantly lower ventilatory requirements than controls over the first 24 hours. However, starting at 6 to 12 hours after the first dose, both surfactant groups showed a deterioration in oxygenation and ventilatory requirements. Multiple doses of surfactant diminished the deterioration in oxygenation but had no effect on diminishing ventilatory requirements or time to extubation. No adverse effects of surfactant therapy were noted.

Bovine surfactant replacement therapy in neonates of 30 to 36 weeks' gestation with RDS is effective in acutely reducing oxygen and ventilatory requirements. Multiple doses of surfactant appear to sustain improvements in oxygenation rather than ventilatory requirements. Further studies are warranted to define the optimal dosage and retreatment protocol.

► Alan Jobe, M.D., Professor of Pediatrics, UCLA Medical Center, and long time investigator in the surfactant arena, comments as follows:

► This small trial from the Toronto group has brought up 2 issues: the efficacy of surfactant in large babies with RDS and the need for retreatment in this group of infants. The "prevention" trials (delivery room treatment) have, in general, focused on infants less than 1,250 g, whereas the treatment trials have included infants up to 2 kg. The mean weight of infants in this trial was 1,900 g. While the incidence of RDS decreases from perhaps 75% of infants at 28 weeks' gestational age to less than 5% of infants at 36 weeks' gestational age, a few of these large and more mature infants have severe disease that is difficult to manage. Such infants can require very high ventilatory pressures and seem prone to oxygenation difficulties because of shunting. A few of these large infants with RDS end up receiving extracorporeal membrane oxygenation therapy, and some infants die from RDS or its complications. Dunn et al. demonstrate improved oxygenation with surfactant, and they said that the infants were much easier to manage. This small trial was not designed to evaluate complications of RDS, which occur at low frequency in this group of infants. However, an Exosurf trial that included over 600 surfactant-treated and 600 air placebo-treated infants with mean birth weights of almost 2 kg documented a decrease in deaths from RDS from 3% in air placebo-treated infants to 1% in surfactant-treated infants (1). The surfactant-treated infants also had less air leak and bronchopulmonary dysplasia, although overall incidences of these complications were low. Thus, the acute gas exchange improvements documented by Dunn et al. seem to translate to better overall outcome when large numbers of infants are studied.

Surfactant did not shorten duration of ventilation or oxygen treatment in this study, although such effects have been reported in trials that have concentrated on smaller infants where overall treatment times are longer for all infants. There are perhaps 3 explanations: (1) Infants with RDS have lung problems associated with prematurity that are not cured by surfactant. The lungs may not be as stable to deflation as the mature lungs and some supplemental oxygen and positive pressure are needed to normalize gas exchange. This possibility is supported by the lack of large effects of surfactant on ventilatory pressures, a general observation in all trials. The explanation for this lack of clear effect on ventilation is not clear but may relate to interstitial edema and immaturities of the basic elasticity and interdependence of tissue elements. (2) The need for retreatment to maintain oxygenation is consistent with surfactant inactivation by ongoing pulmonary edema, assuming surfactant metabolism is similar in humans and preterm animals (2). (3) A third possibility is that the investigators were conservative and did not "push" the infants off ventilatory support. Surfactant was used in a nonrandomized fashion in infants weighing 2 kg with RDS requiring more than 70% oxygen and mechanical ventilation in a unit without ventilation capabilities (3). All infants responded with improved oxygenation and RDS resolved, suggesting that surfactant could be used to avoid mechanical ventilation. Whatever the explanation, it is prudent to observe the large infant closely after surfactant treatment and anticipate a possible deterioration in oxygenation. Infants with RDS are immature both in terms of lung function and overall organ function. Even in these large infants with RDS, surfactant will not necessarily cure all aspects of lung dysfunction and thus shorten the clinical course. However, the clinical experience is that surfactant can decrease the severity and complications of RDS in large infants.—A. Jobe, M.D.

References

1. Exosurf Product Information. Burroughs Wellcome Co, Research Triangle Park, NC.
2. Ikegami M, et al: *J Appl Physiol* 67:429, 1989.
3. Victorin LH, et al: Biol Neonate 58:121, 1990.

Cost of Surfactant Replacement Treatment for Severe Neonatal Respiratory Distress Syndrome: A Randomised Controlled Trial

Tubman TRJ, Halliday HL, Normand C (Royal Maternity Hosp, Belfast; Queen's Univ of Belfast)
Br Med J 301:842–845, 1990   10–5

Replacement treatment with natural surfactant has been effective in neonatal respiratory distress syndrome (RDS). The cost of treating infants with severe RDS with natural porcine surfactant was estimated in a retrospective controlled survey.

Thirty-three preterm infants with severe RDS admitted to a regional neonatal intensive care unit were randomly assigned to treatment with natural porcine surfactant or control group. The cost associated with surfactant replacement treatment per extra survivor was calculated for the treatment group, as well as the cost per quality adjusted life year for each extra survivor.

The proportion of infants surviving in the treated group (79%) was significantly greater than the control group (36%) ($P = 0.01$). The average hospital stay was 20 days for the control group and 61 days for the treatment group, for an additional length of care per extra survivor in the treatment group of 95 days. The total cost per extra survivor in the treatment group was £13,720, which was similar to previously reported costs for very low birth weight infants who survive. Assuming that the surviving infant would live to age 70 with an equal incidence of handicap as the control babies, the cost per additional quality adjusted life year gained by the use of surfactant was about £710. This cost compares favorably with the costs of some established forms of treatment for adults. Surfactant replacement treatment for severe neonatal RDS is fairly inexpensive and cost effective.

▶ With total health care costs for the United States at 12.2% of the gross national product, data such as these will be especially helpful when all health care professions will be asked to prioritize health care interventions for the entire population. Orgeon is the first state to begin the process. With a limited budget they used the following criteria in making priority decisions for any intervention: (1) effect on longevity; (2) quality of life; (3) greatest good for the greatest number; and (4) equity (all citizens to be covered by a basic package). Interestingly, the entire package of interventions proposed by caregivers working in the perinatal period were approved except for in vitro fertilization. In Oregon, with use of the criteria legislated to begin shortly, the care of the mother and fetus will have a high priority.—M.H. Klaus, M.D.

Chronic Respiratory Morbidity After Prolonged and Premature Rupture of the Membranes
Thompson PJ, Greenough A, Nicolaides K (King's Coll Hosp, London)
Arch Dis Child 65:878–880, 1990
10–6

Premature rupture of the membranes can lead to oligohydramnios and, in turn, pulmonary hypoplasia. Many surviving infants have had respiratory problems in the neonatal period. This prospective study followed 21 infants who survived membrane rupture during the second trimester that lasted at least 1 week. The median duration of membrane rupture was 5 weeks (Fig 10–2), and the median follow-up was 15 months.

The 1 death occurring during follow-up was attributed to sudden infant death syndrome at age 6 months. Five (24%) of the survivors had respiratory symptoms at least once a week, most frequently episodic coughing or wheezing. Four of these 5 infants had been ventilated in the neonatal period, compared with 3 of the 16 symptom-free children. The symptomatic infants were younger at delivery, though not at the time of membrane rupture. Three of the infants required admission for chest infection. Symptoms were less frequent in this series than in low and very low birth weight control infants.

Chronic respiratory morbidity occurs in about one fourth of infants

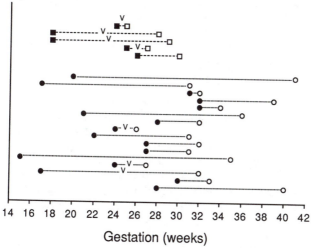

Fig 10–2.—Gestational age at onset of rupture of the membranes *(filled circles and squares)* and delivery *(open circles and squares)* for 21 surviving infants. The data points depicting onset and delivery are linked for each case to show the duration of rupture. (Courtesy of Thompson PJ, Greenough A, Nicolaides K: *Arch Dis Child* 65:878–880, 1990.)

who survive after prolonged premature membrane rupture. It may be especially likely to occur in very preterm deliveries.

▶ This report asks a useful clinical question: are infants born after a prolonged period of ruptured membranes more prone to chronic pulmonary disease? The results are somewhat unexpected since previous reports (1–3) suggested an increased incidence of chronic pulmonary disease. However, there were no long-term studies and many patients were lost to follow-up. The results of this study suggest that morbidity may be reduced by avoiding premature delivery for women with ruptured membranes, and, if possible, avoiding neonatal ventilation, because chronic respiratory morbidity was mainly observed in infants delivered before 30 weeks' gestation.—M.H. Klaus, M.D.

References

1. Taylor J, Garite JJ: *Obstet Gynecol* 64:615, 1984.
2. Beydown MD, Yasin SY: *Am J Obstet Gynecol* 1955:171, 1986.
3. Bengton JM, et al: *Obstet Gynecol* 73:921, 1989.

Maternal Glucocorticoid Therapy and Reduced Risk of Bronchopulmonary Dysplasia
Van Marter LJ, Leviton A, Kuban KCK, Pagano M, Allred EN (The Children's Hosp, Boston; Harvard Univ)
Pediatrics 86:331–336, 1990   10–7

Antenatal maternal glucocorticoid therapy is associated with a reduced incidence of neonatal respiratory distress syndrome in preterm newborns. Maternal antenatal glucocorticoid therapy may also reduce the risk of bronchopulmonary dysplasia (BPD). This hypothesis was evaluated in a sample of 223 intubated infants with birth weights less than 1.751 g. Of these, 76 met diagnostic criteria for BPD as defined by both oxygen requirement and compatible chest radiograph, and 147 had no BPD by day 28 of life (Fig 10–3). Glucocorticoids were given only to enhance fetal lung maturation.

Compared with infants born to mothers who received a complete number of doses and delivered between 24 hours and 7 days after the last glucocorticoid dose, infants whose mothers received a partial course of glucocorticoid were 1.3 times more likely to have BPD. When stratified by gender and birth weight at 1 kg, all subgroups showed a benefit of therapy, except for male infants with birth weight at or less than 1 kg.

A complete course of antenatal maternal glucocorticoid therapy is associated with a lower rate of BPD in very low birth weight infant girls.

▶ David J. Durand, M.D., Neonatologist, Children's Hospital Oakland, California, offers his thoughts on this article.

▶ This is another in a long series of publications documenting the beneficial prenatal glucocorticoid treatment on the outcome of the preterm infant. Not

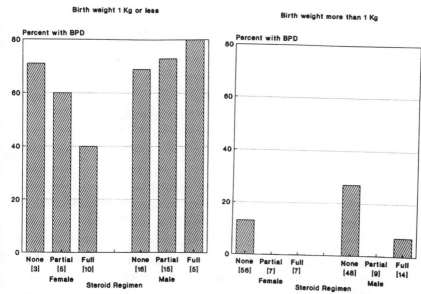

Fig 10–3.—Percent of infants with BPD at 28 days of life for glucocorticoid treatment groups, stratified by birth weight and sex (N = denominator). (Courtesy of Van Marter LJ, Leviton A, Kuban KCK, et al: *Pediatrics* 86:331–336, 1990.)

only does glucocorticoid treatment decrease the incidence of hyaline membrane disease, it decreases the incidence of BPD in those infants with hyaline membrane disease that was severe enough to require mechanical ventilation. This is not surprising information, but it is reassuring to see what most of us have suspected documented in a well-done study. Although this was not a randomized trial, the authors are to be commended for doing an excellent job of analyzing for confounding variables, and showing that they did not account for the difference in incidence of BPD.—D.J. Durand, M.D.

Early Postnatal Dexamethasone Therapy in Premature Infants With Severe Respiratory Distress Syndrome: A Double-Blind, Controlled Study

Yeh TF, Torre JA, Rastogi A, Anyebuno MA, Pildes RS (Cook County Hosp; Univ of Illinois; Hektoen Inst of Med Res, Chicago)
J Pediatr 117:273–282, 1990
10–8

Oxygen toxic effects and barotrauma occur very early in the course of respiratory distress syndrome (RDS). Hence, any therapy, to be effective in reducing lung injury, has to be administered shortly after birth and during this early period of highest risk. In a double-blind, placebo-controlled study, the effect of early (≤12 hours) postnatal dexamethasone therapy in facilitating removal of the endotracheal tube and improving outcome was investigated in 57 premature infants with birth weights <2,000 g and severe RDS. Twenty-eight infants were treated with intravenous dexamethasone at a dose of 1 mg/kg/day for 3 days with the dose reduced progressively for 12 days; the other 29 infants received placebo. Both groups were comparable in birth weight, gestational age, postnatal age, and pulmonary function at the start of the study.

Infants treated with dexamethasone had significantly higher pulmonary compliance, tidal volume, and minute ventilation, and required lower mean airway pressure for ventilation than infants in the placebo group. The proportion of infants whose endotracheal tube was successfully removed was significantly higher in the dexamethasone group (57%) than in the placebo group (28%). The number of infants with lung injuries was significantly lower in the dexamethasone group (39%) than in the placebo group (66%), and the placebo group required significantly longer duration of high oxygen therapy than the dexamethasone group. Mortality rate did not differ between groups because of small sample size. Compared with the placebo group, the dexamethasone group had significantly higher temporary increases in blood pressure and plasma glucose concentrations, as well as delayed somatic growth.

Early administration of dexamethasone shortly after birth and during the first 12 postnatal days improves pulmonary compliance and facilitates weaning from mechanical ventilation, and minimizes lung injuries in premature infants with severe RDS.

▶ There is a wry wisdom to this double-blind placebo-controlled study. The hypothesis that early intervention with steroids would accelerate the course of recovery from RDS and reduce the degree of lung injury is based on the premise that steroids ameliorate the course of bronchopulmonary dysplasia. The few controlled trials published to date support this contention. The study was well planned, flawlessly executed, and carefully analyzed. The investigators concluded that administration of dexamethasone to premature infants with severe RDS improved pulmonary compliance and facilitated weaning from the ventilator. They also suggested that lung injury was reduced. Notable side effects of dexamethasone included hypertension and temporary cessation of growth. The big twist is that this study was completed as surfactant was released for general use for RDS. The dramatic impact of surfactant on the early course of RDS makes the early use of dexamethasone irrelevant. Surfactant has not significantly reduced chronic lung disease and steroids appear to have a role in this disorder. The preferred dose and timing of steroid therapy have yet to be determined.—A.A. Fanaroff, M.B.B.Ch.

Late Pulmonary Sequelae of Bronchopulmonary Dysplasia

Northway WH Jr, Moss RB, Carlisle KB, Parker BR, Popp RL, Pitlick PT, Eichler I, Lamm RL, Brown BW Jr (Stanford Univ Med Ctr; Children's Hosp at Stanford)

N Engl J Med 323:1793–1799, 1990   10–9

Time present and time past
Are both perhaps present in time future
And time future contained in time past.—T.S. Eliot

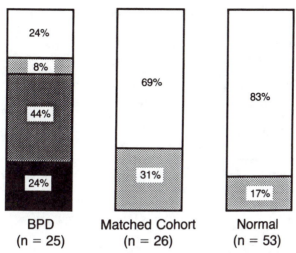

Fig 10–4.—Reactive airway disease in the subjects with BPD in infancy, the matched cohort controls, and the normal controls. Most infants with BPD (52%) had reactive airway disease ($P = .001$ for the comparison between subjects with BPD and normal controls). The *unshaded* areas indicate the absence of the disease, the *lightly shaded* areas a positive response to methacholine provocation, the heavily shaded areas reversible airway obstruction, and the *completely shaded* areas fixed airway obstruction. (Courtesy of Northway WH Jr, Moss RB, Carlisle KB, et al: *N Engl J Med* 323:1793–1799, 1990.

About 40% of infants with bronchopulmonary dysplasia (BPD) die, and those who survive have morbidity from respiratory disease more often than unaffected infants. The lung function in 26 adolescents and young adults aged 14 to 23 years, who had had BPD in infancy was estimated. These subjects were compared with 26 age-matched subjects of similar birth weight and gestational age who had not undergone mechanical ventilation and 53 age-matched normal subjects.

Sixty-eight percent of study subjects tested had airway obstruction, 24% had fixed airway obstruction, and 52% had reactive airway disease (Fig 10–4). Hyperinflation was more frequent in subjects with BPD in infancy than in either control group. Six study subjects had severe pulmonary dysfunction or current symptoms of respiratory difficulty.

Pulmonary dysfunction is common in most adolescents and young adults with a history of BPD in infancy, but symptoms usually are absent. Although most of these subjects may lead normal lives, there is concern over vulnerability to progressive obstructive lung disease with advancing age. They should be strongly discouraged from smoking.

▶ Northway's original description of BPD is one of the landmark papers in neonatology. Bronchopulmonary dysplasia has become the leading cause of morbidity and mortality for low birth weight infants beyond the neonatal period. It is thrilling to see a follow-up report, which includes the original subjects with BPD, from the same author, in the same prestigious journal, 23 years later. For the romantics, anticipating a Hollywood ending, and the survivors, now adolescents and young adults, all surfing off the coast of California demonstrating normal lung function, there is some disappointment. The subjects, now aged

14 to 23 years old, have more evidence of airway obstruction and reactive airway disease than nonventilated preterm infants and control subjects born at term. Those in the BPD group were more likely to wheeze, have limited exercise capacity, develop pulmonary infections, and require medication. The pulmonary dysfunction overall was not severe and they were leading normal lives. Subjects not included in the original report were more likely to be smaller and less mature at birth, manifested more pulmonary dysfunction. We look forward to continuing progress reports concerning this distinctive group of subjects.— A.A. Fanaroff, M.B.B.Ch.

Early Randomized Intervention With High-Frequency Jet Ventilation in Respiratory Distress Syndrome
Carlo WA, Siner B, Chatburn RL, Robertson S, Martin RJ (Rainbow Babies and Childrens Hosp; Case Western Reserve Univ, Cleveland)
J Pediatr 117:765–770, 1990   10–10

Several studies suggest that high-frequency jet ventilation (HFJV) reduces airway pressures and barotrauma in neonates with severe respiratory failure. Using a sequential study design, the effects of early intervention with HFJV on neonatal mortality or pulmonary morbidity rates were studied in 42 randomly selected infants with severe respiratory distress syndrome. Patients were randomly assigned to either conventional ventilation (begun at a mean age of 14 hours) or HFJV (begun at a mean age of 15.5 hours).

Enrollment was stopped when the combined analysis of major outcome measures, including mortality rate, air leaks, bronchopulmonary dysplasia, intraventricular hemorrhage, and assignment crossover, indicated no difference between treatment groups (Fig 10–5). Although early

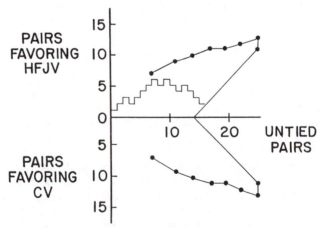

Fig 10–5.—Sequential analysis of combined outcome measures, including mortality rate, air leaks, bronchopulmonary dysplasia intraventricular hemorrhage, and assignment crossover according to method of Armitage. Abscissa indicates number of untied pairs. Study was completed when boundary indicated that no difference was reached. (Courtesy of Carlo WA, Siner B, Chatburn RL, et al: *J Pediatr* 117:765–770, 1990.)

HFJV resulted in improved carbon dioxide elimination and reduced airway pressure, it did not prevent or substantially reduce mortality or morbidity rates associated with assisted ventilation.

Early use of HFJV does not prevent barotrauma or substantially improve overall outcome in neonates with severe respiratory failure.

▶ I am precluded from objectively commenting on this paper because of my emotional involvement. Nonetheless my biased comments will follow. I was monitoring the sequential analysis and at one point only 1 more discordant pair in favor of the jet was necessary to demonstrate its superiority. However, the next pair favored conventional ventilation and the study concluded with no advantage to either form of ventilation. Close, but no cigar. This leaves the high frequency ventilators somewhere out in the cold. The HIFI study reported last year (1) also failed to establish superiority for high frequency ventilation; in fact, the oscillator group had more intraventricular hemorrhage, resulting in a greater incidence of hydrocephalus (see Abstract 8–5). There remain many ardent fans, even some fanatics, for the use of high frequency ventilators, which do have a role in supporting neonatal respiratory disorders. The problem is that the role is ill defined. Some infants with hyaline membrane disease, air leaks, including pulmonary interstitial emphysema, pneumonia, and pulmonary hypertension respond dramatically to jet ventilation. Selection criteria for high frequency ventilation will for the moment remain arbitrary and the reaction between surfactant and the high frequency ventilators needs to be evaluated. A formal study to evaluate hyperventilation (including the jet ventilators) is at an advanced stage of planning. Perhaps the role of the jet will emerge.

Time is that wherein there is opportunity, and opportunity is that wherein there is no great time.—Hippocrates

A.A. Fanaroff, M.B.B. Ch.

Reference

1. 1990 Year Book of Neonatal and Perinatal Medicine, Abstract 8–5.

Percutaneous Carbon Dioxide Excretion in the Newborn Infant
Cartlidge PHT, Rutter N (Royal Hosp for Sick Children, St Michael's Hill, Bristol; City Hosp, Nottingham, England)
Early Hum Dev 21:93–103, 1990
10–11

Preterm infants' skin is more permeable to gases than skin of adults and term infants. Percutaneous oxygen delivery makes a potentially useful contribution to the infants' oxygen requirements. Percutaneous gas exchange was therefore studied to establish its contribution to total CO_2 excretion in newborn infants.

Forty-two newborn infants, aged 25 to 39 weeks' gestation, were studied. Percutaneous CO_2 excretion was investigated using a closed skin cell attached to the infants' abdomens. The rate of excretion in the first few

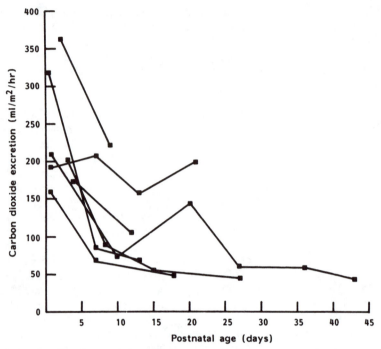

Fig 10–6.—Effect of postnatal skin maturation on rate of percutaneous carbon dioxide excretion in infants of less than 31 weeks' gestation. (Courtesy of Cartlidge PHT, Rutter N: *Early Hum Dev* 21:93–103, 1990.)

days of life was inversely related to gestation. It increased from a mean of 31 mL/m²/hr at term to 198 mL/m²/hr below 30 weeks' gestation. In very preterm infants, there was a rapid decline postnatally in the excretion rate to values about twice those found at term. The excretion rate was linearly related to the CO_2 diffusion gradient. Zero diffusion would be expected when there was no diffusion gradient. Up to 15% of resting CO_2 excretion occurs through the skin of very preterm infants, more if the tissue partial pressure of carbon dioxide is increased (Fig 10–6).

The rate of CO_2 excretion was considerably higher in preterm than in term infants, especially in infants born before 30 weeks' gestation. The linear relationship seen between this excretion rate and the diffusion gradient suggests that the diffusion of CO_2 through the skin is a passive process.

▶ This report continues a long-term interest by these investigators in the permeability of neonatal skin to various gases, noxious substances, and water. As the skin matures and the stratum corneum increases in thickness, the loss of CO_2 and H_2O decrease. Both the loss of CO_2 and H_2O are linearly related to their diffusion gradients; thus, with hypercapnia there will be an increased loss of CO_2. In a very immature infant (25 weeks' gestation) in the first days of life diffusion through the skin surprisingly could account for 15% to 20% of the CO_2

excreted by the neonate. With hypercapnia this could rise to 30%. As the authors note, the use of a sheet of impermeable polythene to reduce evaporative heat and water loss should be avoided since it would also limit the excretion of CO_2. In addition, any study of energy balance in young immature infants should consider the gases lost or gained through the skin.—M.H. Klaus, M.D.

Skin Blood Flow Changes During Apneic Spells in Preterm Infants

Suichies HE, Aarnoudse JG, Okken A, Jentink HW, de Mul FFM, Greve J (Univ Hosp Groningen; Twente Univ of Technology, AE Enschede, The Netherlands)
Early Hum Dev 20:155–163, 1989   10–12

Cardiovascular changes related to apneic spells in preterm infants have been reported, but little is known about the changes in peripheral blood flow during apneic spells. Changes in skin blood flow were measured during apneic spells in 18 preterm infants using a diode laser Doppler flow meter without light conducting fibers. Mean gestational age was 30.7 weeks, and mean birth weight was 1,365 g. In addition to the laser Doppler skin blood flow, heart rate, nasal air flow, impedance pneumography, and skin and incubator temperatures were recorded simultaneously in each infant.

A total of 212 apneic spells with a mean duration of 11.6 seconds were analyzed. In all but 1 child, 73% of the apneic spells were associated with a significant decrease in skin blood flow. The average decrease in skin blood flow was considerably greater for obstructive apneic spells (28.5%), compared with central apenic spells (16.7%); for mixed spells, the average decrease in skin blood flow with mixed apneic spells was 18.9%. The decrease in skin blood flow coincided with the onset of apneic spells in 71%, but was delayed by a mean 3.4 seconds in the remaining apneic spells. There was no correlation between the duration of an apneic spell and the decrease in skin blood flow. Bradycardia accompanied 34% of the apneic spells, but the decrease in skin blood flow was not related to the fall in heart rate.

The majority of apneic spells in preterm infants are associated with a decrease in skin blood flow. The onset of the decrease in skin blood flow coincides with the onset of apnea, but the decrease in skin blood flow is independent of the presence of bradycardia.

▶ What is of special interest is that regardless of the origin of the apnea—central, mixed, or obstructive—the skin blood flow decreases immediately. Clinically, this will alter skin color but more importantly it is probably part of a physiologic defense mechanism to reduce circulation to nonessential areas of the body, conserving oxygen for the vital organs—the heart and brain. Interestingly, the reduced skin blood flow was not always associated with bradycardia. This reduction of skin blood flow is probably a remnant of the dive response.—M.H. Klaus, M.D.

Effects of Nasal CPAP on Supraglottic and Total Pulmonary Resistance in Preterm Infants

Miller MJ, DiFiore JM, Strohl KP, Martin RJ (Rainbow Babies and Childrens Hosp; Case Western Reserve Univ, Cleveland)

J Appl Physiol 68:141–146, 1990   10–13

Nasal continuous positive airway pressure (CPAP) is an effective treatment for apnea in premature infants, but the mechanism by which CPAP exerts this selective effect remains unknown. In the present study, the effect of CPAP on supraglottic resistance (Rsg) and total pulmonary resistance (RL) was evaluated in 10 healthy premature infants with a history of idiopathic apnea of prematurity.

Nasal airflow was measured with a mask pneumotachograph, and pressures in the esophagus and oropharynx were measured with a 5-Fr Millar or fluid-filled catheter. Total Rsg, RL, and Rsg in expiration and inspiration were measured on increasing CPAP, from 1 to 5 cm H_2O, then decreased back to 0 over consecutive 30-second intervals.

Nasal CPAP correlated well with oropharyngeal pressure. Total Rsg decreased significantly by 63% between 0 and 5 cm H_2O CPAP, and a delay in return of Rsg to the previous level was seen as CPAP was reciprocally decreased to 0 (Fig 10–7). There was a 66% decrease in Rsg during inspiration and a 70% decrease during expiration. Likewise, RL decreased by 40% between 0 and 5 cm H_2O CPAP. Thus, the decrease in Rsg on CPAP contributed 60% (range, 25% to 84%) of the change in RL, which occurred on CPAP of 5 cm H_2O.

It appears that CPAP may decrease Rsg resistance directly by mechanical splinting of the airway. This effect of CPAP may be the primary mechanism by which CPAP reduces apnea with an obstructive component in premature infants.

▶ Though low pressure CPAP (5 cm H_2O) was observed 15 years ago to reduce the number of apneic periods, it has taken a long time to understand the

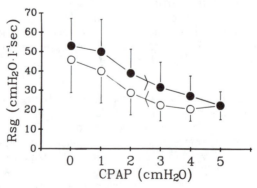

Fig 10–7.—As CPAP was increased from 0 to 5 cm of H_2O and then reciprocally decreased to 0, Rsg remained lower at 3, 2, and 1 cm of H_2O CPAP. Number = 6. Error bar, standard error. (Courtesy of Miller MJ, DeFiore JM, Strohl KP, et al: *J Appl Physiol* 68:141–146, 1990.)

physiology explanation for its effects. Though CPAP increases lung volume and may improve oxygenation it also alters airway dimensions. The data suggest that mechanical splinting of the airway and a reduction in airway resistance may be most significant. This fits with the observation that airway collapse at the pharyngeal level accompanies 90% of apneas in premature infants (1) and would also explain why CPAP is only effective in infants with obstructive apnea and has little or no effect in central apnea. The authors suggest that by preventing upper airway obstruction, CPAP may also decrease inhibitory afferent input that results from increasing negative airway pressure below the obstruction, and thus prevent or shorten an apneic period.—M.H. Klaus, M.D.

Reference

1. Mathew OP, et al: *J Pediatr* 100:964, 1982.

A Blinded, Randomized, Placebo-Controlled Trial to Compare Theophylline and Doxapram for the Treatment of Apnea of Prematurity
Peliowski A, Finer NN (Royal Alexandra Hosp; Univ of Alberta, Edmonton, Alberta)
J Pediatr 116:648–653, 1990   10–14

In a prospective placebo-controlled trial theophylline and doxapram were compared in 31 infants born at 34 weeks' gestation or earlier with significant apnea of prematurity. Significant apnea was defined as a central or mixed event lasting at least 20 seconds, associated with a 25% fall in heart rate and a decline of at least 10% in oxygen saturation, a fall of at least 5 mm Hg in transcutaneous oxygen pressure, or both.

The loading dose of theophylline was 8 mg/kg, followed by an infusion of 0.5 mg/kg/hr. Doxapram was given in a loading dose of 3 mg/kg, followed by 1.5 mg/kg/hr. Eight of 10 infants had a short-term response to theophylline, and 7 of 11 had a short-term response to doxapram. Two of 10 placebo recipients had a short-term response. Both active treatments were significantly more effective than placebo. There was no significant long-term difference in the response to theophylline and doxapram. Neither drug produced significant side effects.

Theophylline and doxapram are both effective treatments for apnea of prematurity, but responses may be short-lived. Continuous monitoring is an appropriate part of managing these infants.

▶ Richard J. Martin, Professor of Pediatrics at Case Western Reserve University and Co-Director of Neonatology at Rainbow Babies and Childrens Hospital, Cleveland, a long-time investigator of apnea, comments as follows:

▶ Peliowski and Finer have made a useful contribution to the apnea literature by comparing the relative efficacy of theophylline and doxapram as different pharmacologic therapies for apnea of prematurity. Previous studies of doxapram have largely used this drug after failure of xanthine therapy. Using doxapram as primary therapy, the authors of the current study failed to document any clear advantage for this drug. Although the latter did not cause any significant side effects (hypertension has been a concern with doxapram) it now appears impossible to justify its use as initial pharmacologic therapy for neonatal apnea.

Since its introduction into neonatal care in the mid 1970s, theophylline has become 1 of the most widely used drugs administered to preterm infants in this setting. Interestingly, caffeine is still less frequently used than its close relative theophylline, despite the greater ease of administration and smaller likelihood of toxicity associated with caffeine therapy. Considerable interest focuses on the mechanism of action, whereby the xanthines enhance respiratory control both at a physiologic and biochemical level. Several studies have focused on the central action of these agents in inhibiting adenosine, which acts as a respiratory depressant in the brain stem. It has been documented that hypoxic depression of breathing is partially reversed by theophylline (1) and recent data from our own research group suggest that this action of theophylline requires the presence of intact peripheral chemoreceptors (2). This line of investigation is clearly worth the effort for a drug that continues to be universally prescribed for low birth weight infants.—R.J. Martin, M.D.

References

1. Darnall RA Jr: *Pediatr Res* 19:706, 1985.
2. Cattarossi L, et al: *Am Rev Respir Dis* 1991. In press.

Autoimmune Hypothesis of Acquired Subglottic Stenosis in Premature Infants
Stolovitzky JP, Todd NW (Emory Univ)
Laryngoscope 100:227–230, 1990   10–15

Acquired subglottic stenosis has been reported in 4% of premature infants who received neonatal intensive care, and prolonged intubation was an important etiologic factor. Not all premature infants acquire subglottic stenosis, and infants with similar characteristics and care have varying laryngeal outcomes. The subglottic stenosis often manifests months after removal of the causative factor.

An autoimmune mechanism to type II collagen may explain the varying laryngeal outcomes in these premature infants. Trauma to the endotracheal mucosa causes mucosal inflammation and cartilaginous matrix degradation. As a result, type-II collagen is exposed to the afferent arm of the immune system, becomes immunogenic, and stimulates the synthesis of anticollagen-II antibodies. The activation of the immuno-inflammatory cells at the site of trauma may play a role in extending the damage and establishing a chronic process.

To test this hypothesis, a retrospective study of premature infants of comparable birth weight, gestational age, and duration of endotracheal intubation was conducted. Antibodies to collagen II were found in the serum of 3 of 5 infants who had subglottic stenosis and none of the 8 control infants who did not have subglottic stenosis. Mean onset of subglottis stenosis after removal of the endotracheal tube was 5 months (range, 3–7 months).

An autoimmune process is suggested in the etiology of subglottic stenosis, and further investigation is warranted that may lead to new diagnostic and therapeutic measures for these infants.

▶ Contributing her commentary is Martha J. Miller, M.D., Ph.D., Assistant Professor of Pediatrics, Rainbow Babies and Childrens Hospital, Case Western Reserve University School of Medicine, Cleveland:

▶ The paucity of immune function in the premature infant has been thought to be directly proportional to the degree of immaturity. The discovery of circulating collagen II antibodies in infants with subglottic stenosis suggests that the premature infants' ability to mount destructive autoimmune responses should be seriously reassessed. Indeed, the remarkable improvement of infants with bronchopulmonary dysplasia (BPD) treated with corticosteroids may be in part because of inhibition of the same class of responses. These observations raise the possibility that a decrease in the incidence of subglottic stenosis may be a fortuitous additional benefit of steroid therapy in infants with BPD.—M.J. Miller, M.D., Ph.D.

Evaluation of Neonatal Subglottic Stenosis: A 3-Year Prospective Study
Nicklaus PJ, Crysdale WS, Conley S, White AK, Sendi K, Forte V (Hosp for Sick Children, Toronto)
Laryngoscope 100:1185–1190, 1990   10–16

Subglottic stenosis is the most frequent cause of chronic airway obstruction in pediatric patients, and it leads to prolonged tracheal cannulation. The incidence has risen since the widespread use of prolonged intubation for respiratory support of neonates. This 3-year prospective study acquired data from 289 infants (mean follow-up, 18 months).

The overall incidence of subglottic stenosis was 2.6%. Younger and smaller infants, who had more attempts at intubation, were likelier to have subglottic stenosis. Girls, those who had difficult intubations, and nonwhites also were at increased risk. No tracheotomies were required and there were no significant long-term sequelae of subglottic stenosis. The most prominent autopsy findings were inflammation and ulceration over the vocal process of the arytenoid and the posterior aspect of the true cords.

Modern taping techniques may help limit the development of subglottic stenosis. It may also help not to change endotracheal tubes on a routine basis.

▶ Add this prospective evaluation of neonatal subglottic stenosis to your reprint files. A well-disciplined team was assembled to daily record the factors relating to intubation, such as tube size, extubations, difficulty with intubation such as popping and hemorrhage, together with a host of other demographic and medical factors concerning all intubated neonates. Subglottic stenosis was established by means of a rigid bronchoscope (diameter < 4mm). Strikingly, the overall incidence of subglottic stenosis was low (2.6%), and none of the infants required a tracheotomy. Factors associated with stenosis were exhaustively searched for and identified. More significantly, the factors responsible for the low incidence are elaborated. Their technique of stabilizing the endotracheal tube with a suture through the tube is worth noting, as is the careful selection of a tube size appropriate for gestational age to prevent subglottic stenosis (1). Routine endotracheal tube changes are not encouraged, and correct stabilization of the tubes minimizes accidental extubations, thus reducing the need for multiple intubations. This is as good as it gets from a single institution. I hope that their plea for a multicenter study to evaluate risk factors for subglottic stenosis does not fall on deaf ears.—A.A. Fanaroff, M.B.B.Ch.

Reference

1. Sherman JM: *J Pediatr* 109:322, 1986.

Maternal Smoking and Childhood Asthma

Weitzman M, Gortmaker S, Walker DK, Sobol A (Boston City Hosp; Boston Univ; Harvard Univ)
Pediatrics 85:505–511, 1990   10–17

Maternal smoking has been correlated with increased respiratory infection and diminished pulmonary function in children, especially in those younger than age 2 years. While adverse effects of passive smoking seem to diminish as children grow older, there may be negative long-term consequences. To study the relationship of parental smoking and childhood asthma in a large sample, data from the Child Health Supplement to the 1981 National Health Interview Survey were analyzed.

Approximately 4,331 children, aged 5 years or younger, were studied for the relationship of maternal smoking and the prevalence and age of onset of childhood asthma. Use of asthma medication in children and the number of overnight hospitalizations were also studied for a link with maternal smoking. Odds ratio of 2.1 for asthma was shown among children of maternal smokers compared with children of nonsmokers. The risk of asthma developing in the first year of life and the likelihood of taking asthma medication were higher for children of smokers (table). Maternal smoking is associated with increased numbers of child hospitalizations independent of asthma. However, maternal smoking did not increase the number of hospitalizations in children with asthma.

Maternal smoking, especially during pregnancy and the first 5 years of life, is associated with higher rates and earlier onset of childhood asthma and an increased likelihood of using asthma medication. Maternal smoking was not associated with increased hospitalizations among children

Prevalence of Asthma and Current Use of Asthma Medications Among Children
Aged 0 to 5 Years by Maternal Smoking Status, 1981 National Health
Interview Survey (n = 4331)

Maternal Smoking Status	No. of Mothers	Prevalence of Asthma (%)	P Value	% of Children Currently Using Asthma Medications	P Value
No maternal smoking	3210	2.3		0.5	
Maternal smoking <½ pack/d	574	2.9	.68	*	
Maternal smoking ≥½ pack/d	547	4.8	.001	2.0	.0003
All children	4331	2.7		0.7	

*Estimate not reported because number in cell is less than 5 observations.
(Courtesy of Weitzman M, Gortmaker S, Walker DK, et al: *Pediatrics* 85:505–511, 1990.)

with asthma. Efforts to discourage smoking in families should be continued.

▶ This report adds further evidence to the large amount of data already available concluding that infants and children of mothers who smoke have a significantly increased incidence of major health problems, including asthma. Surprisingly, not only postnatal passive smoking is injurious to infants, but studies in a rat model (1) reveal that maternal smoking during pregnancy is associated with fetal lung hypoplasia, with decreased numbers of alveoli and a reduced lung volume. In infants of nonallergic parents maternal smoking during pregnancy is also associated with an increased cord blood IgE (2). With many effective programs now available to stop smoking we must continue to strongly support clinical and community efforts to reduce this dangerous practice.—M.H. Klaus, M.D.

References

1. Collins MH, et la: *Pediatr Res* 19:408, 1985.
2. Magnussen CGM: *J Allergy Clin Immunol* 78:898, 1986.

11 The Heart and Blood Vessels

Prenatal Measurement of Cardiothoracic Ratio in Evaluation of Heart Disease

Paladini D, Chita SK, Allan LD (Guy's Hosp, London)
Arch Dis Child 65:20–23, 1990

11–1

Cardiac disease can often be detected by examining the ratio of the size of the heart to that of the thorax on a plain chest radiograph. Because many forms of congenital heart disease are detected by abnormal measurements of individual chambers rather than by cardiac enlargement, cardiologists have used echocardiography to evaluate the fetal heart. To acquire normal data for the prenatal cardiothoracic ratio, the ratio in 410 normal fetuses and 73 fetuses with functional or structural heart disease was measured.

Measurements were obtained when the whole thorax was seen on the

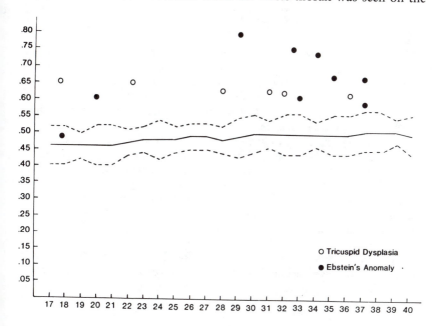

CARDIOTHORACIC RATIO vs GESTATIONAL AGE

Fig 11–1.—The cardiothoracic ratio in 15 patients with tricuspid valve abnormality compared with the normal range. (Courtesy of Paladini D, Chita SK, Allan LD: *Arch Dis Child* 65:20–23, 1990.)

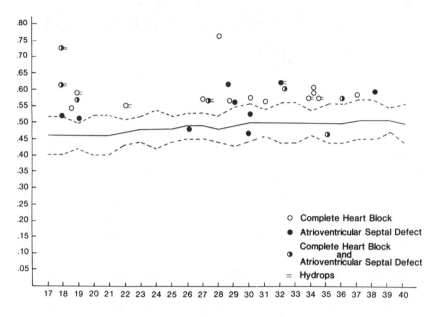

CARDIOTHORACIC RATIO vs GESTATIONAL AGE

Fig 11–2.—With only 1 exception, all patients with complete heart block showed cardiomegaly on the cardiothoracic ratio whether or not thre was associated fetal hydrops. (Courtesy of Paladini D, Chita SK, Allan LD: *Arch Dis Child* 65:20–23, 1990.)

screen, a good 4-chamber view was obtained, and a complete rib and no abdominal contents were in the frame. The ratio was obtained from a mean of 2 different measurements in 2 different frames. There were 4 groups of abnormalities: Ebstein's anomaly or tricuspid dysplasia; complete heart block and/or atrioventricular septal defect, atrial tachycardias, and a variety of other defects.

The cardiothoracic ratio was fairly constant throughout pregnancy, with a slight increase from .45 at 17 weeks' to .50 at term. Of the 15 fetuses with tricuspid valve abnormality, 14 had a high cardiothoracic ratio (Fig 11–1). In the second group, 24 of 29 fetuses had an increased cardiothoracic ratio (Fig 11–2). No clear pattern of cardiac size was characteristic of all forms of congenital heart disease. In some fetuses the cardiothoracic ratio was within the normal range.

Measurements of this index may provide useful information about secondary lung compression or cardiac failure. The cardiothoracic ratio is essential in the evaluation of fetal hydrops because an increased value may indicate an intermittent fetal tachycardia if the fetus is assessed during a period of sinus rhythm.

▶ Our quest for a complete view of the fetus continues. Based on the examination of 410 normal fetuses, this report provides, for the first time, normative data on the cardiothoracic ratio in the fetus. Fetuses studied had normal intrauterine growth and a normal uneventful neonatal course. The ratio was derived from measurements of the circumference of the heart and thorax. Of interest is how little this ratio changes in normal pregnancy and how significantly it increases with such disorders as tricuspid atresia, heart block, and arrhythmias, resulting in heart failure or hydrops. The ratio may decrease dramatically with correction of an arrhythmia in the fetus. The authors claim that the technique is simple and the diameters are always available. Measurement of the cardiothoracic ratio is recommended when evaluating the fetus for congenital heart disease or congestive heart failure. Note that conditions such as hypoplastic left heart will not be identified in this manner. See also Abstract 4–12.—A.A. Fanaroff, M.B.B.Ch.

The Timing of Spontaneous Closure of the Ductus Arteriosus in Infants With Respiratory Distress Syndrome

Reller MD, Colasurdo MA, Rice MJ, McDonald RW (Oregon Health Sciences Univ, Portland)
Am J Cardiol 66:75–78, 1990   11–2

Healthy premature infants without respiratory distress syndrome (RDS) undergo spontaneous closure of the ductus arteriosus in the first 4 days of life similar to that observed in full-term infants. Thus, ductal patency within this time frame appears to be "physiologic." Because sick premature infants are already known to be at risk for persistent ductal patency, the actual impact that RDS has on duration of ductal shunting was evaluated. The timing of spontaneous functional closure was assessed in 36 premature infants (30–37 weeks' gestational age) with uncomplicated RDS, and the presence of ductal shunting was detected using echocardiographic color-flow Doppler techniques.

Of the 36 infants, 17 required either oxygen therapy only or transient

Comparison of Group 1 and Group 2					
	Group 1 (n = 19)			Group 2 (n = 17)	
Birthweight (g)	1,760 ± 373			2,088 ± 614	
Gestational age (weeks)	31.8 ± 2.1			32.6 ± 1.7	
Outborn referral	9*			1	
	Age (hrs)	No. closed (%)		Age (hrs)	No. closed (%)
Day 1	9 ± 4	0 (0)		10 ± 5	2 (12)
Day 2	33 ± 7	7 (37)		33 ± 8	9 (53)
Day 3	58 ± 7	14 (74)		57 ± 8	13 (76)
Day 4	83 ± 6	17 (89)		82 ± 9	15 (88)

Values are mean ± SD.
*$P < .01$ using chi-square analysis and Fisher's exact test.
(Courtesy of Reller MD, Colasurdo MA, Rice MJ, et al: *Am J Cardiol* 66:75–78, 1990.)

nasal prong continuous positive airway pressure, and 19 required endotrachial intubation and ventilatory assistance. The 17 less sick infants had a tendency for earlier spontaneous ductal closure on days 1 and 2 of life than did the severely sick infants. However, by the fourth day of life, only 4 (11.1%) infants continued to have evidence of ductal patency, whereas the remaining 89% had spontaneous functional ductal closure within the time frame of "physiologically normal" patency in healthy infants (table). In the majority of premature infants at or more than 30 weeks' gestational age, uncomplicated RDS does not appear to alter the usual timing of functional ductal closure.

▶ The natural history of patency of the ductus arteriosus becomes a semantic debate. To participate you need to arm yourself with the terms patency, functional patency, physiologic patency, functional closure, and pathologic patency or closure. At times the ductus closes prematurely and innopportunely, making it necessary to restore patency pharmacologically or via a surigal conduit. At other times persistence of the patency results in cardiorespiratory compromise. Reller et al. have methodically studied term and preterm infants and documented when the ductus closes "physiologically" and when patency should be considered pathologic. In the present survey 89% of infants had spontaneous functional closure of the ductus within the time frame of physiologically normal patency in healthy infants. The infants were more than 30 weeks' gestation and moderately ill. It remains for him to now collect similar data from smaller, less mature, sicker infants.

Stop Press.

Prolonged courses of indomethacin have been used to close the ductus when short courses fail (1, 2).—A.A. Fanaroff, M.B.B.Ch.

References

1. Reller MD, et al: *Pediatr Cardiol* 6:17, 1985.
2. Reller MD, et al: *J Pediatr* 112:441, 1988.

Abnormal Renal and Splanchnic Arterial Doppler Pattern in Premature Babies With Symptomatic Patent Ductus Arteriosus
Wong S-N, Lo RN-S, Hui P-W (Queen Mary Hosp, Hong Kong)
J Ultrasound Med 9:125–130, 1990   11–3

Premature infants with patent ductus arteriosus (PDA) are at risk for heart failure, respiratory distress, and other complications. These problems may result from the shunting effect of the patent ductus that reduces blood flow to major organs. The pulsed Doppler technique was used to compare flow velocity patterns in infants with symptomatic PDA and normal infants.

Two-dimensional echocardiography and Doppler study confirmed the diagnosis of PDA in 8 premature infants with bounding peripheral pulses and/or a heart murmur, usually systolic, over the upper left sternal edge. Nine infants without PDA were also evaluated. Blood flow patterns were

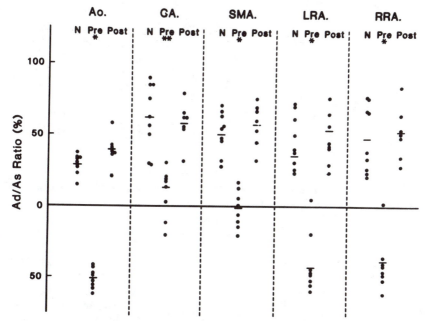

Fig 11–3.—The diastolic to systolic flow ratio (Ad/As) in the descending aorta (Ao.) and celiac (CA.), superior mesenteric (SMA.), left renal (LRA.), and right renal (RRA.) arteries in the group of normal infants (N) and infants with PDA before (Pre) and after (Post) closure (*P < .001 by Student's *t* test when compared with the N and Post groups; **P < .05 by Student's *t* test when compared with the N and Post groups). (Courtesy of Wong S-N, Lo RN-S, Hui P-W: *J Ultrasound Med* 9:125–130, 1990.)

studied in the descending aorta, renal arteries, and celiac and superior mesenteric arteries.

In the control infants, the blood flow pattern in the descending aorta consisted of forward systolic flow and absent or minimal diastolic flow. Abdominal arteries showed a similar systolic peak followed by a continuous diastolic flow. A characteristically different pattern was observed in infants with symptomatic PDAs. In the aorta, a retrograde flow in the diastolic phase indicated diastolic runoff. Patterns in the superior mesenteric and both renal arteries were similar. Repeat Doppler studies after treatment showed the disappearance of diastolic reversal of flow in all major arteries when the PDA closed. The Ad/As ratios in infants with PDAs were significantly reduced compared with premature infants without PDAs and the posttreatment values of those infants with PDAs who had been treated (Fig 11–3).

The diastolic steal phenomenon described here—not previously demonstrated in the abdominal arteries—may contribute to ischemic damage of abdominal organs in infants with PDA. Pulsed Doppler imaging was able to document the absence or reversal of diastolic blood flow to major abdominal arteries in these infants.

▶ This is a small but closely monitored group of infants with PDA. The characteristic flow pattern in the aorta of the control infants consists of forward flow during systole, with absent or minimum diastolic flow. The abnormal arteries have a similar systolic peak, followed by a continuous diastolic flow. In infants with PDA, there is reversal of flow in the aorta during diastole and in the mesenteric vessels reduced to absent flow in late diastole. The technique provides some semiquantitative flow data and confirms a disturbance in the splanchnic circulation in infants with PDA. It does not establish cause and effect between PDA and necrotizing enterocolitis. Ultrasound and flow Doppler are useful in establishing the presence of major occlusions in the aorta and its branches, a not infrequent complication of catheterization of these vessels.—A.A. Fanaroff, M.B.B.Ch.

Two-Dimensional and Doppler Echocardiographic and Pathologic Characteristics of the Infantile Marfan Syndrome
Geva T, Sanders SP, Diogenes MS, Rockenmacher S, Van Praagh R (The Children's Hosp, Boston; Harvard Univ; Dartmouth-Hitchcock Med Ctr, Hanover, NH)
Am J Cardiol 65:1230–1237, 1990   11–4

Marfan's syndrome is rarely diagnosed in the first year of life or in utero. The clinical, 2-dimensional and Doppler echocardiographic and pathologic findings in 9 infants who were diagnosed as having Marfan's syndrome during the first year of life are evaluated. The records of 86 previously reported cases of infantile Marfan's syndrome were also studied.

There were 5 boys and 4 girls, with a mean age at diagnosis of 2.7 months (range, birth to 12 months). Mitral valve prolapse was present in all infants, and mitral regurgitation occurred in 8. Tricuspid valve prolapse was present in 8, with regurgitation in 6. Two-dimensional echocardiography of mitral and tricuspid valve prolapse showed holosystolic prolapse associated with markedly elongated and redundant chordae tendineae and redundant valve leaflets herniating into the left and right atrium, respectively. Marked aortic root dilatation was a characteristic and prominent feature in all infants and assumed a "clover leaf" appearance in the parasternal short-axis view. Aortic root dimensions increased progressively compared to that in normal children. Aortic regurgitation was present initially in 1 patient and developed in another 4 infants during follow-up. Pulmonary artery dilatation and regurgitation were present in 3 infants.

During a mean follow-up of 41 months (range, 10–103 months), 7 infants had congestive heart failure associated with mitral or tricuspid regurgitation. Four infants died during infancy. The salient pathologic features were myxomatous thickening and redundancy of the mitral and tricuspid leaflets, marked elongation of the chordae tendineae, and prominent dilatation of the aortic and pulmonary roots. Histologically, there was disruption, disarray, and fragmentation of collagen and elastic fibers with increased interstitial ground substance.

These data and those from 86 previously reported cases suggest that infantile Marfan's syndrome is phenotypically and prognostically different from the classic syndrome seen in adolescents and adults. Infantile Marfan's syndrome is characterized by prominent mitral and tricuspid valve involvement associated with significant cardiovascular morbidity. Prognosis is poor and most fatalities are related to severe, intractable congestive heart failure associated with mitral or tricuspid regurgitation.

▶ Offering commentary on this selection is Christian Hardy, M.D., Associate Director, Division of Cardiology, Children's Hospital Oakland, California.

▶ Overall this is an excellent paper describing the echocardiographic pathologic syndrome of infantile Marfan's syndrome. The paper is well-organized and the information well-presented. The authors clearly depict the differences between the presentation, progressions, and prognosis of Marfan's syndrome with infantile versus adolescent/adult onset. There are, however, a few questions still unanswered.

The authors leave us guessing as to whether they support cardiac catheterization in this patient population. In all 3 patients taken for catheterization, the aortic root dimension was not measured, making it impossible to determine the aortic root to aortic annulus ratio. Additionally 2 of the 3 patients at the time of the catheterization had no determination of absence or presence of aortic or pulmonary insufficiency. It is not clear why 2 patients failed to have echocardiographic evaluation and were taken for cardiac catheterization. It appears evident from the discussion of the clear echocardiographic delineation of the various components of the disease that this noninvasive evaluation is preferable to cardiac catheterization and at least should be performed in conjunction with the invasive studies.

The morbidity and mortality of infantile Marfan's syndrome is quite high related to the severe mitral insufficiency. This often results in severe congestive heart failure and occasionally the need for mitral valve replacement. This report does not help the reader in determining the best mode of therapy for these children. Did the medical management consist of digoxin and diuretics alone? Was afterload reduction attempted in any patient? If so, was it helpful? Perhaps with aggressive afterload reduction the prognosis will be improved.

This paper also raises the question of whether these are truly 2 separate syndromes or a variation in the severity. As indicated, genetic or biomechanical differences between these syndromes are not known. It would be very interesting to see a prospective study of infants born with a strong family history of Marfan's syndrome and compare the echocardiographic findings in these children to those in the population with infantile Marfan's syndrome. Perhaps the adolescent/adult form of Marfan's would not seem quite so different if the at-risk population were more carefully followed from infancy.

The authors are to be applauded for this clearly written, well-researched, and long overdue review, and I look forward to reading further as they investigate this syndrome with its multiple forms.—C. Hardy, M.D.

Evaluation of Complex Congenital Ventricular Anomalies With Magnetic Resonance Imaging

Kersting-Sommerhoff BA, Diethelm L, Stanger P, Dery R, Higashino SM, Higgins SS, Higgins CB (Univ of California Med Ctr, San Francisco; Childrens Hosp Med Ctr, Oakland, Calif)

Am Heart J 120:133–142, 1990   11–5

Complex ventricular anomalies are frequently associated with abnormalities of the thoracic and abdominal situs, arterioventricular connection, and venous connection. The effectiveness of ECG gated spin-echo MRI in defining the components of these anomalies was compared to that of cardiac angiography in 29 patients with a clinical diagnosis of single or common ventricle or complete atrioventricular (AV) septal (canal) defect. The MRI studies and angiograms were evaluated independently using a sequential approach to define 9 anatomical components.

There were 261 observations with ECG gated MRI and 209 observations with angiography. Of the 209 mutual observations, 17 discrepancies were found between MRI and angiography. The MRI studies were as precise as angiography in the depiction of ventricular anomalies, including determination of morphology and evaluation of size of the ventricles, the orientation of the ventricular septum relative to the AV valves, and the origins and spatial relationships of the great arteries. Furthermore, MRI was more effective than angiography in determining thoracic and abdominal situs, and systemic and venoatrial connections. All but 1 of the discrepancies occurred in the evaluation of ventricular outflow tracts and semilunar valves; MRI studies were not as effective as angiography in evaluating these features. These findings indicate that ECG gated MRI effectively defines most anatomical components of complex ventricular anomalies. Its major limitation is the evaluation of semilunar valves and ventricular outflow tracts.

▶ Newer technology results in constant challenges to the gold standards. The role of MRI in an evaluation of complex congenital heart disease is explored in this comparative study. The study design was highlighted by the a priori agreement on definitions for the complex congenital heart disorders. Furthermore, the panel of readers was unaware of the results of the other imaging study, as MRI and angiography were evaluated independently by different teams. The report card on MRI is excellent, with deficiencies only in evaluation of the semilunar valves. It was superior to angiography in the determination of abdominal and thoracic situs, as well as the systemic and pulmonary venoarterial connections. Angiography and MRI are complementary, providing the cardiothoracic team with precise information on the anatomical relationships in permitting optimal planning for interventional procedures.—A.A. Fanaroff, M.B.B.Ch.

Pulmonary Vascular Resistance in Neonatal Swine: Response to Right Pulmonary Artery Occlusion, Isoproterenol, and Prostaglandin E₁

Crombleholme TM, Adzick NS, Longaker MT, Bradley SM, Duncan BW, Jennings R, Verrier ED, Harrison MR (Univ of California, San Francisco)
J Pediatr Surg 25:861–866, 1990   11–6

Unilateral pulmonary artery (PA) occlusion in an adult results in a decrease in the pulmonary vascular resistance, allowing the pulmonary vascular bed to accommodate twice its normal flow while maintaining a normal pulmonary artery pressure. In newborns, the pulmonary circulation response to unilateral pulmonary artery occlusion has not been characterized. Persistent pulmonary hypertension in newborns (PPHN) results in increased pulmonary vascular resistance, inadequate pulmonary blood flow, and right-to-left shunting.

To study newborn pulmonary circulation response and modulation of response by a vasodilator or an inotropic agent, unilateral pulmonary artery occlusion was induced in 20 piglets by left lateral thoracotomy. After left lateral thoracotomy, measurement of the pulmonary artery and left atrial pressures, cardiac output and pulmonary vascular resistance were taken with the right pulmonary artery open and with the pulmonary artery occluded. The experiment was repeated with infusions of the vasodi-

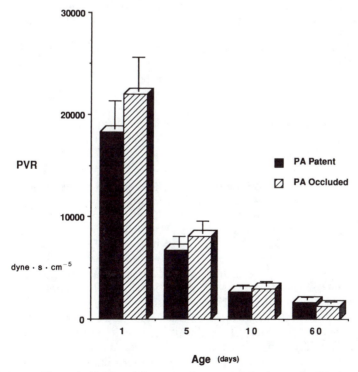

Fig 11–4.—The graph plots the pulmonary vascular resistance (dyne/sec/cm^{-5}) of the left lung in piglets aged 1, 5, 10, and 60 days at baseline and during right pulmonary artery (PA) occlusion. The values plotted represent the mean ± 1 SEM. (Courtesy of Crombleholme TM, Adzick NS, Longaker MT, et al: *J Pediatr Surg* 25: 861–866, 1990.)

lator and the inotropic agent. The response to pulmonary artery occlusion similar to that of a human adult first appeared at 60 days in the pig (Fig 11–4).

The vascular capacity of the neonatal lung is fixed. Unilateral pulmonary occlusion results in a dramatic increase in pulmonary vascular resistance that is not altered by either a vasodilator or an inotrope. The results may have implications for the treatment of newborns with pulmonary hypertension.

▶ The following comment was contributed by David J. Durand, M.D., Neonatologist, Children's Hospital Oakland, California.

▶ Pulmonary artery hypertension continues to fascinate researchers and frustrate clinicians. This study seems to confirm the suspicion of many of us that the neonatal pulmonary vascular bed is basically uncooperative; it refuses to (or is unable to) dilate in response to drugs that have been shown to be potent pulmonary vascular dilators in adults. The obvious conclusion is that the neonatal pulmonary vascular bed is maximally dilated.

However, extrapolating from the healthy piglet model to the neonate with PPHN may not be accurate. The pulmonary hypertension in this model was caused by extrinsic constriction of normal pulmonary vessels. In many, if not all, infants with PPHN there is extensive in utero remodeling of the pulmonary arteries, resulting in pulmonary artery morphology different than that of the normal infant. The real question for clinicians is whether the pulmonary vessels of infants with PPHN are maximally dilated at birth, as in the healthy piglet, or whether there are effective strategies for dilating them. Until this is answered, researchers will continue to search for the elusive pulmonary vasodilator, and clinicians will continue to use extracorporeal membrane oxygenation for those infants who do not respond to them.—D.J. Durand, M.D.

Effect of Extracorporeal Membrane Oxygenation on Cerebral Blood Flow and Cerebral Oxygen Metabolism in Newborn Sheep
Short BL, Walker LK, Gleason CA, Jones MD Jr, Traystman RJ (George Washington Univ, Washington, DC; Johns Hopkins Univ)
Pediatr Res 28:50–53, 1990   11–7

There are concerns regarding the risks associated with extracorporeal membrane oxygenation (ECMO) used for respiratory support to term or near-term infants with refractory respiratory failure. The possibility that the procedure itself may worsen or cause neurologic injury in infants that may have already sustained significant hypoxia and/or ischemia has been raised. To address this, the effects of ECMO on normal neonatal cerebral circulation were studied in 13 healthy newborn lambs 1- to 7-days old. Measurements of regional cerebral blood flow (CBF), using the radiolabeled microsphere technique, cerebral oxygen consumption, fractional oxygen extraction, and oxygen transport, were taken at 30 and 120 minutes after initiation of normothermic venoarterial ECMO at 150 mL/kg/min flow.

Neither CBF nor cerebral oxygen consumption was significantly changed after ECMO. There were no right-left or regional differences in CBF during ECMO.

▶ There is a crying need for more physiologic investigations on the impact of ECMO. This report addresses that need and provides some reassuring data on the immediate effects of ECMO on the brain. In the healthy 1- to 7-day old lambs initiation of bypass under normothermic conditions did not alter CBF or cerebral oxygen metabolism. Previous studies had suggested that cerebral blood flow would increase with the initiation of ECMO. It is important to note that these studies were short-term and in a healthy animal model with different anatomy from the human infant. The insightful discussion speculates on the various mechanisms coming into play with the onset of bypass. Rapid correction of hypocarbia, alterations in blood pressure, nonpulsatile flow, and the overall hemodynamic and biochemical changes associated with bypass are all taken into consideration. The measurement of CBF and cerebral oxygenation was accomplished without a major hitch, and ECMO was well-tolerated by these animals, who serve as excellent models for training ECMO teams. Preliminary data suggest that the vertebral circulation, which is insignificant in the lamb, plays a major role in compensating for carotid ligation in human neonates. We look forward to more data on the pathophysiologic impact of ECMO.—A.A. Fanaroff, M.B.B.Ch.

Extracorporeal Membrane Oxygenation and Conventional Medical Therapy in Neonates With Persistent Pulmonary Hypertension of the Newborn: A Prospective Randomized Study
O'Rourke PP, Crone RK, Vacanti JP, Ware JH, Lillehei CW, Parad RB, Epstein MF (Children's Hosp, Boston; Harvard Univ)
Pediatrics 84:957–963, 1989   11–8

The use of extracorporeal membrane oxygenation (ECMO) in the treatment of persistent pulmonary hypertension of the newborn (PPHN) has increased dramatically. The effectiveness of ECMO was compared to that of conventional medical therapy (CMT) in 39 newborn infants with severe persistent pulmonary hypertension and respiratory failure who met criteria for 85% likelihood of dying. In this prospective study, an adaptive design with both a randomized and a nonrandomized phase was used. Initially, the first 19 neonates were randomly assigned to ECMO or CMT therapy (phase 1). Randomization was continued until the fourth death occurred in either group, and all subsequent patients were enrolled in the group with less than 4 deaths (phase 2). All patients were comparable in severity of illness and mechanical ventilator support.

In phase 1, 4 of 10 patients in the CMT group died, whereas all 9 patients in the ECMO group survived (table). After the fourth death, the next 20 patients were assigned to ECMO treatment and 19 survived.

Survival Experience of Patients Randomly Assigned
to ECMO and Conventional Therapy During Phase I,
Randomized, and Phase II, Nonrandomized

	Phase I		Phase II	
	ECMO	CMT	ECMO	CMT
Lived	9	6	19	0
Died	0	4	1	0

Abbreviations: CMT, conventional medical therapy. Results represent numbers of children.
(Courtesy of O'Rourke PP, Crone RK, Vacanti JP, et al: *Pediatrics* 84:957–963, 1989.)

Overall survival rates were 97% (28 of 29) for the ECMO group and 60% (6 of 10) in the CMT group; the difference was significant. Except for the 1 patient who died in phase 2, there were no serious acute complications in the ECMO group.

Extracorporeal membrane oxygenation significantly improves survival in neonates with PPHN, as compared to CMT. The survivors in this study are currently being followed to determine the long-term outcome of ECMO.

▶ To reverse paraphrase famous statesman and former British Prime Minister Sir Winston Churchill, "Never in the history of medicine has so much grief been hurled by so many at so few for such a minor infraction." This article was first commented on in the Boston Globe with banner headlines suggesting that potentially life-saving therapy was being withheld from some babies. Publication in *Pediatrics* was followed by some scathing, other more tongue-in-cheek, eloquently humorous commentaries and editorials. The statistical design is what was drawing the bulk of the fire. The National Institutes of Health responded by slapping a technical foul on Harvard University, threatening withdrawal of research funds if research involving human subjects was not better controlled by the Institutional Review Board. The study design and method of randomization has been the focus of the criticism. The central point of discussion is whether it is now possible to perform a truly randomized trial to determine the efficacy of ECMO. My humble opinion is that such a study is doomed before it starts and will not be attempted. The only published randomized trials of ECMO have involved unconventional statistical maneuvering (1). Proponents of ECMO, and there are many, point to the data from the ECMO registry, containing more than 4,000 patients at the time of writing, with marvelous survival rates. The equally vociferous opponents of ECMO will argue that the therapy was unnecessary in the first place. Indications for ECMO remain a moving target and suggesting that a set of numbers, such as Aa gradients or oxygenation indices, predict mortality, oversimplifies the evaluation. Nonetheless, extremely ill babies are being selected for ECMO and the vast majority are surviving. Although the precise number of infants treated with ECMO who would have survived with conservative management will always remain unknown, the quality of the ECMO survivors followed to date has been encouraging. Furthermore, the ECMO technology has advanced the pathophysiologic understanding of cardiorespiratory disorders. I subscribe to the school advocating ECMO for carefully selected patients. We must strive to attempt to make these selection criteria extremely rigorous and to ensure that maximal conservative therapy has been offered before initiation of ECMO. Sophocles said it all many years ago:

Knowledge must come through action; you can have no test which is not fanciful, save by trial.— Sophocles

A.A. Fanaroff, M.B.B.Ch.

Reference

1. Bartlett RH, et al: *Pediatrics* 76:479, 1985.

Hidden Mortality Rate Associated with Extracorporeal Membrane Oxygenation

Boedy RF, Howell CG, Kanto WP Jr (Med College of Georgia, Augusta)
J Pediatr 117:462–464, 1990

11–9

Extracorporeal membrane oxygenation (ECMO) is increasingly used for the treatment of neonatal respiratory failure not responsive to conventional therapy. However, significant mortality has been observed during transport of these critically ill infants. Because these deaths should be considered in the evaluation of an ECMO program, the outcomes in all infants referred to and accepted in an ECMO program during a 52-month period were reviewed. Data were reviewed in 167 referrals, including 9 mothers who had not yet delivered.

The overall mortality rate was 27.5% (46 of 167); 18 infants, representing 11.3% of all neonates transported, died before leaving the referring hospital, during transport, or shortly after admission. These 18 transport-related deaths represented 39.1% of all deaths (18 of 46); death was caused by meconium aspiration syndrome in 8 infants, congenital diaphragmatic hernia (CDH) in 5, persistent fetal circulation in 4, and group B streptococcal sepsis in 1.

Because of contraindications to ECMO 17 (10.7%) referrals were excluded. Another 62 (37.1%) infants initially failed to meet ECMO criteria, and 2 died before ECMO could be started. Of the infants, 68 (40.7%) underwent ECMO, and 11 (16.1%) died. Congenital diaphragmatic hernia occurred in 22 infants, 14 (63.6%) of whom died. Of these 14 deaths, 5 occurred during transport, respresenting 27.7% of all transport deaths.

These data suggest a hidden mortality rate within referral and transport of critically ill infants referred for ECMO therapy. It is recommended that infants with meconium aspiration syndrome be transported to an ECMO center when an oxygenation index of 25 is reached. Early transport is also recommended for infants with CDH, in utero transport with delivery at an ECMO center, or during the postoperative period. Transport-related mortality should be considered in the evaluation of an ECMO program outcome.

▶ Contributing her thoughts on this selection is Eileen K. Stork, M.D., Assistant Professor of Pediatrics, C.W.R.V. Director of E.C.M.O. Program, Rainbow Babies and Childrens Hospital, Cleveland:

▶ This title is somewhat misleading, as the hidden mortality lies not with the ECMO procedure, but with the newborn population at risk for respiratory failure. The message contained in this article is an important one, however. Eighteen infants died during transport who might otherwise have survived with more timely referral to an ECMO center. An equal number (n = 17) were not suitable ECMO candidates for a variety of reasons, especially cyanotic congenital heart disease. Conversely, 59 infants routed to an ECMO center were successfully managed with conventional medical support alone. Fewer than half (64 of 158) of the infants transported were ultimately treated with ECMO.

The referring hospital faces a difficult task in identifying those at risk for death because of respiratory failure early enough in the clinical course to allow safe dispatch to an ECMO center. The fact that many babies improve rather than worsen following transfer reflects the dynamic nature of respiratory disease in the neonate, not the poor clinical acumen on the part of referring physicians. Early transports will always mean that some babies never need ECMO, but for others the decision may well be lifesaving.—E.K. Stork, M.D.

12 The Blood

Risks to the Fetus of Anticoagulant Therapy During Pregnancy
Ginsberg JS, Hirsh J, Turner DC, Levine MN, Burrows R (McMaster Univ, Hamilton, Ontario)
Thromb Haemost 61:197–203, 1989   12–1

Anticoagulant therapy during pregnancy has potential adverse effects for both the mother and fetus. In a recent report heparin was said to be as risky as oral anticoagulant therapy in pregnancy, even though heparin

	Summary of Adverse Outcomes in Patients With Venous Thromboembolic Disease		
	Group A Heparin alone (%)	Group B Oral anticoagulants alone (%)	Group C Both heparin and oral anticoagulants (%)
First analysis Adverse outcomes (all pregnancies included)	37/279 (13.3%)	36/193 (18.7%)	30/156 (19.2%)
Second analysis Adverse outcomes (after excluding pregnancies with maternal comorbid conditions)	24/266 (9.0%)	32/189 (16.9%)	25/151 (16.6%)
Third analysis Adverse outcomes (after excluding pregnancies with maternal comorbid conditions and prematurity with normal outcomes)	8/266 (3.0%)	32/189 (16.9%)	25/151 (16.6%)
Fourth analysis Deaths (abortions, stillbirths and neonatal deaths after excluding pregnancies with maternal comorbid conditions)	7/266 (2.6%)	16/189 (8.5%)	12/151 (7.9%)

(Courtesy of Ginsberg JS, Hirsh J, Turner DC, et al: *Thromb Haemost* 61:197–203, 1989.)

does not cross the placenta. One hundred eighty-six studies presented in the literature that described the fetal and infant outcomes in 1,325 pregnancies associated with anticoagulant therapy were analyzed, and the rates of death, prematurity, and congenital malformations after treatment with heparin or oral anticoagulants, or both, were determined (table).

The previously reported high rate of adverse fetal and infant outcomes after heparin therapy could be accounted for by the frequent use of heparin in women with comorbid conditions independently associated with adverse outcomes and by reports of uncomplicated prematurity. When such pregnancies were excluded from the analysis, outcomes in heparin-treated women were comparable to those in the normal population.

Women should be offered heparin therapy if anticoagulants are indicated during pregnancy for preventing or treating thromboembolic disease. If anticoagulants are indicated for the entire pregnancy and patients cannot tolerate subcutaneous injections, oral anticoagulants may be used in the second trimester and early part of the third trimester. However, patients should be warned that oral anticoagulants may be fetopathic even in the second trimester.

▶ How do you resolve the question as to the best anticoagulant to use during pregnancy? Answer—a novel approach—a statistical analysis of the available literature. Truly an example of strength in numbers. The verdict: although initially judged as guilty, then guilty by association, the final verdict is innocent and still drug of choice—heparin. Recognize that the underlying condition requiring anticoagulant therapy renders the pregnancy high risk de novo.

Genius is an infinite capacity for taking pains.—Jane Ellice Hopkins

A.A. Fanaroff, M.B.B.Ch.

Postnatal Changes in Serum Immunoreactive Erythropoietin in Relation to Hypoxia Before and After Birth
Ruth V, Widness JA, Clemons G, Raivio KO (Univ of Helsinki; Women and Infants' Hosp of Rhode Island, Providence; Univ of California, Berkeley)
J Pediatr 116:950–954, 1990   12–2

There is yet no gold standard for perinatal hypoxia. Tissue hypoxia is the only known stimulus for the production of erythropoietin (EP). To assess the immediate postnatal changes of serum immunoreactive EP in infants born after acute or chronic fetal hypoxia and to estimate the rate of EP disappearance, EP concentration was measured by double-antibody radioimmunoassay in cord venous blood and in serum at a mean age of 8 hours in 10 infants with polycythemia; 22 infants born to mothers with preeclampsia of pregnancy, including 22 without and 11 with acidosis at birth; 19 infants with acute birth asphyxia, including 7 with postnatal hypoxia; and 9 healthy term infants.

Compared with the control group, cord venous EP concentrations were

Serum EP Concentration at Birth and at a Mean
Age of 8 Hours

	Cord venous EP (mU/ml)	EP at 8 hr (mU/ml)	Change; *p*
Polycythemia	123† (23-2016)	24 (11-316)	Decrease; <0.001
Preeclampsia, no birth asphyxia	78‡ (19-2350)	26 (9-995)	Decrease; <0.001
Preeclampsia, birth asphyxia	176‡ (28-1364)	38* (14-496)	Decrease; <0.001
Acute asphyxia, no postnatal hypoxia	58* (9-374)	30* (7-94)	Decrease; <0.001
Acute asphyxia, postnatal hypoxia	122† (28-44000)	72* (9-987)	No change
Control values	20 (6-39)	16 (12-26)	No change

Note: Data are expressed as the geometric mean, with range in parentheses.
Significance compared with control values are as follows:
*P < .05.
†P < .01.
‡P < .001.
(Courtesy of Ruth V, Widness JA, Clemons G, et al: *J Pediatr* 116:950–954, 1990.)

significantly increased in all infants born after acute or chronic fetal hypoxia. Serum EP levels did not change significantly from birth to 8 hours of age in control infants and in asphyxiated infants with continuing postnatal hypoxia, whereas serum EP levels decreased significantly in infants with polycythemia, infants in the preeclampsia group with or without acidosis, and infants with acute birth asphyxia without postnatal hypoxia (table). The mean half-life of EP disappearance was 2.6 hours in infants with polycythemia and 3.7 hours in infants in the preeclampsia group.

Except for asphyxiated infants with postnatal hypoxia, a postnatal decrease of increased EP concentrations is present in infants with chronic or acute hypoxia in utero. It appears that acute or chronic hypoxia in utero is quickly relieved subsequent to birth, provided postnatal hypoxemia does not occur. This postnatal decrease in EP concentration most likely results from improved oxygenation, as the lung becomes the organ of gas exchange. The neonatal disappearance rate of plasma EP is about twice that in adults. These data can be applied to clinical trials of human recombinant EP to correct neonatal anemia, suggesting that higher doses of EP should be administered relative to that in adults.

▶ The goal of this cross-cultural American-Finnish investigation was to establish a gold standard for which perinatal asphyxia could be clearly defined, indisputably a noble motivation and worthy of close consideration. Erythropoietin is the newest kid on the block to come under careful scrutiny. Erythropoietin levels are elevated from the cord blood in a number of clinical situations, including hypertension, diabetes, Rh disease, and perinatal asphyxia. Furthermore, the hypoxic stimulus associated with normal labor may be sufficient to elevate cord blood levels as values are lower in infants delivered electively by cesarean section. In neonates with polycythemia, the elevated cord EP levels may indicate acute or chronic fetal hypoxia. Erythropoietin levels decline after birth unless there is sustained hypoxia. Notably, the rate of decline is far more rapid than in adults, which may have implications for dosing with EP in the correction of anemia of prematurity (see Abstract 12–4). The lack of correlation between cord EP levels and cerebral damage was in accord with previous work by this group (1). Thus, EP cord blood levels cannot distinguish acute from chronic hypoxia, are not predictive of outcome, and therefore cannot be considered as the gold standard in defining perinatal asphyxia.—A.A. Fanaroff, M.B.B.Ch.

Reference

1. Ruth Y, et al: *J Pediatr* 113:880, 1988.

Erythroid "Burst Promoting" Activity in Serum of Patients With the Anemia of Prematurity

Ohls RK, Liechty KW, Turner MC, Kimura RE, Christensen RD (Univ of Utah, Salt Lake City)
J Pediatr 116:786–789, 1990   12–3

The pathogenesis of anemia of prematurity remains to be defined. Erythroid "burst promoting" activity (BPA) is a collective term for growth factors, such as interleukin-3 (IL-3) and granulocyte-macrophage colony-stimulating factor (GM-CSF), that are needed to support the maturation of primitive erythroid progenitors into clones of normoblasts in vitro. To define the role of BPA in anemia of prematurity, serum erythroid BPA concentrations were measured in 15 patients with anemia of prematurity and in 9 patients with anemia of end-stage renal disease. For comparison, erythroid BPA levels were also measured in the sera of 12 healthy adults and 8 term cord blood samples. Serum from each subject was incubated with normal adult marrow progenitor cells, and if BPA was present, erythroid burst-forming units would develop into clones of normoblasts.

Erythroid BPA concentrations in patients with anemia of prematurity were significantly greater than concentrations in cord blood or adult sera. Likewise, BPA concentrations in patients with anemia of end-stage renal disease were significantly greater than in the sera of normal adults. When the test sera were incubated with antibodies raised against the hematopoietic growth factors with known BPA, BPA was completely ablated by anti-GM-CSF antibody in patients with anemia of end-stage renal disease. In contrast, neither anti-GM-CSF, anti-IL-3, nor the combination completely ablated the activity. There was no evidence to suggest that IL-6 was responsible for the residual BPA.

Erythroid BPA is present in the sera of patients with anemia of prematurity as well as in patients with anemia of end-stage renal disease. These findings suggest that these anemias are not the result of an overall deficiency of erythropoietin (EP) growth factors but are secondary to a specific deficiency of EP.

▶ This commentary was contributed by Wade Clapp, M.D., Assistant Professor of Pediatrics, Case Western Reserve University School of Medicine, Cleveland:

▶ The regulation of hematopoiesis is dependent on complex interrelationships between hematopoietic progenitors, the bone marrow microenvironment, and glycoprotein hormones such as EP. The bone marrow microenvironment serves as a source of regulatory molecules known as hematopoietic growth factors. Erythropoietin is elaborated in the fetal liver and adult kidney.

Three critical factors involved in the production of red blood cells in the neonate include: (1) the responsivity of hematopoietic progenitors to hematopoietic growth factors; (2) the production of a group of growth factors collectively known as BPA that support the proliferation of primitive hematopoietic progenitors; and (3) the elaboration of EP to hematopoietic tissues where it stimulates the proliferation and differentiation of erythroid precursors.

Shannon (1) has previously demonstrated that primitive erythroid progenitors, BFU-E (burst forming unit-erythroid), cultured from cord blood are actually more sensitive to EP than are BFU-E from the bone marrow of adults. Subsequently, Rhondeau et al. (2) determined that the differentiated erythroid progenitor (CFU-E) cultured from bone marrow cells of preterm infants responded as well to EP as CFU-E cultured from adult bone marrow. This interesting report by Ohls et al. demonstrates that the supportive BPA factors found in sera of preterm infants are sufficient to maintain support for the proliferation and differentiation of BFU-E. All of the above studies demonstrate that the critical questions to be answered in understanding the physiology of "anemia of prematurity" concern the regulation of EP production in the preterm infant.—W. Clapp, M.D.

References

1. Shannon: *N Engl J Med* 317:728, 1987.
2. Rhondeau SM, et al: *J Pediatr* 112:935, 1988.

Effects of Recombinant Human Erythropoietin in Infants With the Anemia of Prematurity: A Pilot Study
Halpérin DS, Wacker P, Lacourt G, Félix M, Babel J-F, Aapro M, Wyss M (Hôpital Cantonal Univ, Geneva)
J Pediatr 116:779–786, 1990   12–4

The anemia of prematurity is characterized by reduced bone marrow erythropoietic activity and low serum levels of erythropoietin (EP). Because bone marrow and circulating erythroid progenitors in premature infants display normal proliferation and differentiation in vitro in the presence of recombinant human erythropoietin (rHuEP), a clinical trial was designed to stimulate production of endogenous EP in infants with anemia of prematurity and thereby provide a new therapeutic alternative to potentially hazardous transfusions of EP.

Beginning at 21 to 33 days of life 7 infants with the anemia of prematurity received rHuEP in doses of 75 to 300 U/kg/wk for 4 weeks. All patients received elemental iron and vitamin E oral supplements.

Baseline serum level of EP was low in all patients (mean, 9.9 mU/mL). After rHuEP therapy the number of reticulocytes increased significantly from a mean baseline count of 75×10^9/L to 165×10^9/L on day 14 of treatment. Six patients had correction or stabilization of anemia, with an estimated increase in total volume of erythrocytes of 49% during therapy versus a predicted increment of 18% in the absence of rHuEP. One patient showed a decline in hematocrit during treatment. Three of the responders showed a secondary fall in hematocrit during or after therapy was discontinued. Serum levels of iron and ferritin decreased rapidly during therapy. A transient early thrombocytosis was noted in most patients, as well as a slight decline in absolute neutrophil count. Treatment was well tolerated.

Treatment with rHuEP may correct or stabilize the anemia of prematurity, but its effects may be limited by a variety of factors, including iron availability. Controlled clinical trials are needed to confirm this limited but encouraging experience.

▶ Anemia of prematurity has proved refractory to iron, folic acid, and vitamin E. It is characterized by low serum EP levels relative to the anemia. Erythropoietin has been used successfully in adults and children with renal failure. The logical step was therefore to evaluate EP in anemia of prematurity. This pilot study on a carefully selected group of infants would have to be characterized as only encouraging. It in no way had the same impact as penicillin on a strep throat. Most of the patients responded in the predicted manner. Of some concern was the significant drop in neutrophil counts and thrombocytosis in many of the infants. There are, however, flickers of hope that EP may reduce the need for transfusions. Iron supplementation may be necessary as iron deficiency may be the limiting factor in the EP response.

It was the Rainbow gave thee birth,
And left thee all her lovely hues—W.H. Davies

A.A. Fanaroff, M.B.B.Ch.

Prevention of Iron Deficiency in Preterm Neonates During Infancy
Heese H de V, Smith S, Watermeyer S, Dempster WS, Jakubiec L (Univ of Cape Town; Red Cross War Meml Children's Hosp, Cape Town)
S Afr Med J 77:339–345, 1990

Iron deficiency will inevitably occur in preterm infants unless supplementary iron is given. Although oral iron supplementation is recommended, intramuscular administration of iron dextran may be more effective when maternal compliance is uncertain and where poor social and economic circumstances are prevalent. The effectiveness of these 2 methods of preventing iron deficiency of prematurity was evaluated in 61 infants aged 1 week to 24 weeks. The infants were born at gestational ages of 30 to 35 weeks and with birth weights appropriate for gestational age. Infants were followed up until 52 weeks of age.

Thirty-two infants were given ferrous lactate orally at a dose of 2 mg/kg/day until the age of 6 months and the remaining 29 infants received iron dextran, 100 mg, intramuscularly between the ages of 6 and 8 weeks. Breastfeeding was encouraged; otherwise a modified formula fortified with 6 mg iron/L, vitamins, and trace metals was given.

Infants given iron dextran were largely protected against iron deficiency up to age 24 weeks. On the other hand, infants given oral iron were protected to a lesser extent with an increasing incidence of iron deficiency (serum ferritin <12 μg/L) by 24 weeks.

Hematologic values were significantly higher at 16 and 20 weeks in infants given iron dextran; mean reticulocyte count did not differ between groups. By 52 weeks, iron deficiency was evident in 59% of the infants in the oral iron group compared with 35% in the iron-dextran group. Both groups demonstrated satisfactory physical growth. Administration of iron dextran did not affect the incidence of morbidity and mortality from infection.

Intramuscularly administered iron dextran appears to be superior to oral iron supplementation as prophylaxis against iron deficiency in premature infants. However, the recommended dose of iron of 2 mg/kg body weight in North American infants appears to be inadequate for premature infants from lower socioeconomic groups in Cape Town; the recommended dose for the latter should be at least 4 mg/kg after the age of 2 months. A further injection of 100 mg of iron dextran should be considered during late infancy when iron deficiency still exists.

▶ We tend to focus on the esoteric disorders in premature infants and often neglect the mundane important problems. Boet Heese, my former chief and mentor, rivets our attention to iron deficiency, a universal affliction among preterm infants in the developing world. To overcome the problem of noncompliance he has for many years insisted on administering intramuscular iron before discharge. Despite concerns regarding the toxicity of intramuscular iron his considerable experience has failed to verify such toxicity. The above report suggests that in order to prevent iron deficiency a repeat dose of intramuscular iron may be required, and furthermore, the current recommendations of 2 mg/kg/day orally are inadequate in the population under consideration. Preterm infants are already developmentally vulnerable, and iron deficiency may aggravate the situation by contributing to impaired psychomotor development and learning. Iron may also play a critical role in the response to exogenous erythropoietin (see Abstract 12–4). Iron status and close monitoring of hematologic values should be an integral part of the follow-up of preterm infants. A universal cheap solution to prevention of iron deficiency is needed for the developing countries.

Gold is for the mistress—silver for the maid
Copper for the craftsman cunning at his trade,
"Good!" said the Baron, sitting in his hall,
But Iron, Cold Iron is master of them all.—Rudyard Kipling

A.A. Fanaroff, M.B.B.Ch.

Deficient Collagen-Induced Activation in the Newborn Platelet
Israels SJ, Daniels M, McMillan EM (Univ of Manitoba, Winnipeg)
Pediatr Res 27:337–343, 1990   12–6

Differences exist between neonatal and adult platelet function. The impaired secretion response of neonatal platelets was examined, and the response of washed neonatal and adult platelets to thrombin, collagen, specific activators of calcium flux, and protein kinase C activation was investigated.

Neonatal platelets demonstrated no impairment of aggregation, secretion of serotonin, or phosphorylation of specific intracellular proteins in response to thrombin, activators of calcium flux, or protein kinase C activation. However, the response of neonatal platelets to collagen was significantly less than that of adult platelets.

There was no difference between adult and neonatal platelets in adhesion to collagen-coated dishes. There was no difference in binding to antibody against GPIa/IIa, a collagen receptor. Phosphoinositide hydrolysis was normal in response to thrombin, but it decreased in response to collagen in neonatal platelets. Neonatal platelets released more arachidonic acid in response to thrombin, but they released less in response to collagen than adult platelets. Thromboxane B_2 production was decreased in response to collagen in neonatal platelets (table).

Neonatal platelets are deficient in their response to collagen. This deficiency may involve the transduction of the collagen signal to phospholipases A_2 and C.

▶ In my estimation the platelet continues to grow in stature. The cytokines that modulate the platelet and the factors released by the platelet form an ever-expanding list. Always regarded as the ugly duckling within the hematopoietic system the scanning electron microscope has revealed beauty and grace in motion as the platelets plug breaches in the vascular integrity. The above report highlights differences in the functional responses between the adult and neonatal platelet. One can either be concerned at the impaired

Thromboxane B_2 Production in Neonatal and Adult Platelets

Agonist	% AA converted to TxB_2		Quantity TxB_2 produced (ng/mL)	
	Adult	Neonate	Adult	Neonate
Thrombin 0.2 U/mL	17 ± 3*	11 ± 4	382.5 ± 101.5†	319.0 ± 93.4 (NS)
Collagen 10 µg/mL	15 ± 4	10 ± 2	101.4 ± 18.7	52.7 ± 12.6 ($p < 0.05$)

*Mean ± 1 SD of 7 experiments.
†Mean ± SE of 8 experiments.
(Courtesy of Israels SJ, Daniels M, McMillan EM: *Pediatr Res* 27:337–343, 1990.)

response of the newborn platelet to collagen activation or marvel at all the responses that equal the adult. I chose the latter course. The question is whether this diminished response to collagen is merely a developmental delay or is in some manner protective for the fetus and newborn?—A.A. Fanaroff, M.B.B.Ch.

13 Endocrine and Metabolic Disorders

Extracellular Dehydration During Pregnancy Increases Salt Appetite of Offspring
Nicolaidis S, Galaverna O, Metzler CH (Collège de France, Paris; Univ of California, San Francisco)
Am J Physiol 258:R281–R283, 1990   13–1

The pathogenic properties of excessive salt intake (natriophilia) are being increasingly acknowledged. Sodium appetite and the associated tendency to prefer and to eat salty foods are unequally distributed between and within subpopulations of human beings, as well as in rats. The synergistic actions of angiotensin and aldosterone have been assumed to indicate that these are primary mechanisms responsible for the induction of salt appetite. However, the factors that stimulate these mechanisms in some subjects but not in others are not well understood. Extracellular dehydration occurs in human beings after vomiting and diarrhea, and is generally noted during pregnancy.

It was hypothesized that extracellular dehydration during pregnancy may increase the tendency of offspring to consume salt. Pregnant rats were treated with polyethylene glycol, which produces extracellular dehydration and exaggerates sodium appetite. The offspring of these treated pregnant rats demonstrated an increase in salt appetite when compared with the offspring of control untreated dams.

It can be assumed that human beings who are particularly disposed to prefer salty ingestants are the offspring of mothers who experienced some kind of extracellular dehydration. Preliminary information demonstrates that children who prefer salty solutions tended to descend from mothers who vomited during pregnancy. Cognizance of a prenatal mechanism that increases salt appetite indicates that earlier intervention should be considered in patients with dehydration during pregnancy so as to decrease the possibility of inducing natriophilia in the offspring and perhaps reducing the incidence of hypertension. In addition, data regarding the incidence of dehydration during pregnancy should be obtained from patients with diseases characterized by disorders of fluid and electrolyte balance.

▶ This report has interesting implications. The authors note that unpublished preliminary data reveal that children who prefer salty solutions tended to be born to mothers who vomited during pregnancy. If this is true in humans it would be an interesting example of how the mother's internal environment altered the later behavior of the child. Is this why some children like pickles?—M.H. Klaus, M.D.

Transabdominal Villus Sampling in Early Second Trimester: A Safe Sampling Method for Women of Advanced Age
Jahoda MGJ, Pijpers L, Reuss A, Brandenburg H, Cohen-Overbeek TE, Los FJ, Sachs ES, Wladimiroff JW (Erasmus Univ, Rotterdam, The Netherlands)
Prenat Diagn 10:307–311, 1990   13–2

Transabdominal chorionic villus sampling (TA-CVS) has been reported to be safer and simpler than transcervical CVS. In a retrospective study the outcome of TA-CVS performed between March 1987 and October 1988 in 707 viable singleton pregnancies of mothers of advanced age was reviewed. Maternal age ranged from 36 to 49 years.

In each case TA-CVS was carried out as an office procedure without local anesthesia under continuous ultrasound monitoring. In 121 women TA-CVS was performed between 10.2 and 11.6 weeks' gestation, 477 women underwent TA-CVS at 12.0 to 14.6 weeks' gestation, and 109 women underwent TA-CVS between 15.0 and 18.3 weeks' gestation.

In 90.3% of women only 1 needle insertion was required to obtain sufficient chorionic tissue (at least 10 mg); in 9.3%, 2 insertions were required. In 19 cases (2.9%) an abnormal karyotype was established. Bleeding or spotting was reported by 1.5% of patients, and transient lower abdominal discomfort was reported by 10.2%. Among the 688 chromosomally normal pregnancies the overall fetal loss rate was 2.6% before 28 weeks' and .9% thereafter.

In women who were sampled before 12 weeks' gestation the fetal loss rate was 6.6%, compared to 1.8% for those who were sampled after 12 weeks'. This difference was statistically significant. Seventy-five percent of women who experienced fetal loss after a TA-CVS performed before 12 weeks' gestation suffered the loss within 2 weeks of the procedure; only 30% of women sampled after 12 weeks' gestation who experienced fetal loss did so within 2 weeks of TA-CVS. The fetal loss rate was unrelated to the number of needle insertions.

When performed after the natural decrease in fetal loss rate (after 12 weeks' gestation), TA-CVS appears to be a safe option for women of advanced age.

▶ The technique was described as recently as 1986 and is now refined and appears especially useful in older mothers when used after the 12th week of gestation. A much larger trial would be useful to fully evaluate its risks and benefits.—M.H. Klaus, M.D.

Hypothalamic-Pituitary-Adrenal Axis Function in Very Low Birth Weight Infants Treated With Dexamethasone

Alkalay AL, Pomerance JF, Puri AR, Lin BJC, Vinstein AL, Neufeld ND, Klein AH (Ahmanson Pediatric Ctr, Los Angeles; Cedars-Sinai Med Ctr, Los Angeles; Univ of California, Los Angeles)
Pediatrics 86:204–210, 1990   13–3

Dexamethasone is currently used in respirator-dependent very low birth weight infants with bronchopulmonary dysplasia (BPD). Because the initial dexamethasone dose in the current therapeutic regimen is significantly higher than the physiologic secretory rate of hydrocortisone, and the tapering period extends over several weeks, the potential of causing suppression of the hypothalamic-pituitary-adrenal axis (HPAA) function exists. Using the metyrapone test, the effects of dexamethasone therapy on the HPAA was evaluated prospectively in 10 very low birth infants with BPD who had a mean birth weight of 825 g, mean gestation of 25.8 weeks', and postnatal age of 33.1 days. Dexamethasone, 0.5 mg/kg/day, was given intravenously for 3 days, and then tapered off over a mean period of 45 days to a replacement dose.

Five infants had normal metyrapone test results (group A) and 5 had abnormal test results (group B); the 2 groups did not differ in birth weight, gestational age, and age when entered into the study. Compared with group B, group A infants had significantly higher basal plasma cortisol levels, higher postmetyrapone 11-deoxycortisol levels, and larger differences between basal and postmetyrapone levels of cortisol and 11-deoxycortisol. Duration of dexamethasone therapy was longer in group A than in group B. The metyrapone test eventually became normal in group B infants when they continued to receive low-dose dexamethasone therapy after a period of 36.8 days. Side effects of dexamethasone therapy were transient and easy to manage.

Dexamethasone therapy is associated with suppression of HPAA function in a substantial number of very low birth weight infants with BPD. The HPAA function should be evaluated before discontinuation of dexamethasone therapy to ensure proper adrenal secretory response.

▶ The following comment was contributed by Art D'Harlingue, M.D., Neonatologist, Children's Hospital Oakland, California:

▶ Although prenatal steroids have been clearly shown to be safe and efficacious in the prevention of respiratory distress syndrome (RDS), the same statement cannot yet be made for the use of steroids for BPD. Several published randomized control studies of the use of steroids to treat BPD have shown improvement in oxygen requirements and ventilator settings. However, steroids do not appear to have much effect on the long-term pulmonary outcome. All of these studies have been relatively small in size, so the true incidence of complications as a result of steroids for BPD treatment is not yet defined. The present study demonstrates that some premature infants with BPD have significant suppression of adrenal function after the prolonged use of steroids. Hence, these infants would be at risk for adrenal crisis. Other complications of steroids include hypertension, infection, gastrointestinal bleeding, impaired growth, and hyperglycemia. Steroids have been proposed for the treatment or prevention of several other neonatal diseases (perinatal asphyxia, necrotizing enterocolitis, severe RDS). Although some benefit has been reported for some of these problems, very little is known about the mechanism of effects. Steroids should be used with caution in the treatment of BPD. There should be close monitoring for complications of steroids both during and (as this study shows) after treatment.—A.D'Harlingue, M.D.

Changes in Vasopressin, Atrial Natriuretic Factor, and Water Homeostasis in the Early Stage of Bronchopulmonary Dysplasia
Kojima T, Fukuda Y, Hirata Y, Matsuzaki S, Kobayashi Y (Kansai Med Univ, Osaka; Tokyo Med and Dent Univ)
Pediatr Res 27:260–263, 1990   13–4

Edema, oliguria, hyponatremia, and increased plasma levels of arginine vasopressin (AVP), have been reported in some children with chronic bronchopulmonary dysplasia (BPD). To determine if these changes also occur in the early stage of BPD, water and sodium balance, renal function, and plasma AVP and atrial natriuretic factor (ANF) concentrations were determined during the first 4 weeks of life in 9 infants in the early stage of BPD secondary to respiratory distress syndrome and 5 healthy low birth weight infants.

At the fourth week of life, arterial carbon dioxide pressure was increased more in infants with BPD compared with low birth weight infants. Both plasma AVP and ANF levels were also higher in infants with BPD. Urine osmolality was increased and free water clearance was decreased in infants with BPD at the fourth week of life compared with those in low birth weight infants.

Increased plasma AVP levels may be related to pulmonary abnormalities in the early stage of BPD. Water retention established in response to hypersecretion of AVP may stimulate the secretion of ANF; hence, ANF may compensate the effect of AVP in the early stage of BPD.

▶ This is a sequel to the studies of Hazinski (1) that confirms the elevated levels of AVP in infants with early stages of BPD. It has been postulated that AVP is secreted in response to pulmonary hypovolemia secondary to air trapping, which in turn decreases left atrial filling and reduces pressures in the left atrium. There was an attenuated response to AVP in the preterm infants, thus, changes in plasma osmolality were not demonstrated. An added wrinkle was the documentation that ANF was also elevated, presumably as a counter-regulatory response to AVP. Atrial natriuretic factor has potent natriuretic and diuretic activities and may also suppress AVP release. Disturbances in water regulation appear to be an integral component of BPD. There are no direct clinical implications at this time, but with further elucidation of these complex interactions perhaps a rationale for therapy will emerge.—A.A. Fanaroff, M.B.B.Ch.

Reference

1. 1989 YEAR BOOK OF NEONATAL AND PERINATAL MEDICINE, Abstract 14–10.

Hormonal-Metabolic Stress Responses in Neonates Undergoing Cardiac Surgery

Anand KJS, Hansen DD, Hickey PR (Harvard Univ)
Anesthesiology 73:661–670, 1990

13–5

The process of living is the process of reacting to stress.—Dr. S. J. Sarnoff

Hormonal and metabolic responses were examined in 15 neonates who had repair of complex congenital cardiac defects during standardized anesthesia. Anesthesia included halothane, ketamine, morphine, pancuronium, and an oxygen-air mixture. All infants survived the surgery, but 4 died in the intensive care unit.

All infants had increases in plasma catecholamines, cortisol, glucagon, and β-endorphin. Insulin levels rose at the end of surgery and remained elevated for 24 hours. Hyperglycemia and lactic acidemia developed during surgery and persisted afterward. The infants who died tended to have more marked stress responses during and after surgery, although they were not distinct from the survivors on the usual clinical and hemodynamic grounds. The differences were apparent before cardiopulmonary bypass and the creation of new hemodynamics could have influenced the hormonal and metabolic responses.

The pattern of neonatal stress response differs from that seen in adult cardiac surgery patients. It is associated with a high hospital mortality rate. Whether the catabolic state is a cause or an effect of poor outcome in cases where the operation itself seems adequate remains uncertain, but there is some suggestion that extreme stress responses may underly poor outcomes.

▶ Previous studies in neonates confirmed that like adults the stress responses to surgery correlate with morbidity and mortality. This is another major contribution from Anand et al. to a subject area that has been largely neglected. (See also the 1988 YEAR BOOK OF NEONATAL AND PERINATAL MEDICINE, and Reference 1.) Cardiac surgery is often performed on precarious neonates who have had poor perfusion with metabolic acidosis. Not surprisingly, it carries a high mortality. In light of the limited functional capabilities of immature organ systems, understanding the stress responses, facilitating them, and providing the optimal thermal and metabolic milieu are mandatory to reduce this morbidity and mortality. It is noteworthy that the infants who did not survive were already manifesting a frank catabolic status at the start of the surgery and demonstrated extreme hormonal responses to surgery. Voluminous data from these few subjects merely represent the tip of the iceberg. More patients must be investigated to confirm these patterns. The cardiothoracic surgeons have perfected many of their techniques and can tackle all the anomalies. Evaluation and correction of metabolic status before surgery may be critical to improving survival.—A.A. Fanaroff, M.D.

Reference

1. Anand KJS, et al: *Br Med J* 296:668, 1988.

Accuracy and Reliability of Glucose Reflectance Meters in the High-Risk Neonate

Lin HC, Maguire C, Oh W, Cowett R (Women and Infants Hosp of Rhode Island; Brown Univ, Providence)
J Pediatr 115:998–1002, 1989   13–6

Because glucose reflectance meters have been found convenient and reliable in the maintenance of euglycemia in adults, the accuracy and reliability of 4 currently available glucose reflectance meters were determined in the neonatal intensive care setting. Glucose concentrations were measured by the Glucometer M, Diascan S, Accu-Chek II, and One Touch meters that use whole blood obtained by capillary heelstick in 25 randomly selected neonates. The results were compared to those of cord arterial blood from 25 other neonates as analyzed on the Yellow Springs Instrument (YSI) glucose analyzer and the 4 glucose reflectance meters.

Blood glucose concentrations in heelstick capillary blood and cord arterial blood measured with the glucose reflectance meters exhibited wide variability relative to the values obtained by the YSI analyzer (table). There were significant differences in the correlation between heelstick capillary blood values obtained with the glucose reflectance meters, except the One Touch meter, and the cord blood and the heelstick capillary

Accuracy of Reflectance Meters Versus YSE Glucose Analyzer

Reflectance meter	Cord	Heel	p
Difference between means (%)			
Glucometer M	−9.3	−23.2	
Diascan S	0.4	−0.4	
Accu-Chek II	1.2	16.4	
One Touch	35.2	25.6	
Correlation coefficient (r)			
Glucometer M	0.88	0.64	<0.05
Diascan S	0.96	0.71	<0.01
Accu-Chek II	0.91	0.71	<0.05
One Touch	0.92	0.86	NS

Abbreviations: NS, not significant.
(Courtesy of Lin HC, Maguire C, Oh W, et al: *J Pediatr* 115:998–1000, 1989.)

blood glucose values obtained with the YSI analyzer. Except for the Accu-Chek II, there were no significant differences in the reliability between cord blood and heelstick capillary blood with the various glucose reflectance meters and the YSI analyzer. However, there was no relationship between the accuracy and reliability of the glucose reflectance meters.

Glucose reflectance meters should probably not be used for evaluation of capillary blood glucose concentrations in the high-risk neonate.

▶ Satish Kalhan, M.D., Professor of Pediatrics, Department of Pediatrics, Rainbow Babies and Children's Hosp, Cleveland, comments as follows:

▶ Although blood/plasma glucose is one of the commonest analyses performed in the newborn nursery or the intensive care unit, its measurement remains fraught with multiple errors. The laboratory results are probably influenced by sampling methods, the transport technique, and the analytical method used. For example, blood samples from a polycythemic infant obtained by heelstick are likely to give different results than that from the central venous site. Furthermore, samples obtained by repeated heelstick, and thus inflicted pain, are likely to have higher glucose values than those from indwelling lines. Blood samples transported to the laboratory immediately and on ice to prevent glycolysis by red blood cells are more likely to reflect the true glucose concentration of the infant than those that are transported at room temperature and left lying around before analysis. Finally, the whole blood glucose concentration is somewhat lower than plasma glucose concentration and the different laboratory analytical methods often give different measurements of glucose concentration, which are confusing for the clinician.

The long laboratory turnaround time involved in obtaining blood glucose concentrations and the problems identified above led to the development of rapid bedside chemical strip methods. However, ever since these chemical strips were introduced some 20 years ago, controversy has raged about their accuracy. To decrease the bias of the human eye in the assessment of color change on the chemical strip, bedside reflectance meters were introduced to precisely define the change in color and relate it to glucose concentration. Although these chemical strips have been very useful for the management of adults with diabetes where glucose concentration is maintained around 100 mg/dL, the accuracy of these strips for measurement of blood glucose in low concentration, i.e., less than 50 mg/dL, in newborn infants has been questionable. Thus, the above study by Lin et al. is very timely in pointing out the inaccuracies involved with the use of these methods. As concluded at a recent CIBA Foundation Discussion Meeting, "The use of glucose oxidase reagent sticks in the neonate may be best eliminated and replaced by a glucose analyzer" (1). Conrad et al. have demonstrated that clinical nurses in the intensive care unit can learn these methods with excellent precision (2). However, whether this old habit can ever be discontinued after having once introduced these methods into the nursery remains an open question. It has always been easy to bring new technologies into the nursery, but takes a long time to prove their worthiness. Not only are we continuing to debate the "definition of hypoglycemia," we still argue about how to measure the "true blood sugar." These thorny issues need prompt resolution so that rational clinical management can follow.—S. Kalhan, M.D.

References

1. Cornblath M, et al: *Pediatrics* 85:834, 1990.
2. Conrad PD, et al: *J Pediatr* 114:281, 1989.

Longitudinal Changes in the Bone Mineral Content of Term and Premature Infants

Pittard WB III, Geddes KM, Sutherland SE, Miller MC, Hollis BW (Med Univ of South Carolina, Charleston)
Am J Dis Child 144:36–40, 1990   13–7

Rickets of prematurity is a well-recognized disorder of bone mineralization in very low birth weight neonates. Deficiencies in calcium and phosphorus intake are thought to be important contributing causes. Some have hypothesized that premature infants with minimal illness who received no parenteral nutrition would have improved bone mineralization when compared with very low birth weight neonates who required more medical support.

Photon absorptiometry was used to measure bone mineralization in 12 very low birth weight premature infants at birth and at 8 and 16 weeks

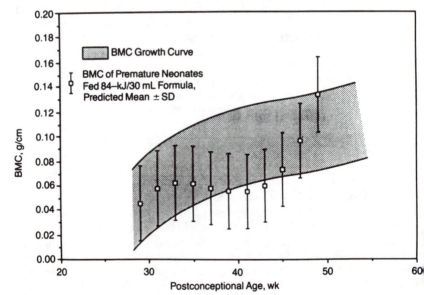

Fig 13–1.—Estimated upper and lower 95% confidence interval limits for normal bone mineral content determined from observations after 29 to 42 weeks of gestation plus 8- and 16-week observed values of term infants. The mean (± standard deviation) predicted bone mineral content (BMC) for preterm infants is superimposed. (Courtesy of Pittard WB III, Geddes KM, Sutherland SE, et al: *Am J Dis Child* 144:36–40, 1990.)

after delivery. These infants had a mean gestational age of 31 weeks and required minimal medical support. Nineteen healthy term infants were studied simultaneously. All infants received modified 84–kJ/30 mL formula without added calciferol throughout the study. Each infant received 400 IU daily of calciferol as an oral supplement. Serum levels of 25-hydroxyvitamin D, calcium, phosphorus, and parathyroid hormone were monitored biweekly and were normal.

At birth bone mineral content and bone width differed significantly between premature and term infants. By 16 weeks, however, premature infants had exceeded the bone mineral status of term infants at birth, and their bone mineral content was not significantly less than that of term infants.

The data indicate a more rapid rate of bone mineralization in premature neonates in this series than has been previously reported in similar infants who required more extensive medical support. After 4 weeks of age, the bone mineral content in these premature infants increased steadily at a rate consistent with that found in term infants (Fig 13–1).

▶ Contributing his comment is Art D'Harlingue, M.D., Neonatologist, Children's Hospital Oakland, California:

▶ This study of the bone mineralization in healthy premature infants, who did not require parenteral nutrition, has 2 important findings. First, the bone mineral content (BMC) of relatively healthy premature infants can increase to normal levels by 16 postnatal weeks while feeding an infant formula containing levels of calcium and phosphorus much below these available in current premature infant formulas. Second, the growth of bone width in the premature infant may be accelerated by premature delivery as compared to normal intrauterine bone growth. However, normal BMC by 16 postnatal weeks in these premature infants was preceded by little change in the BMC over the span of 30 to 43 weeks' postconceptional age. In fact, at about 40 to 43 weeks' postconceptional age the mean BMC of these premature infants was below the lower 95% confidence interval limits for normal intrauterine BMC. This suggests that some nutrient (most likely calcium and phosphorus) was lacking during the postnatal growth of these premature infants. The infants then demonstrated some "catch up" in bone mineralization, so that their BMC was normal by 16 postnatal weeks. This "catch up" in BMC has been seen in other studies. The premature infant must retain about 150 mg/kg/day of calcium and 80 mg/kg/day of phosphorus in order to match the intrauterine accretion of these minerals. Most of this calcium and phosphorus is deposited in bone and contributes to the bone mineral content. Multiple factors can interfere with normal bone mineralization in the premature infant. Inadequate mineral intake is the most important problem, and this is particularly true for the infant who requires prolonged parenteral nutrition. Even with enteral feedings there can be problems. Calcium and phosphorus bind to the plastic tubing during continuous nasogastric feedings. Formulas high in calcium and phosphorus must be thoroughly mixed before feeding, or else mineral salts will be left behind as precipitate in the bottom of the bottle. Calcium losses in the urine are increased by the use of furosemide, phosphorus depletion syndrome, and the use of steroids. The accelerated growth of bone width may exacerbate the problem of osteopenia, as the premature infant must mineralize a rapidly growing bone matrix. All of these problems are greatly enhanced in extremely low birth weight infants of less than 1,000 g. I would recommend that all premature infants of less than 1500 be provided sufficient calcium and phosphorus in their enteral feedings to approximate intrauterine retention of these minerals. Infants fed human milk will require further supplementation with a commercial fortifier or the addition of calcium and phorphorus to the feedings. For those infants not receiving human milk, a premature infant formula high in calcium and phosphorus should be used until the infant is about 1,800 to 2,000 g. Supplemental vitamin D should be provided to all premature infants of less than 1,500 g at a dose of 400 IU per day. Pharmacologic doses of vitamin D (2,000–5,000 IU/day) may actually excerbate osteopenia of prematurity.—A. D'Harlingue, M.D.

14 The Genitourinary Tract

Relation of Rate of Urine Production to Oxygen Tension in Small-for-Gestational-Age Fetuses
Nicolaides KH, Peters MT, Vyas S, Rabinowitz R, Rosen DJD, Campbell S
(King's College School of Medicine, London)
Am J Obstet Gynecol 162:387–391, 1990   14–1

One consequence of redistribution of fetal blood flow in fetal hypoxemia is reduced renal perfusion, which results in decreased urine production. To investigate further the relationship between urine production and fetal blood oxygen tension, the hourly fetal urine production rate (HFUPR) was determined by real-time ultrasonography immediately before cordocentesis for blood gas analysis in 27 small-for-gestational-age (SGA) fetuses at 20–37 weeks' gestation. The results were compared with those in 101 appropriate-for-gestational-age (AGA) fetuses. Fourteen SGA fetuses had associated oligohydramnios.

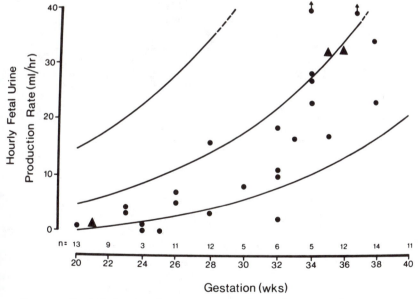

Fig 14–1.—Hourly fetal urine production rate in 27 SGA fetuses (chromosomes abnormal, *filled triangles;* normal, *filled circles*) plotted on reference range (mean and individual 95% confidence intervals) constructed from study of 101 normal pregnancies. (Courtesy of Nicolaides KH, Peters MT, Vyas S, et al: *Am J Obstet Gynecol* 162:387–391, 1990.)

In SGA fetuses the mean HFUPR was significantly lower than in AGA fetuses (Fig 14–1). Furthermore, the decrease in urine production correlated significantly with both the degree of fetal hypoxemia and the degree of fetal smallness. Comparison of the 14 cases with oligohydramnios and the 13 without showed no significant differences in degree of decrease in urine production or degree of fetal hypoxemia.

These data provide further evidence that in fetal hypoxemia there is redistribution in blood flow with a decrease in renal perfusion and a subsequent decrease in HFUPR. It appears that urine production may reflect fetal oxygenation, but further studies are warranted to define its value in assessment of fetal well-being.

▶ There are many theories governing the conditions that result in growth failure in utero. The proliferation of more sophisticated ultrasonographic equipment, together with the increased utilization of umbilical blood sampling from the fetus, forms the background for establishing a relationship between fetal growth, fetal blood gas status, and hourly urinary production. The data presented above suggest that the growth-retarded fetuses produce less urine per hour, presumably because of redistribution of cardiac output in response to chronic fetal hypoxia. The net effect is reduced quantities of amniotic fluid and even gross oligohydramnios. Indomethacin may also reduce fetal urine production (1).

Although we are dazzled with many numbers and the usual statistical manipulations, I accept for the moment only the broad principles enuciated. Measurements of hourly urine production differ considerably from previously published reports and require validation from other investigators. These bladder watchers have contributed another piece to the physiologic puzzle of the fetus that fails to thrive in utero. We will watch for further clinical correlations.

Life is a gamble at terrible odds—if it was a bet you wouldn't take it— Tom Stoppard.

A.A. Fanaroff, M.B.B.Ch.

Reference

1. 1989 Year Book of Neonatal and Perinatal Medicine, Abstract 1–15.

Increased Renal Echogenicity in the Neonate
Chiara A, Chirico G, Comelli L, De Vecchi E, Rondini G (Policlinico San Matteo IRCCS, Pavia, Italy)
Early Hum Dev 22:29–37, 1990   14–2

Ultrasound is a well-established diagnostic tool for assessing renal anatomy. It is particularly valuable in the neonate because it involves no ionizing radiation, it is noninvasive, and it can be done without moving the neonate from the incubator. Data on infants with increased renal echogenicity were evaluated.

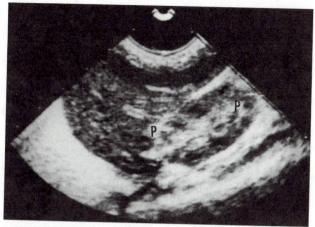

Fig 14–2.—Renal disease secondary to perinatal asphyxia (longitudinal scan): increased pyramids echogenicity. P = pyramid. (Courtesy of Chiara A, Chirico G, Comelli L, et al: *Early Hum Dev* 22:29–37, 1990.)

A review of 1,600 abdominal ultrasonic assessments revealed increased renal echogenicity in 103 newborn infants (56 girls). Birth weights ranged from 560 to 3,700 g, and gestational age ranged from 25 to 42 weeks. Diffuse hyperechogenicity was noted in 3 infants with infantile polycystic kidney disease, 2 with renal candidiasis, 3 with dysplastic kidney, and 2 with renal vein thrombosis. Three infants with hemolytic-uremic syndrome had cortical hyperechogenicity. Ninety infants with renal disease secondary to perinatal asphyxia showed increased medullary echogenicity (Fig 14–2). Renal function and evaluation of renal echogenicity improved in 76 infants; renal changes in the remaining 14 persisted until death.

Ultrasonography is useful in infants with renal failure for assessment of presence, size, morphology, and echogenicity of the kidneys. The most common cause of renal failure is the hypoxia and hypoperfusion that follow a decrease in systemic blood pressure caused by perinatal asphyxia and other disorders.

▶ We have asked Roy A. Cohen, Pediatric Radiologist, Children's Hospital Oakland, Oakland, California, for his thoughts on this article:

▶ Ultrasound is frequently used in the evaluation of renal disease in neonates. As stated in the article, the renal cortex of neonates frequently has the same echogenicity as the liver or spleen, whereas the adult renal cortex is less echogenic. Also, the medullary pyramids are more conspicuous in neonates (not to be confused with hydronephrosis).

Most of the cases of increased echogenicity in the neonates reported in this article were the result of perinatal asphyxia. The cause of the increased echogenicity of the medullary pyramids is not well understood but may be attributable in part to precipitation of Amon Horsfall proteins.

The authors do not include another important cause of increased medullary echogenicity: Neonates receiving chronic diuretic therapy (e.g., furosemide) sometimes exhibit nephrocalcinosis. In this case, ultrasound shows increased medullary echogenicity and/or calcification with acoustical shadowing.—R.A. Cohen, M.D.

Natural History of Pelviureteric Obstruction Detected by Prenatal Sonography

Arnold AJ, Rickwood AMK (Royal Liverpool Children's Hosp, England)
Br J Urol 65:91–96, 1990   14–3

The management of infants with prenatally diagnosed pelviureteric obstruction is not clear, particularly with regard to the role of pyeloplasty. To investigate, the natural history of pelviureteric obstruction was analyzed in 56 infants who had prenatal radiologic or sonographic evidence of pelviureteric obstruction. Operative intervention was advised only when initial renographic assessment of the affected kidney was below 40% of total. Renographic assessment was obtained at a mean age of 3 months (range, 1–9 months), and differential renal function was assessed from estimated glomerular filtration rate (^{99m}Tc-diethylenetriaminepentaacetic acid), effective renal plasma flow (^{123}I hippuran, ^{99m}Tc-mercaptoacetyltriglycine), or differential uptake of isotope (^{99}Tc-dimercaptosuccinic acid).

Pelviureteric obstruction was not confirmed by radiographic criteria in 11 infants but was confirmed in 45 others. Of these, 17 underwent immediate (15) or delayed (2) pyeloplasty, including 6 who had differential renal function <40% of total. All had satisfactory anatomical results. The remaining 28 patients (30 renal units) with renographic evidence of obstruction and differential function exceeding 40% of total were managed nonoperatively. Among the 18 infants (19 renal units) who had follow-up renography at a mean age of 26 months (range, 10–54 months), persistent obstruction was seen in 11. Sonography showed improving hydronephrosis in 8 kidneys, with resolution in 5 others and no change in 6. In the other 10 infants (11 renal units), hydronephrosis improved in 4, resolved in 1, and remained unchanged in 6.

Early pyeloplasty should be restricted to a modest number of infants with impaired renal function. A conservative approach may be adapted in infants with normal renal function in whom the natural history appears essentially benign. These findings do not support the policy of routine pyeloplasty for prenatally diagnosed pelviureteric obstruction.

▶ We chose this paper because the approach differed from that in North America. In the United States it is widely believed that infants with prenatally diagnosed pelvoureteric obstruction should undergo surgery in the neonatal period. The authors deliberately did not do renography in the neonatal period, when renal function is rapidly adapting from a high fetal to low postnatal urinary output. They suggest that this probably explains the spontaneous improvement observed within the first weeks after birth. It also demonstrates how vital it is to know the wide range of normal in the fetus before submitting these infants to surgery. The conservative approach described in this report will probably gradually alter our own management.—M.H. Klaus, M.D.

Peritoneal Dialysis in the First 60 Days of Life

Matthews DE, West KW, Rescorla FJ, Vane DW, Grosfeld JL, Wappner RS, Bergstein J, Andreoli S (Indiana Univ; James Whitcomb Riley Hosp for Children, Indianapolis)

J Pediatr Surg 25:110–116, 1990   14–4

Peritoneal dialysis is technically feasible in very small infants and may decrease the morbidity and mortality associated with renal failure in the newborn. During a 7-year period, 31 neonates and infants less than 60 days old (average age, 23 days) underwent peritoneal dialysis for congenital metabolic disorders, acute tubular necrosis, postcardiopulmonary bypass with renal failure, renal cortical necrosis, obstructive uropathy, renal agenesis, and bilateral renal dysplasia. With Tenckhoff catheters of modified length, hourly exchanges of 20 cc/kg were started immediately after catheter insertion.

Effective dialysis, defined as resolution of hyperkalemia, uremia, hyperammonemia, acidosis, and/or fluid overload in the presence of oliguria or anuria, was possible in all infants. The average duration of catheter use was 16 days (range, 1–73 days). Complications included peritonitis in 4 infants, bowel perforation in 1, exit site infection in 2, inguinal hernias in 3, umbilical hernia in 1, and retroperitoneal hemorrhage in 1. Nineteen (61.3%) patients died between 1 and 90 days post insertion, but all deaths were related to the near-moribund condition of the patients, as evidenced by high scores on the physiologic stability index. Of the 12 survivors, 5 continued to undergo chronic dialysis while awaiting renal transplantation.

Peritoneal dialysis is effective in the management of metabolic derangements and renal failure in the newborn period. Infants who survive the acute illness requiring peritoneal dialysis can generally progress to outpatient chronic ambulatory peritoneal dialysis and possible renal transplantation.

▶ This commentary is contributed by John Stork, M.D., Assistant Professor of Pediatrics, Rainbow Babies and Childrens Hospital, Case Western Reserve University School of Medicine, Cleveland, Ohio.

▶ The need for dialysis in the neonatal period is thankfully rare. Our experience at Rainbow with peritoneal dialysis in infants is similar to that of these authors, with a few caveats. First, despite the increased technical difficulties, hemodialysis remains our therapy of choice in infants with hyperammonemia. A high clearance of ammonia is of paramount importance, and normalization of ammonia levels can be achieved much more rapidly with hemodialysis. Using percutaneous access (internal jugular) and a umbilical venous catheter, we have hemodialyzed infants as small as 1,900 g. Activated clotting time can be used to monitor heparin dosage, and we have not had bleeding complications. I agree that peritoneal dialysis is effective and should be used if hemodialysis is not readily available.

Second, although our complications have been similar with peritoneal dialysis, we have also seen frequent hyperglycemia, necessitating insulin therapy, because of the neonate's limited rate of glucose metabolism. Therapy is required to maintain adequate ultrafiltration. Hernias in our experience may also limit efficacy of dialysis if they are large and trap dialysate. We have seen omental obstruction of the catheter. This seems more common in the neonate, as the omentum is filmy and can migrate into the catheter, obstructing all holes.

Third, I would like to have seen data on the effectiveness of dialysis, rather than simply accept the authors' blanket statement that dialysis is effective. Inadequate ultrafiltration has been a common problem in our postoperative cardiac infants with poor cardiac outputs. I would expect that this is because of poor perfusion of the splanchnic bed, with decreased blood flow to the peritoneal membrane. In our experience, continuous hemofiltration procedures have been more effective in these patients and have not been associated with increased or more serious complications. Such procedures do require technical expertise, as well as increased nursing and physician time. Further, for infants with congenital renal anomalies or uncomplicated acute renal failure, peritoneal dialysis is clearly the method of choice and can be performed successfully for extended periods of time.—J. Stork, M.D.

15 Developmental Pharmacology and Toxicology

Pharmacokinetics of Dopamine in Critically Ill Newborn Infants
Padbury JF, Agata Y, Baylen BG, Ludlow JK, Polk DH, Habib DM, Martinez AM
(Harbor-UCLA Med Ctr; Univ of California at Los Angeles, Torrance)
J Pediatr 117:472–476, 1990   15–1

Inotropic agents are used extensively in the intensive care unit in both neonates and older children. Because there is little pharmacokinetic data on their use, particularly during critical illness, plasma levels of dopamine were measured in 14 critically ill newborn infants whose birth weights ranged from 900 to more than 4,000 g; gestational age was from 27 to 43 weeks. Dopamine was administered through a calibrated infusion pump in stepwise increasing doses up to 8 µg/kg/min. Dopamine concentration and dopamine clearance rates were determined from duplicate samples drawn during each infusion in each patient.

The plasma dopamine concentration increased by .5 ng/mL before infusion to 69.3 ng/mL at an infusion rate of 4–8 µg/kg/min. There was a significant linear correlation between infusion rate and plasma dopamine concentration. Dopamine plasma clearance rate averaged 59 mL/kg/min, and neither plasma dopamine concentration nor infusion rate had any effect on plasma clearance rate over the range of concentrations studied. These data demonstrate a first-order kinetics of dopamine administered to critically ill newborn infants during infusion rates varying from 1 to 8 µg/kg/min.

▶ Despite the fact that inotropic agents are used with almost gay abandon in the intensive care unit, there are very few pharmacokinetic data available. Pharmacokinetics were investigated in of 14 patients first reported in 1986 when a log linear relationship between plasma dopamine level and hemodynamic response was observed. For the nonpharmacologists, and I rank myself in this group, this translates into a need for a logarithmic increase in dopamine level, above threshold, to achieve a linear increase in hemodynamic response (1). The present publication documented first-order kinetics with regard to dopamine infusions and also presented data on dopamine metabolism. A better understanding of the pharmacology of dopamine should assist the clinician striving to sustain a neonate in shock.

There is nothing more productive of problems than a really good solution.—Dr. Nathan S. Kline

A.A. Fanaroff, M.B.B.Ch.

Reference

1. Padbury JF: *J Pediatr* 110:293, 1986.

Pharmacokinetics of a Single Dose of Morphine in Preterm Infants During the First Week of Life

Bhat R, Chari G, Gulati A, Aldana O, Velamati R, Bhargava H (Univ of Illinois; St Joseph's Hosp, Chicago)
J Pediatr 117:477–481, 1990   15–2

Morphine is a commonly used analgesic in the newborn period, but its pharmacokinetics have been evaluated only in children and term infants. The pharmacokinetics of a single parenteral dose of morphine was studied in preterm newborn infants during the first week of life. Pharmacokinetic data obtained after the intravenous administration of a single dose of morphine, .1 mg/kg, were evaluated in 20 newborn infants of 26–40 weeks of gestation who were younger than 5 days. The 10 infants in group 1 were born at 30 weeks of gestation, the 7 infants in group 2

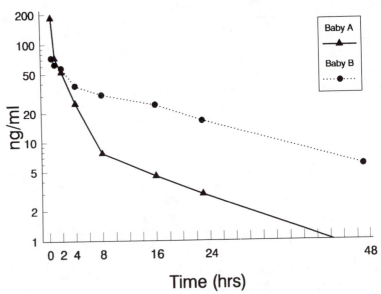

Time (hrs)

Fig 15–1.—Typical examples of serum morphine levels in 2 infants: Infant A, with a birth weight of 2,860 g and a gestational age of 40 weeks, had βt½ of 5.8 hours and a clearance of 6.6 mL/kg/min. Infant B, with a birth weight of 920 g and a gestational age of 28 weeks, had a βt½ and a clearance of 1.452 mL/kg per minute. (Both axes are in log scale.) (Courtesy of Bhat R, Chari G, Gulati A, et al: *J Pediatr* 117:477–481, 1990.)

were born at 31–37 weeks of gestation, and the 3 infants in group 3 were born at 38–40 weeks of gestation.

The mean distribution half-life ($\alpha t\frac{1}{2}$) was 50 minutes in group 1, 41 minutes in group 2, and 19 minutes in group 3. The mean elimination half-life ($\beta t\frac{1}{2}$) was 10 hours in group 1, 7.4 in group 2, and 6.7 hours in group 3. A linear regression model showed a declining trend for both $\alpha t\frac{1}{2}$ and $\beta t\frac{1}{2}$ (Fig 15–1); however, there was marked variation within groups. Serum morphine levels remained at 12 ng/mL or greater 4 weeks after administration in 5 of 10 infants born at 31 weeks or more of gestation. Similarly, the same morphine level was maintained at 8 hours after initial dosing in 8 of 10 infants born at 30 weeks or less of gestation. Total body clearance rate of morphine increased progressively with increasing gestation, from 3.39 mL/kg/min in group 1 to 15.5 mL/kg/min in group 3. Only 18% to 22% of the drug was protein bound in preterm and term infants, respectively.

There is marked variation in the pharmacokinetics of morphine in the neonatal period. Nearly 80% of the intravenously infused drug remains free, which may explain the increased sensitivity to morphine during the neonatal period. In the first week of life, morphine can be administered at intervals of 4–6 weeks in term infants and at less frequent intervals in very premature infants.

▶ The barbaric era wherein painful procedures, including major surgery, were performed on newborn babies without benefit of analgesia has thankfully passed. Unfortunately, there is a paucity of information concerning the pharmacokinetics, metabolism, and appropriate doses of analgesics for both term and preterm infants. Furthermore, there is a singular lack of objective measures of pain response in this population.

Studies of narcotic dependency in adults suggest that imprinting may result from exposure to narcotics in utero. This raises serious concerns about their use in the neonatal period. The optimal agents for analgesia in newborns, as well as their short- and long-term side effects must be established.

There is an increased experience, but still limited knowledge, with respect to powerful narcotics such as morphine. It is opportune that the above investigators provide us with some insights into the pharmacokinetics of a single dose of morphine in preterm infants. A few subjects yield a flurry of calculations and linear regression equations. In summary, guidelines for morphine administration to achieve analgesia are suggested, but like all good investigators who strive to perpetuate both careers and research funding, these authors conclude that more studies are needed. They will not get any argument from this corner.—A.A. Fanaroff, M.B.B.Ch.

Gentamicin in Neonates: The Need for Loading Doses

Gal P, Ransom JL, Weaver RL (Moses H. Cone Mem Hosp, Greensboro, NC; Univ of North Carolina)
Am J Perinatol 7:254–257, 1990   15–3

Gentamicin is frequently chosen for initiating antibiotic therapy for neonates. Target gentamicin peak concentrations are 5–10 μg/mL and target trough concentration are less than 2 μg/mL. Initial gentamicin dosing guidelines use doses of 2.5 mg/kg at varying dosing intervals of 12–24 hours.

A series of 184 neonates with a gestational age of 25–44 weeks and with a birth weight from 660 to 4,786 gm were admitted to the neonatal intensive care unit (NICU) with possible sepsis. The initial gentamicin loading dose was 5 mg/kg administered intravenously. No gentamicin had been administered before admission to the NICU or as maternal treatment. Gentamicin therapy was begun on day 1 in 145 neonates; therapy was started in only 1 neonate after day 4 and that was on day 10. The neonates were categorized in 4 gestational age groups based on Ballard examination: less than 28 weeks, 28–30 weeks, 31–34 weeks, and more than 34 weeks.

Comparison of calculated immediate postinfusion concentrations revealed no dependency of extrapolated peak concentrations on timing of the initial gentamicin concentrations, consequently permitting data from all patients to be combined. Mean extrapolated, postinfusion, peak gentamicin concentrations were as follows: group 1, 7.81 μg/mL; group 2, 8.08 μg/mL; group 3, 8.46 μg/mL; and group 4, 9.37 μg/mL. In only 4 patients (2.2%) were the peak levels less than 5 μg/mL, and 7 (3.8%) had extrapolated peaks above 12 μg/mL, with the highest being 15 μg/mL.

When a proportional relationship between peak concentrations attained and dose is assumed, an initial dose of 2.5 mg/kg would have failed to attain initial peak concentrations of 5 μ/mL in 18 of 19 neonates of less than 28 weeks' gestation, 44 of 49 neonates of 28–30 weeks' gestation, 49 of 55 neonates of 31–34 weeks' gestation, and 39 of 61 neonates of more than 34 weeks' gestation.

These data support the need for greater loading doses of gentamicin in newborns. The recommended dose of gentamicin of 5 mg/kg achieves concentrations known to be safe and effective.

▶ Gentamicin remains one of the drugs of choice in initiating antibiotic therapy in neonates. Concerns for toxicity have resulted in careful monitoring of trough and peak levels at steady state with little attention paid to early peak levels. The authors present compelling data for using a larger loading dose. Peak levels achieve desired therapeutic ranges more than 90% of the time, and a relationship between gentamicin concentrations early in treatment and toxicity has not been established, nor is it likely on theoretical considerations. In fact, transient peak concentrations above 12 μg/mL are less hazardous than the risks of gram-negative infection when inadequate peak concentrations are achieved during the first 24 hours of therapy. Watterberg (1) reported that 19% of infants achieved peak gentamicin levels of less than 5 μg/mL after 3 maintenance doses. In adults, Moore (2) reported an increased mortality in patients with gram-negative infections who did not achieve early adequate peak gentamicin levels. The important message is not only should larger loading doses be used, but gentamicin levels must also be closely monitored in order to walk the fine line between attaining optimal therapeutic levels and avoiding toxicity (3,4).—A.A. Fanaroff, M.B.B.Ch.

References

1. Watterberg KL, et al: *Ther Drug Monit* 11:16, 1987.
2. Moore RD, et al: *J Infect Dis* 149:443, 1984.
3. 1987 YEAR BOOK OF NEONATAL AND PERINATAL MEDICINE, Abstract 16–4.
4. 1988 YEAR BOOK OF NEONATAL AND PERINATAL MEDICINE, Abstract 15–11.

Pharmacokinetics, Outcome of Treatment, and Toxic Effects of Amphotericin B and 5-Fluorocytosine in Neonates
Baley JE, Meyers C, Kliegman RM, Jacobs MR, Blumer JL (Rainbow Babies and Children's Hosp, Cleveland; Case Western Reserve Univ)
J Pediatr 116:791–797, 1990   15–4

Current antifungal drug dosing in very-low-birth-weight and term infants is based on studies performed on older infants and children. The pharmacokinetics, therapeutic response, and toxic effects of amphotericin B and 5-fluorocytosine (5-FC) were evaluated in 13 neonates (mean birth weight, 1.2 kg; range, .6 to 3.3 kg), including 11 born at 27 weeks' gestation and 2 born at 36 and 40 weeks' gestation.

The dose of amphotericin B was serially increased from .1 to .5 mg/kg/day in 10 infants; in 3 infants the dose of .8 to 1 mg/kg/day was subsequently reduced to .5 mg/kg/day. Treatment with 5-FC was begun on the same day as amphotericin B at a dose of 25 to 100 mg/kg/day. Serum

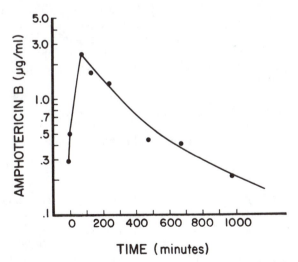

TIME (minutes)

Fig 15–2.—Serum concentration-time curve of steady-state amphotericin B level showed drug elimination in 9 infants between doses. (Courtesy of Baley JE, Meyers C, Kliegman RM, et al: *J Pediatr* 116:791–797, 1990.)

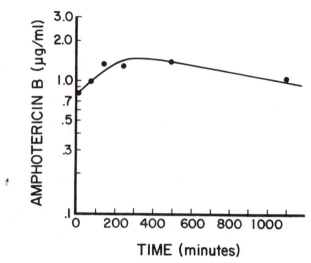

TIME (minutes)

Fig 15–3.—Serum concentration-time curve of steady-state amphotericin B level showed minimal drug elimination in 4 infants during dosing interval. (Courtesy of Baley JE, Meyers C, Kliegman RM, et al: *J Pediatr* 116:791–797, 1990.)

concentrations were measured at first dose and after 5 days of therapy by high-performance liquid chromatography.

Amphotericin B was detectable only in infants who received .8 to 1 mg/kg/day, but not in those who received .1 mg/kg/day. Drug elimination between doses was detectable in 9 infants (Fig 15–2), whereas minimal or no drug elimination between doses was observed in 4 (Fig 15–3). The latter was associated with increases in serum levels of creatinine (more than .4 mg/dL, 40 μmol/L) and blood urea nitrogen (more than 10 mg/dL, 3.6 mmol/L). Drug concentration in the CSF was 40% to 90% of serum concentrations. With 5-FC, all infants had detectable serum concentrations after the oral dose. There was remarkable interindividual variability for the half-life, volume of distribution, and clearance for both amphotericin B and 5-FC.

It is recommended that the initial dose of amphotericin B be .5 mg/kg/day to achieve a therapeutic level quickly, and the initial dosing interval be at least 24 hours for both amphotericin B and 5-FC. Serum concentrations of the drugs should be monitored in high-risk, low-birth-weight infants.

▶ With increased frequency, fungal infections intrude during the sojourn of low-birth-weight infants in the intensive care unit. My colleagues have attempted to fill a long-standing void by establishing data concerning the pharmacokinetics of amphotericin and 5-FC. Amphotericin remains the primary drug for the treatment of systemic fungal infections, whereas the role of 5-FC remains controversial. Regrettably, the total cumulative effective dose of amphotericin remains unknown. Nonetheless, it was definitively demonstrated that a dose of less than .5 mg/kg/day did not achieve significant serum levels, but commencing with such a dose had no adverse effects. The recommendation for .5 mg/kg/day as the initial dose to quickly achieve therapeutic levels appears justified. Thereafter, amphotericin should be administered once every 24 hours. Because of the unpredictable pharmacokinetic response in the immature infant, with no drug elimination between doses a frequent finding, serum levels should be monitored to avoid toxicity. Admittedly, these are not earth-shattering recommendations, but they are now based on some foundation. Newer antifungal agents such as fluconazole have been introduced successfully in adults with systemic fungal infections. Unfortunately, no data are yet available for neonates regarding these drugs.

Humor is a drug which it's the fashion to abuse.—*Sir William S. Gilbert*

A.A. Fanaroff, M.B.B.Ch.

Determination of Gestational Cocaine Exposure by Hair Analysis
Graham K, Koren G, Klein J, Schneiderman J, Greenwald M (The Hosp for Sick Children, Toronto)
JAMA 262:3328–3330, 1989   15–5

"It is easy to get hooked, it is difficult to break the habit."

Reports of pregnancy outcome after gestational cocaine use are increasing, but there is little consensus about the effects of gestational cocaine exposure, probably because of inaccurate identification of drug users. Maternal self-reported drug history is often unreliable, and standard blood and urine tests detect only recent cocaine use.

Because cocaine is deposited in the hair, hair samples were obtained from 16 admitted cocaine users who were participating in treatment programs, 21 adult controls with a cocaine-free history and negative urine screening tests, and 7 infants with known or suspected in utero exposure to cocaine. Hair extracts were analyzed by radioimmunoassay for the cocaine metabolite benzoylecgonine.

Hair from 16 adult cocaine users was positive for benzoylecgonine in the presence of negative findings from urine screening tests. The concentration of benzoylecgonine in hair samples was consistent with self-reported drug histories (Fig 15–4). The average concentration of benzoylecgonine in the 3 occasional users was 624 ng/g of hair, compared to an average of 8,775 ng/g of hair in the 13 heavy users. In contrast, none of the 21 control adults tested positive for benzoylecgonine. Hair from 7 neonates with a confirmed maternal history of cocaine use was positive for benzoylecgonine, with a mean concentration of 5,430 ng/g of hair. Hair from 2 infants aged 2.5 and 3.5 months contained benzoylecgonine, 4,300 and 7,800 ng/g of hair, respectively. However, hair from 3 infants aged 1 year and older contained no benzoylecgonine, corresponding to loss of fetal hair in the first few months after birth.

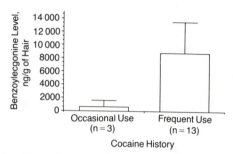

Cocaine History

Fig 15—4.—Detection of benzoylecgonine in hair of 3 occcasional and 13 frequent users of cocaine (95% confidence interval shown). (Courtesy of Graham K, Koren G, Klein J, et al: *JAMA* 262:3328–3330, 1989.)

Hair analysis may remedy the disadvantages of currently used methods for detecting cocaine use and may identify intrauterine exposure to cocaine in infants when a maternal drug history is not available or doubtful. Hair analysis cannot replace urine testing, because the former cannot detect recent cocaine use. In addition, its usefulness in defining in utero exposure is limited to the neonatal period.

▶ Drug use during pregnancy has assumed epidemic proportions despite the President's "war on drugs." The ability to establish fetal drug exposure has been refined. A combination of analyses, including hair, urine, and meconium (1) may now be used to document recent and remote cocaine use by the mother. Positive hair, but negative urine and meconium, would be consistent with fetal exposure during the first trimester. The above report includes a small patient sample. Currently, hair analysis is of limited value, as it provides no information about recent exposure. It may be used to distinguish occasional from heavy users. This is a simple and painless procedure. Further exposure will establish the role of hair analysis in the overall evaluation of cocaine use during pregnancy (See also Abstract 2–13).—A.A. Fanaroff, M.B.B.Ch.

Reference

1. 1990 YEAR BOOK OF NEONATAL AND PERINATAL MEDICINE, Abstract 16–1.

Effects of Indomethacin on Cerebral Haemodynamics in Very Preterm Infants
Edwards AD, Wyatt JS, Richardson C, Potter A, Cope M, Delpy DT, Reynolds EOR (Univ College and Middlesex School of Medicine, London)
Lancet 335:1491–1495, 1990   15–6

Intravenously administered indomethacin in adults may cause reductions in cerebral blood flow and its response to changes in arterial carbon dioxide tension. When indomethacin is used in infants for patent ductus arteriosus, cerebral blood flow may fall to unacceptably low levels. To study the effects of indomethacin on cerebral blood flow and to test

Group Mean (SD) Values of Cerebral Circulation Variables
Before and After Indomethacin

—	Rapid (n = 7)		Slow (n = 6)	
	Before	After	Before	After
Cerebral blood flow (ml.100 g^{-1}.min^{-1})	34 (12)	20 (12)	32 (6)	21(4)
Cerebral oxygen delivery (ml.100 g^{-1}.min^{-1})	3·8 (1·1)	2·2 (1·1)	3·5 (0·6)	2·2 (0·5)
Cerebral blood volume (ml/100 g)	2·7 (1·0)	2·3 (1·1)	3·1 (0·7)	2·8 (0·8)
Volume response to change in PaCO$_2$ (ml.100 g^{-1}.kPa^{-1})	0·20 (0·05)	0·05 (0·05)	0·11 (0·03)	0

All values after indomethacin were significantly ($P < .005$, paired t test) lower than those before.
(Courtesy of Edwards AD, Wyatt JS, Richardson C, et al: *Lancet* 335:1491–1495, 1990.)

whether the rate of administration changes these effects, studies were made in 13 infants with patent ductus arteriosus.

Of the 13 preterm infants treated with indomethacin, 7 received indomethacin by rapid injection and 6 received it by slow infusion. Near infrared spectroscopy showed that cerebral blood flow, oxygen delivery, blood volume, and the reactivity of blood volume to changes in arterial carbon dioxide tension fell sharply in all infants (table). There were no differences in effects whether drug administration was fast or slow.

Levels of the decrease in cerebral blood flow in infants after indomethacin administration require further study. To prevent an oxygen deficit, especially in areas of precarious arterial supply, optimum cerebral oxygen delivery should be insured before indomethacin is given to preterm infants.

► The following comment was contributed by David K. Stevenson, M.D., Professor of Pediatrics; Chief, Division of Neonatal and Developmental Medicine; Director of Newborn Nurseries, Stanford Medical Center, Palo Alto, California:

► Edwards and co-workers describe an interesting bedside application of near-infrared spectroscopy. Although the information about cerebral blood flow and cerebral blood volume is derived indirectly, the changes observed with the administration of indomethacin raise interesting questions that cannot be answered by this study. Is there a measurable, permanent, long-term, adverse neurologic consequence of indomethacin treatment in the premature infant? The apparent changes in hemodynamics suggest a rationale for the protective effects of indomethacin against intracranial hemorrhage but raise the possibility of a potential critical reduction in global cerebral oxygen supply, which could cause injury in the boundary zones that are the site of periventricular leukomalacia in premature infants.

If, in fact, the authors are correct, it is important to recognize what their recommendations about ensuring optimal cerebral oxygen delivery before indomethacin is given mean to the clinician. For example, the administration of oxygen will do little to correct the changes caused by indomethacin if the oxygen-carrying capacity, saturation, and cardiac output are normal. Specifically, increasing the Fio_2 does not necessarily represent a preventive solution to the threat imposed by indomethacin, because the side effect is one of decreased cerebral blood flow or compromised O_2 delivery. A blood transfusion to increase the oxygen-carrying capacity, cardiotonic enhancement of cardiac output, or avoidance of hyperventilation might provide better insurance but still could be insufficient to protect against the effect of indomethacin on cerebral blood flow. In fact, cerebral blood flow in the human neonate is a difficult phenomenon to study, and indirectly derived estimates may be the only ones that can be made clinically. Near-infrared spectroscopy seems promising in this regard.

Nonetheless, further validation of these findings by independent measures is required, which would set the stage for other studies to evaluate long-term, neurologic consequences of such drug exposure independent of effect modifiers and other contributing causes of neurologic injury. Indomethacin may close the door on one kind of problem and open the door on another.—D.K. Stevenson, M.D.

Cerebral Lesions in Preterm Infants After Tocolytic Indomethacin

Baerts W, Fetter WPF, Hop WCJ, Wallenburg HCS, Spritzer R, Sauer PJJ (Erasmus Univ Hosp; Sophia Children's Hosp; Dykzigt Hosp, Rotterdam)
Dev Med Child Neurol 32:910–918, 1990   15–7

Indomethacin is a potent tocolytic agent, but its use has been limited by its potential adverse effects on the fetus and newborn infant. To determine the incidence and type of cerebral lesions in very preterm infants exposed antenatally to indomethacin, 159 infants born before 30 weeks' gestation were studied using 2-dimensional ultrasound. Indomethacin was given to 76 mothers as part of tocolytic management; the other 83 did not receive indomethacin or tocolysis was limited to fenoterol (control).

Except for the lower incidence of patent ductus arteriosus in infants exposed prenatally to indomethacin, the early neonatal courses were similar in both groups. The incidence and types of periventricular and intraventricular hemorrhages did not differ significantly between groups. There was a trend toward a higher incidence of periventricular leukomalacia (PVL) in the indomethacin group, and the difference was statistically significant for PVL II (table). Multivariate analysis showed that prenatal administration of indomethacin was independently and significantly related to PVL II.

These data show that tocolytic indomethacin may have negative effects on the severity of hypoxic-ischemic cerebral lesions in very preterm infants with gestational ages of less than 30 weeks. Considering the particularly poor prognosis of PVL II, tocolytic indomethacin should be used only after weighing the benefits of prolonging gestation.

Incidence of Cerebral Lesions vs. Tocolysis

	Group 1 (N = 83 (28*)) (no indomethacin)		Group 2 (N = 76) (indomethacin)		
	N	%	N	%	p
Normal	24 (6)*	29	22	29	NS
PIVH I	3	4	5	7	NS
PIVH II	17	20	9	9	NS
PIVH III	7	8	9	12	NS
PIVH IV	8	10	3	4	NS
All haemorrhages	35 (11)*	42	26	34	NS
PVL I	12	14	10	13	NS
PVL II	6	7	16	21	0·03**
All leukomalacias	18 (8)*	22	26	34	NS
Other lesions	17 (1)*	20	9	12	NS

*N, infants in group 1 exposed to tocolysis with fenoterol
**χ^2 analysis (2 df) = 64.
PVL I = periventricular flaring followed by ventricular dilatation; PVL II = cystic periventricular leukomalacia.
(Courtesy of Baerts W, Fetter WPF, Hop WCJ, et al: *Dev Med Child Neurol* 32:910–918, 1990.)

▶ What we have here, ladies and gentlemen, is an association, an extremely ugly association. Infants who were born prematurely and who had been exposed to indomethacin in utero were more likely to have PVL. Clinical conditions associated with PVL include asphysia, shock, anemia, apnea, endotoxemia, and prematurity. It is more common with advancing gestational age. Note that indomethacin was administered antenatally without randomization or control as part of obstetric management, and the results do not establish cause and effect. However, even if this proves to be a chance association it will in the interim furrow many a brow and produce much acid indigestion.

On the one hand, every attempt is made to inhibit premature labor and birth to eliminate such major complications as intracranial hemorrhage. On the other, we are confronted with a situation wherein the very agent used to inhibit premature labor may alter cerebral blood flow so that the PVL ensues. This is truly sitting between a rock and a hard place.

Previously reported major studies with tocolytic agents have not highlighted PVL as a complication, but how diligently was this specific problem looked for? There is thus a paradoxical situation wherein indomethacin reduces the risk for IVH postnatally but may increase the chance for PVL when administered to inhibit labor. A similar situation exists which phenobarbital. Antenatal administration reduces the incidence of intraventricular hemorrhage (see Abstract 15–8), but postnatal administration may increase the risk of hemorrhage in the most immature infants (1). One can only conclude that premature infants are unreliable subjects to work with. Would that we could reduce their numbers!—A.A. Fanaroff, M.B.B.Ch.

Reference

1. 1987 YEAR BOOK OF NEONATAL AND PERINATAL MEDICINE, Abstract 16–2.

Antenatal Phenobarbital for the Prevention of Periventricular and Intraventricular Hemorrhage: A Double-Blind, Randomized, Placebo-Controlled, Multihospital Trial

Kaempf JW, Porreco R, Molina R, Hale K, Pantoja AF, Rosenberg AA (Univ of Colorado; AMI St Luke's Hosp, Denver; St Joseph's Hosp, Denver)

J Pediatr 117:933–938, 1990.   15–8

"Sometimes a fool makes a good suggestion."—Nicholas Boileau.

Because hypoxia and ischemia play major roles in the pathogenesis of periventricular-intraventricular hemorrhage (PVH-IVH) in premature infants, it was hypothesized that agents would be more effective in reducing PVH-IVH when given before birth rather than postnatally. Two previous studies suggest that the antenatal administration of phenobarbital, an agent shown to be neuroprotective after cerebral hypoxic-ischemic insults in animals, significantly reduces the incidence and severity of PVH-IVH in premature infants.

To investigate further, 110 women at 31 weeks of gestation in whom delivery appeared imminent because of premature labor or with premature rupture of membranes or maternal-fetal complications necessitating elective delivery were randomly assigned to receive intravenous infusion of phenobarbital 10 mg/kg or placebo for 30 minutes in a blinded fashion before delivery. Infants were studied within the first 4 days of life with real-time ultrasonography.

Maternal demographics, pregnancy complications, antenatal management, and route of delivery did not differ significantly between the phenobarbital and placebo groups. The overall incidence of PVH-IVH was 20.4% among the 54 infants in the active drug group and 28.4% among the 67 in the placebo group; the difference was not significant. Similarly,

Periventricular-Intraventricular Hemorrhages

	Placebo (n = 67)		Phenobarbital (n = 54)	
	No.	%	No.	%
Normal	48	71.6	43	79.6
Grade 1	9	13.4	8	14.8
Grade 2	0	0	1	1.9
Grade 3	5	7.5 ⎤	0	0 ⎤
		⎥ 15%		⎥ 3.7%*
Grade 4	5	7.5 ⎦	2	3.7 ⎦
All grades	19	28.4	11	20.4

Results presented in this table represent the highest grade of hemorrhage noted on scans performed before 7 days of age.
*P < .05 compared with placebo.
(Courtesy of Kaempf JW, Porreco R, Molina R, et al: *J Pediatr* 117:933–938, 1990.)

the incidence of grade 1 or 2 PVH-IVH was about the same in the 2 groups. However, the frequency of grades 3 and 4 hemorrhage was significantly lower in the phenobarbital group (3.7%), compared to the placebo group (15%) (table). There were no differences in the severity of associated conditions in the infants to account for the difference in incidence of severe hemorrhage. These findings confirm previous reports of the efficacy of antenatal administration of phenobarbital in reducing the severity of PVH-IVH in infants delivered at 31 weeks' gestation.

▶ Add another chapter to the ongoing saga involving phenobarbital and IVH. The verdict on the postnatal administration of phenobarbital was negative (1). The phenobarbital group had a greater incidence of more severe hemorrhage in the more immature, lighter infants. Phenobarbital appeared ready for disposal to the wastelands of the therapeutic armamentarium as far as prevention of hemorrhage goes. However, there is some evidence, weakly supported by the present study, that the antenatal administration of phenobarbital reduces the incidence of severe IVH (2,3). This study by Kaempf et al. was prospective and fully blinded, and the incidence of hemorrhage in the control group (28.4%) was not greater than anticipated. The fetuses who had been exposed to barbiturate were sleepier, had lower Apgar scores, and were more likely to need assisted ventilation, certainly not a ringing endorsement for its administration. Also, the exclusion of infants who died on the first day of life may, however, have influenced the outcome data. My impression is that even these authors are not very confident with their results and only barely promote the use of phenobarbital. They plead the old standby, "More work is needed." We agree.—A.A. Fanaroff, M.B.B.Ch.

References

1. 1987 YEAR BOOK OF NEONATAL AND PERINATAL MEDICINE, Abstract 16−2.
2. Shankaran S, et al: *Am J Obstet Gynecol* 154:53, 1986.
3. Morales WJ, et al: *Obstet Gynecol* 68:295, 1986.

Effect of Intramuscular Vitamin E on Mortality and Intracranial Hemorrhage in Neonates of 1000 Grams or Less

Fish WH, Cohen M, Franzek D, Williams JM, Lemons JA (Indiana Univ, Indianapolis)
Pediatrics 85:578−584, 1990   15−9

Recent investigations indicate that vitamin E supplementation can effectively reduce the incidence of intracranial hemorrhage (ICH) and mortality in premature neonates. In a double-blind randomized study, the effects of the intramuscular administration of vitamin E on ICH and mortality were investigated in 149 neonates with birth weights of ≤1,000 g and age of 24 hours or less. The neonates were stratified into 2 groups by weight, 501−750 g and 751−1,000 g, and then randomly assigned to receive either placebo or vitamin E (*dl*-α-tocopherol) at doses of 15, 10, 10, and 10 mg/kg given intramuscularly on days 1, 2, 4, and 6 of life, respec-

Total and Severe Intracranial Hemorrhage

	Treatment	Placebo
All ICH		
501–750 g	7/24 (29%)*	15/25 (60%)
751–1000 g	17/44 (39%)	20/44 (45%)
All neonates	24/68 (35%)	35/69 (51%)
Severe ICH		
501–750 g	1/24 (4%)	8/25 (32%)
751–1000 g	10/44 (23%)	11/44 (25%)
All neonates	11/68 (16%)	19/69 (27%)

*$P = .045$.
†$P = .023$.
(Courtesy of Fish WH, Cohen M, Franzek D, et al: *Pediatrics* 85:578–584, 1990.)

tively. All neonates initially received vitamin E, 100 mg/kg/day *dl*-α-tocopherol acetate orally; this dose was subsequently adjusted to keep serum levels at .5–3.5 mg/dL. Ultrasound examinations of the head were performed on days 1, 5–7, and 12–14, when possible.

Neonatal or total hospital mortality rates did not differ significantly between placebo-treated and vitamin-E-treated neonates. Overall, there were no significant differences between groups in the incidence of all ICH or severe ICH. However, among the neonates weighing ≤750 g, all ICH, as well as severe ICH, was significantly less in the vitamin-E-treated group than in the placebo group (table). Among survivors, the incidence of severe ICH was significantly less in the vitamin-E-treated infants who weighed ≤750 g at birth. Except for mild induration at injection sites in 2 infants, no other serious side effects of vitamin E treatment were observed. Further, there was no significant increase in the incidence of necrotizing enterocolitis or sepsis in the vitamin-E-treated infants.

Previous findings that the supplemental intramuscular administration of vitamin E may play a role in preventing severe ICH in extremely premature infants were supported. Additional studies, however, are necessary before parenteral vitamin E can be recommended routinely for these infants.

▶ This represents another valiant, if not necessarily successful, effort to find a role for vitamin E in the treatment or prevention of a significant disorder in neonates. All of the ingredients for success are present. The study is prospective, randomized, blinded, and there is appropriate stratification. The diagnosis of intraventricular hemorrhage, the primary outcome variable, is reliably established with multiple ultrasound examinations. The study is accomplished with reasonably strict adherence to protocol and minimal side effects attributable to the intramuscular vitamin E administration with no increase in sepsis or necrotizing enterocolitis. Well, where is the catch? The problem emerges with the results. Vitamin E is really only effective for infants with birth weights below 750 g and not for those between 751 and 1,000 g. The difference in the low-weight group is powerful enough so that when the groups are combined there is a significant reduction in hemorrhage among the survivors. However, if all infants weighing less than 750 g who died and were not studied by ultrasound/autopsy had bleeds, this difference would disappear. The results, however, are moot. There is no available approved preparation of intramuscular vitamin E, nor is there a sufficient market to galvanize the pharmaceutical industry to remedy this deficiency.

Whereas the conclusions from the study are in accordance with those of other clinical studies, they only "suggest" that vitamin E may be efficacious. Vitamin E prevents intraventricular hemorrhage allegedly by reducing lipid oxidants, stabilizing membrane lipids, and quenching oxygen radicals. Previous studies have suggested optimal tissue levels of vitamin E. However, the best product, timing of first dose, dosage, and the target population have yet to be clearly delineated. Vitamin E therefore remains on the sidelines, rooted to the bench, but eager to be a player in the neonatal arena.

The approach to preventing intraventricular hemorrhage is once again covered in this YEAR BOOK (see Abstracts 7–13 and 10–3).—A.A. Fanaroff, M.B.B.Ch.

16 Miscellaneous Topics

The Scars of Newborn Intensive Care
Cartlidge PHT, Fox PE, Rutter N (City Hosp, Nottingham, England)
Early Hum Dev 21:1–10, 1990   16–1

Many techniques used in neonatal intensive care are invasive, and the risk of producing skin damage is high. One hundred consecutive newborns discharged from neonatal intensive care between March and December 1985 were studied. The group included all infants who received assisted ventilation, parenteral nutrition, and major surgery. Gestational age was less than 32 weeks in 48 infants and between 32 and 36 weeks in 36; 16 were term infants. Birth weight was a median of 1,700 g. Ninety-seven children were white, 2 were Asian, and 1 was black. Eighteen infants were admitted for a surgical condition, and surgery was also

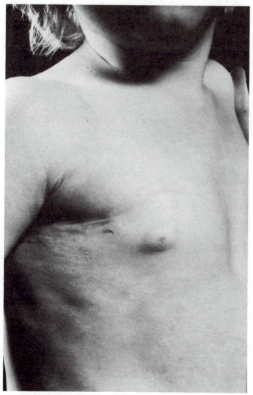

Fig 16–1.—Disfiguring scars on chest of girl aged 2 years. Upper puckered scars are caused by thoracocentesis tubes. Scar below this and extending laterally follows stripping of skin by removal of adhesive tape. (Courtesy of Cartlidge PHT, Fox PE, Rutter N: *Early Hum Dev* 21:1–10, 1990.)

required to treat complications in 14 infants admitted primarily for medical reasons.

Each child was examined by the same observer between 16 and 29 months of age to assess the incidence and severity of iatrogenic skin damage. The severity of lesions was graded on a 4-point scale. Seventy children had also been examined immediately before discharge to allow assessment of the predictive power of early examination in recognizing scar severity.

Each child had scars attributable to invasive procedures during neonatal intensive care. The number of lesions was inversely related to the child's gestational age and directly related to the duration of intensive care. Eleven children had cosmetically or functionally important scars (grade 3 or 4) caused by central venous catheter insertion, extravasation of intravenous fluid, or by chest drains (Fig 16–1). Four of these children and 7 others also had grade 3 scars caused by thoracic or abdominal surgery for congenital defects or necrotizing enterocolitis. Most children, however, had very minor scarring. Fifty-nine children had grade 1 lesions, but many were so inconspicuous parents had not noticed them. Early examination was able to predict scarring from cosmetically and functionally important lesions but not from minor lesions caused by needles or burns from transcutaneous oxygen monitoring. These lesions were rarely evident before age 6 months.

In this series all infants had some, generally trivial, scarring. To reduce the frequency and severity of skin damage in neonates, the staff should be aware that many routine procedures may lead to long-term scarring. Careful wound closure after removal of chest drains is particularly important.

▶ Although the parents accepted uncritically the disfiguring scars, in the future the children will not be as tolerant. Skin stripping at the dermoepidermal junction (as noted in Figure 16–1) should not occur in the future as less adherent tape is used in conjunction with various barriers between the tape and the skin. Greater precautions are required in the care of smaller and more fragile infants because they have even thinner and more easily damaged skin. With anterior chest wall tube insertion, additional caution is also advised to prevent damage to the developing breast tissue.—M.H. Klaus, M.D.

Congenital Neuroblastoma: Evaluation With Multimodality Imaging
Forman HP, Leonidas JC, Berdon WE, Slovis TL, Wood BP, Samudrala R (Schneider Children's Hosp, Long Island Jewish Med Ctr, New Hyde Park, NY; Babies Hosp, Columbia Presbyterian Med Ctr, New York; Children's Hosp of Michigan, Detroit; Univ of Rochester Med Ctr, NY)
Radiology 175:365–368, 1990 16–2

The efficacy of the newer imaging modalities in the diagnosis of neonatal neuroblastoma was evaluated in a retrospective study involving 12 patients with histologically proven congenital neuroblastoma. Prenatal ultrasound was performed in 4 patients; findings were nonspecific in 2 and consistent with a cystic or solid suprarenal mass in the other 2. Postnatal ultrasound in 11 infants accurately defined the adrenal tumor in 10; the tumors were solid in 8, cystic in 1, and mixed in appearance in 1. Postnatal ultrasound confirmed 5 of 7 (71%) liver metastases and was falsely negative in 2. Computed tomography accurately defined all tumors in 6 patients, as well as the presence or absence of liver metastases. Magnetic resonance imaging helped to define the correct diagnosis in 3 patients.

At an average follow-up of more than 3 years, 10 patients were alive and well. Of 6 patients with stage IV-S disease, 5 (83%) were alive. One infant with stage IV disease died, and another died of complications.

This study confirms the benign course of congenital neuroblastoma. Considering this, aggressive diagnostic imaging modality is less desirable. Despite its limitations, ultrasound may be the only procedure needed to establish the diagnosis. Magnetic resonance imaging may be a good alternative in some cases.

▶ This report attempts to make sense of new clinical data and to define how to evaluate and utilize information on a tumor that has often up to now appeared discretely and disappeared without worrying anyone. The large screening trials for catecholamine metabolites in 57,000 infants from Quebec studies at 3 weeks and 6 months will intensify efforts to learn how to manage this elusive tumor without injuring the patients (1).—M.H. Klaus, M.D.

Reference

1. Tackman M, et al: *Pediatrics* 86:765, 1990.

Intrauterine Spermatic Cord Torsion in the Newborn: Sonographic and Pathologic Correlation
Brown SM, Casillas VJ, Montalvo BM, Albores-Saavedra J (Univ of Miami—Jackson Mem Med Ctr, Miami)
Radiology 177:755–757, 1990   16–3

The radiologic findings of spermatic cord torsion that occurs as a scrotal mass in the neonate were reviewed. Five full-term newborns had a firm, enlarged, nontender scrotal mass. Sonography revealed an enlarged and globular testis, skin thickening, and hydrocele in all patients. The presence of fibrosis within the infarcted testis suggests that infarction may have resulted from in utero torsion in at least 4 patients. Surgery confirmed the diagnosis of spermatic cord torsion. A normal testis and epididymis with hydrocele in a newborn is shown.

Extravaginal torsion may occur because the testicular tunics are loosely attached to the scrotum in the in utero period. After birth, the scrotal attachments form rapidly and make extravaginal spermatic cord torsion unlikely beyond the newborn period.

The differential diagnosis of a scrotal mass in a newborn may include neoplasm and infection. However, radiologists should be aware that neonatal spermatic cord torsion presents as a mass. The radiologist should recognize the distinctive sonographic appearance of an enlarged and globular testis, hydrocele, and skin thickening in this entity.

▶ It brings a lump to my throat to even think about torsion of the testis in utero. That is the ultimate in bad luck. The testis is doomed even before it starts to function. The paper is written from a radiologic perspective and even suggests that radiologists may examine patients. That is obviously farfetched. The clinician performing the newborn physical must be aware that the presence of a mass in the scrotum may indicate spermatic cord or testicular torsion. Ultrasonography provides a definitive diagnosis, and exploration by the surgeon is merely administration of last rites for what would have been a noble organ. Lest I be accused of sexism, I am equally empathetic with the rare condition of torsion of the ovary.

"A phrase is born into the world both good and bad at the same time. The secret lies in a slight, an almost invisible twist."—Isaac Babel.

A.A. Fanaroff, M.B.B.Ch.

How Do Parents of Babies Interpret Qualitative Expressions of Probability?
Shaw NJ, Dear PRF (St James's Univ Hosp, Leeds, England)
Arch Dis Child 65:520–523, 1990   16–4

"Of that there is no matter of doubt—
No probable, possible shadow of doubt—
No possible doubt whatever."—Sir William S. Gilbert.

Qualitative expressions of probability, such as "probably" and "likely," are used by the medical profession to express views about diagnosis and prognosis. Because their meaning may be critical to the correct interpretation of the information being transmitted, 100 mothers and 50 medical students and physicians were interviewed to examine their understanding of 8 common probability expressions. Each respondent was asked to translate the expression of probability in 8 statements, given in the context of an imagined setting with an infant, into numerical value on a scale of 0 to 10.

For the mothers there was a wide range of interpretation for each expression of probability, as well as considerable overlap of values for the expressions. For the physicians and medical students, there was a wide range of interpretation for 4 expressions such as "probably," "possible," "sometimes," and "occasionally," but not for extremes of the scale (Fig 16–2). In all but 1 expression, significant differences in interpretation were evident between the professional and nonprofessional group. Most mothers preferred to receive information in numerical terms.

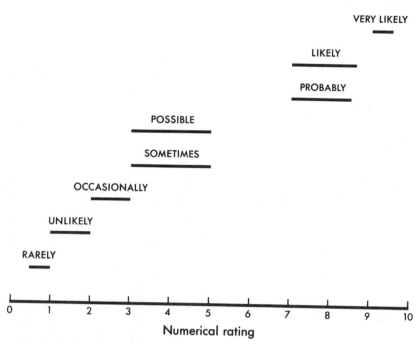

Fig 16–2.—Numerical interpretation of probability expressions by doctors and students (interquartile ranges). (Courtesy of Shaw NJ, Dear PRF: *Arch Dis Child* 65:520–523, 1990.)

There was wide variation in the interpretation of common expressions of probability not only by mothers but also among the medical profession. Qualitative expressions of probability should be restricted, and more information should be presented in numerical terms. It is essential that verbal expressions of probability be avoided when the information being given is to be used as a basis for making a decision.

▶ This is an interesting manuscript. Frequently used terminology was "quantitated" by lay parents, pediatricians, and medical students. The recommendation is that instead of using "vague" terms, specific numbers and risks be presented. I take exception to that as a global recommendation. There are times when precise numbers are indeed helpful and should be quoted; at other times specific numbers only add a layer of anxiety to an already stressful situation for the family. My own preference is to use numbers so that the infant's course can be described semiquantitatively. The tendency for caretakers to dazzle families with sophisticated terminology and complex numbers must be avoided.

Presentations should be simple and repetitive so that the family is brought up to speed at a pace they are comfortable with and can comprehend.—A.A. Fanaroff, M.B.B.Ch.

17 Outcome—Postnatal Growth and Development

Phototherapy for Neonatal Hyperbilirubinemia: Six-Year Follow-Up of the National Institute of Child Health and Human Development Clinical Trial
Scheidt PC, Bryla DA, Nelson KB, Hirtz DG, Hoffman HJ, and Principal Investigators (Natl Inst of Child Health and Human Development; Natl Inst of Neurological Disorders and Stroke, Bethesda, Md)
Pediatrics 85:455–463, 1990

17–1

The long-term effects of phototherapy used for the treatment of neonatal hyperbilirubinemia remain to be defined. To address this, the National Institute of Child Health and Human Development undertook a multicenter, randomized, collaborative study to assess whether phototherapy used to control the serum bilirubin level is safe and is as effective in preventing brain injury as exchange transfusion. The neurosensory, neuromotor, and cognitive development of the children at ages 1 year and 6 years was evaluated.

The Randomized, Controlled Trial of Phototherapy for Neonatal Hyperbilirubinemia was conducted at 6 neonatal care centers where 1,339 newborn infants were randomly assigned to phototherapy or control groups by the following subgroups: (1) birth weight <2,000 g; (2) birth weight 2,000–2,499 g and bilirubin level >171 μmol/L (10 mg/dL); or (3) birth weight ≥2,500 g and bilirubin level >222 μmol/L (13 mg/dL). Phototherapy was administered for 96 hours, and exchange transfusion was administered to both groups when serum bilirubin levels reached predetermined levels.

At follow-up, 83% of the patients returned for 1-year and 58% for 6-year examinations. Mortality and diagnosed medical conditions did not differ significantly between phototherapy and control groups. At 6 years the phototherapy and control groups had similar rates of cerebral palsy (5.8% vs. 5.9%); other motor abnormalities, including clumsiness and hypotonia (11.1% vs. 11.4%); and sensorineural hearing loss (1.8% vs. 1.9%). Similarly, overall scores on the Wechsler Intelligence Scale for Children-Revised were not significantly different between groups. These findings were consistent in each of the birth weight groups, ethnic groups, and 6 centers individually.

Phototherapy can effectively control neonatal hyperbilirubinemia without evidence of adverse outcome at 6 years of age and in this series was at least as effective as management with exchange transfusion alone. Still, phototherapy should be used with the same concerns for possible unknown adverse effects as for any therapeutic intervention in the newborn infant.

▶ M. Jeffrey Maisels, M.B.B.Ch., Professor of Pediatrics, Wayne State University School of Medicine, University of Michigan Medical School, and Chairman, Department of Pediatrics, William Beaumont Hospital, our resident bilirubin commentator, offers the following insightful remarks on this paper:

▶ This is an important study because it is a detailed 6-year follow-up of infants who were entered into a randomized controlled trial. Although only 58% of survivors were examined at age 6 years, this study provides some reassurance about the overall safety of phototherapy. Perhaps more interesting is the fact that, although phototherapy reduced peak serum bilirubin levels and the duration of hyperbilirubinemia, it had *no effect* on neurologic or developmental outcome. Thus the primary effect of phototherapy was to *reduce the bilirubin level and the risk of exchange transfusion, rather than the risk of brain injury.* The authors conclude: "With respect to the outcome measures assessed in this study, we believe that phototherapy is a safe and effective treatment," We should recognize that the treatment referred to is the reduction of serum bilirubin. But hyperbilirubinemia in infants is a possible risk factor, not a disease, and reduction of the serum bilirubin level should be seen as a means of improving the developmental outcome rather than an end in itself. It is also a pity that the study protocol required exchange transfusions in nonhemolyzing full-term infants in both the phototherapy and control groups when the bilirubin level reached 20 mg/dL (342 μm/L). Thus we are no wiser about the crucial question of whether serum bilirubin concentrations above these limits are dangerous for these infants.—M.J. Maisels, M.B.B.Ch.

High-Frequency Oscillatory Ventilation Compared With Conventional Intermittent Mechanical Ventilation in the Treatment of Respiratory Failure in Preterm Infants: Neurodevelopmental Status at 16 to 24 Months of Postterm Age
HIFI Study Group (Natl Heart, Lung and Blood Inst, Bethesda, Md; Univ of California, San Diego; Case Western Reserve Univ; Univ of Manitoba, Winnipeg; Univ of Miami; et al)
J Pediatr 117:939–946, 1990   17–2

Ten centers participated in a controlled clinical trial to compare the efficacy and safety of the new technology of high-frequency oscillatory ventilation (HFO) with intermittent mechanical ventilation (IMV) in low-birth-weight, premature infants with respiratory failure. Infants were assigned randomly to 2 groups, with 327 in the HFO group and 346 in the IMV group. Psychometric evaluations that used the Bayley Scales of Infant Development and a detailed neurologic examination were performed at 16–24 months of postterm age.

At follow-up, the proportion of children with a normal neurodevelopmental status was significantly less in the HFO than in the IMV group.

There was no difference in growth or respiratory status at follow-up. Cerebral palsy was diagnosed in 10% of the HFO-treated infants and 11% of the IMV-treated infants. There was a significantly higher incidence of hydrocephalus (12% vs. 6%) in the HFO group. In both groups there was a strong association between the presence of intraventricular hemorrhage and the development of major CNS or cognitive defects.

There were no significant long-term beneficial or deleterious effects in the use of HFO vs. IMV in the treatment of respiratory failure in low-birth-weight, premature infants. Because the HFO group had a higher proportion of survivors with intraventricular hemorrhage, there was an accompanying trend of more neurologic deficits.

▶ When the original production fails to reach Broadway, the odds against the sequel hitting the big time are even greater. The original report comparing oscillatory ventilation with conventional ventilators failed to show any difference in survival rates or incidence of biparietal diameter (BPD) (1). This manuscript details the neurodevelopmental follow-up status of the ventilated infants during infancy. As was eminently predictable from the increased incidence of intraventricular hemorrhage (IVH) among the oscillator group, they now had more hydrocephalus. Regrettably, many of the survivors with IVH in the conventional group were lost to follow-up. The incidence of cerebral palsy was approximately 10% in both groups, lower than in infants with BPD requiring prolonged ventilation (2,3), but nonetheless greater than in most premature infants.

This excellent study produced a negative result. The critics are harsh, searching for and finding blemishes and flaws. My contention is that the study was fundamentally sound, well designed, and well carried out. Studies are designed to answer questions—preconceived notions and well-thought-out hypotheses are often incorrect, thus results don't always meet expectations, yielding unanticipated findings. That does not detract from the quality of the study. That is the saga of the HIFI trial.

"The great secret of doctors, known only to their wives, but still hidden from the public, is that most things get better by themselves; most things are better in the morning."—Dr. Lewis Thomas.

A.A. Fanaroff, M.B.B.Ch.

References

1. 1990 YEAR BOOK OF NEONATAL AND PERINATAL MEDICINE, Abstract 11–5.
2. Skidmore MD, et al: *Dev Med Child Neurol* 32:325, 1990.
3. Vohr BR, et al: *Am J Dis Child* 136:443, 1982.

Prematures With and Without Regressed Retinopathy of Prematurity: Comparison of Long-Term (6–10 Years) Ophthalmological Morbidity
Cats BP, Tan KEWP (Univ Children's Hosp, Utrecht, The Netherlands; Royal Dutch Eye Hosp, Utrecht)
J Pediatr Ophthalmol Strabismus 26:271–275, 1989

17–3

Most follow-up ophthalmologic studies of premature infants have been limited to 1–3 years. At age 6–10 years long-term ophthalmologic sequelae in 42 exprematures with regressed forms of retinopathy of prematurity (ROP) in the neonatal period were compared with sequelae in 42 matched non-ROP infants.

Ophthalmologic disorders were identified at follow-up in 55% of the ROP group and 36% of the control group. The duration of supplemental oxygen in the neonatal period did not relate to the risk of later eye disease. Six of 7 patients who had stage III ROP had subsequent problems, compared with 17 of 35 who had stage I or II ROP. All 3 children with stage III disease who underwent cryotherapy of the avascular retina had subnormal vision at follow-up. Both children with late retinal detachment had had stage I or II ROP.

Regular follow-up and ophthalmologic assessment is necessary in children who have had ROP. Premature infants without ROP also should be followed, regardless of the presence or absence of CNS sequelae. Strabismus and astigmatism are frequent in both groups.

▶ The ongoing toll of prematurity is exemplified by this report, which comprises a follow-up of 6–10 years of premature infants admitted from April 1977 to March 1981. The primary objective of this study was to compare the overall incidence of ocular problems in children with and without ROP in the neonatal period. The ophthalmologic investigation consisted of inspection and cover tests for squint, visual acuity tests, and refraction by streak retinoscopy. The ophthalmologic problems were defined as intermittent heterotropia (manifest squint), amblyopia, myopia, or astigmatism. Decreased vision in at least 1 eye was a prominent feature in the ROP group. The presence of eye abnormalities in 55% of the infants with ROP was higher than anticipated but not entirely unexpected; however, the detection of eye problems in 36% of the non-ROP group mandates close ophthalmologic follow-up of all low-birth-weight graduates from the intensive care unit. Visual disturbances may compound any learning disability. We can only speculate as to the outcome for current graduates who are the beneficiaries of earlier aggressive cryotherapy for retinopathy. This may be offset by the survival of smaller, less mature infants who are at greater risk for other eye abnormalities (1).

For I dipped into the future, far as human eye could see, Saw the Vision of the world, and all the wonder that would be.—Alfred Lord Tennyson.

A.A. Fanaroff, M.B.B.Ch.

Reference

1. 1990 YEAR BOOK OF NEONATAL AND PERINATAL MEDICINE, Abstract 18–8.

Neurodevelopmental Performance of Very-Low-Birth-Weight Infants With Mild Periventricular, Intraventricular Hemorrhage: Outcome at 5 to 6 Years of Age

Lowe J, Papile L (Univ of New Mexico, Albuquerque)
Am J Dis Child 144:1242–1245, 1990   17–4

The introduction of noninvasive cranial imaging techniques has resulted in the recognition that periventricular intraventricular hemorrhage (PIVH) occurs often in very low-birth-weight (VLBW) infants. The long-term developmental outcome of such infants with PIVH was examined.

Thirty-eight VLBW neonates were followed prospectively from birth to 5 or 6 years of age. All neonates were screened for PIVH within 5–10 days after birth. Eleven had mild PIVH and 27 had none. All children were developmentally normal at 1–2 years of age. The 38 children were matched by race, age, gender, and socioeconomic status with a group of children born at term. At 5 and 6 years of age, all of the children who had been born with VLBWs scored significantly lower than the normal control group on combined test measurements and on 3 of 4 individual measurements (table). The VLBW group with PIVH scored significantly lower than the VLBW group without PIVH on the combined test measures only.

Infants of VLBW are at risk for subsequent learning problems. Although VLBW children with mild PIVH did not have a significant deficit on individual test scores, the significant difference on the combined battery of tests suggests that PIVH may adversely affect global performance.

▶ Although we continue to observe the adverse effects of mild PIVH on school performance in LBW infants with a normal IQ, there are beginning to be reports of improvement in the number of VLBW babies (500–750 g) who survive and of a possible reduction in the number of major handicaps they have (see Abstract 4–2). Because of the small number of survivors between 500 and 700 g, many further studies will have to be evaluated to determine whether this is truly an improvement in the quality of survival.—M.H. Klaus, M.D.

Outcome Measurements for Very Low—Birth-Weight Infants and Matched Control Children Born at Term

	Term (n = 22)	VLBW (n = 38)	P
Postnatal age, mo	72.7 (60-85)	72.0 (60-84)	...
McCarthy Scales of Children's Ability	117 (89-141)	97 (71-123)	<.01
Test of Early Reading Ability	104.1 (79-139)	84.9 (55-126)	<.01
Developmental Test of Visual-Motor Integration	11.9 (9-16)	9.8 (4-15)	NS
Benton Finger Localization			<.01
R	9.2 (8-10)	7.5 (3-10)	
L	9.1 (7-10)	7.1 (3-10)	

Note: Values are means with range in parentheses.
Abbreviations: VLBW, very low–birth-weight; *NS,* not significant.
(Courtesy of Lowe J, Papile L: *Am J Dis Child* 144:1242–1245, 1990.)

Six Year Follow Up of Infants With Bacteriuria on Screening

Wettergren B, Hellström M, Stokland E, Jodal U (Gothenburg Univ, East Hosp, Sweden)
Br Med J 301:845–848, 1990   17–5

Several studies indicate that pyelonephritic renal scarring commonly occurs early in life. In a prospective 6-year study, 3,581 infants in a defined area in Gothenburg underwent screening for bacteriuria to determine whether screening for bacteriuria in infancy may identify individual children at risk of sustaining renal damage. Of these, 50 (14 girls, 36 boys) had bacteriuria confirmed by suprapubic aspiration. Regular checkups for at least 6 years included urine culture and determinations of C reactive protein concentrations, evaluation of renal concentrating capacity with a desmopressin test, and radiologic studies that included measurement of renal parenchymal thickness and renal surface area. Children with asymptomatic bacteriuria and normal findings on initial urography were not treated, although other infections were treated.

Of the 50 infants with screening bacteriuria, 37 were followed for at least 6 years. In 2 infants pyelonephritis developed within 2 weeks after bacteriuria was diagnosed; the remaining 48 infants were asymptomatic. Forty-five infants were not treated; bacteriuria cleared spontaneously in 36 and after antibiotic treatment for other infections in 8.

Bacteriuria recurred in 10 children, including 1 with pyelonephritis, but none of these children had more than 1 recurrence. Follow-up urography in 36 children after a median 32 months showed no renal damage in terms of caliceal deformity or renal parenchymal thickness. First samples tested for renal concentrating capacity showed significantly higher values in infants with bacteriuria, compared with a reference population. However, analysis of the last samples showed no significant difference. These data suggest that mass screening for bacteriuria in infancy results in detection of innocent bacteriuric episodes and is not recommended.

▶ It should be emphasized that the initial screening of the 3,581 infants was with a bag urine. Superpubic aspiration was performed in infants with more than 50,000 bacteria in 2 successive bag samples. This thorough, long-term study from Sweden demonstrates that mass screening for a symptomatic bacteriuria in infants is not a useful tool for preventing renal disease. It also makes us reconsider the significance of bacteriuria in healthy infants.—M.H. Klaus, M.D.

Survival and Outcome of Infants Weighing <800 Grams at Birth

Lipper EG, Ross GS, Auld PAM, Glassman MB (New York Hosp-Cornell Univ, New York; Yeshiva Univ)
Am J Obstet Gynecol 163:146–150, 1990   17–6

Several previous studies have examined the influence of perinatal factors on survival of infants with birth weights of less than 1,000 g. Neo-

Long-Term Outcome of 28 Infants Weighing Less Than 800 g at Birth

Mental development/intelligence quotient score

	≥85	71-84	≤70
Neurologic classification			
Normal (*n* = 16)	8	8	0
Suspect (*n* = 9)	5	2	2
Abnormal (*n* = 3)	0	0	3
Attention-deficit hyperactivity disorder		11	
Visual impairment		10	
Sensorineural hearing loss		1	
Rehabilitation, special education		17	
Weight < 10th percentile		17	
Height < 10th percentile		16	
Microcephaly		3	

(Courtesy of Lipper EG, Ross GS, Auld PAM, et al: *Am J Obstet Gynecol* 163:146–150, 1990.)

natologists have reported improved survival rates of infants weighing less than 800 g at birth, but most studies have reported outcomes for infants this small who were born between 1975 and 1980. Data were reviewed on 184 infants with birth weights of 500–799 g born from 1980 through 1985. The effects of maternal and early neonatal variables on survival were analyzed and the neural development of surviving infants was assessed at follow-up from 7 months to 7 years.

Stepwise linear regression analysis was used to predict mortality using 21 independent variables. Only 5-minute Apgar scores and the initial pH of neonatal umbilical arterial blood were significant predictors of mortality. Analysis of the neurodevelopmental outcome of 28 children showed that only 8 (28%) were completely normal at follow-up (table). Seventeen children (61%) had an IQ of between 71 and 84 or suspect results of neurologic examination, or both; 3 children (11%) had an IQ of 70 or less and cerebral palsy (table). Seventeen of these children had received special educational or therapeutic services.

These findings show that the physiologic maturity of the infant, as reflected in Apgar score and initial pH, predicted survival of these extremely low-birth-weight infants. The high rates of neurologic and intellectual impairment in these children make it imperative that they be followed through school age. As the survival rate of extremely low-birth-weight infants increases, special education facilities will require expansion.

▶ David K. Stevenson, M.D., Professor of Pediatrics; Chief, Division of Neonatal and Developmental Medicine, and Director of Newborn Nurseries, Stanford Med Ctr, Palo Alto, California, offers his thoughts on this selection:

▶ Lipper and colleagues juxtapose observations about the prediction of mortality and the quality of survival in a provocative discussion about the survival and outcome of infants weighing <800 g at birth, commenting on both issues separately, but carefully avoiding a recommended course of action that would link them in practice. The interpretation that "For each unit increase in Apgar score, controlling for initial pH, the odds of dying decrease 1.38-fold or by 27%; for each 0.1 increase in pH, controlling for Apgar score, the odds of dying decrease 1.85-fold or by 46%," tempts one to believe that initial pH and the 5-minute Apgar score could be used to predict on an individual basis who, among infants weighing <800 g, could have resuscitative efforts or intensive care withheld or withdrawn because death is inevitable or at least very probable. This temptation is enhanced by coupling the prediction of mortality with the finding of a 72% overall handicap rate and a 9.8% mortality rate after neonatal care unit discharge.

One seems justified in concluding that progress has been little or, at least, uneven with respect to the outcome of extremely low-birth-weight infants through the 1980s. This is supported by the experience at Stanford as well (1), which revealed no change in the survival rate (34%), while doubling the number of survivors reported since an earlier report (2), and no change in the relative proportions of infants dying in the delivery room (31%) and in the Intensive Care Nursery (35%). Moreover, we found that, whereas 32% of all nonsurvivors died before 24 hours of age, an additional 36% died before 1 week of age, and 12% died between 1 week and 1 month of age; still, 20% of infants who ultimately died, died after 1 month of age (range, 37 days to 11 months).

With respect to permanent injuries, the prospects are largely uncertain. For comparison, of 51 survivors at Stanford, 45% had moderate handicaps and 15% were severely disabled, with both statistics being higher than we reported before. However, most of the moderately delayed children (34%) had slow motor development, with normal muscle tone and mental development scores. Another important point is that cerebral palsy remained uncommon among survivors, with only 4 infants having spastic diplegia.

Lipper and colleagues make the comment that "Higher survival rates of infants of increasingly smaller birth weight signify that a greater number of infants will have neurologic and intellectual impairments. . . ." When their mortality data are compared to those of others, the rationale for this claim is not apparent because overall mortality has not declined. Nonetheless, because the absolute number of very-low-birth-weight babies is increasing proportionately with the absolute number of live births (a reflection of no improvement in the prevention of prematurity), the absolute number of actual or possible neurologic and intellectual impairments is also increased and seems to justify the ". . . imperative that they be followed up carefully through school age."

Predictors of mortality, however, must remain generally idle tools in practice, because their application to decision-making about withholding or withdrawing care for individual patients is limited (3). Predictors are derived from the analysis of populations of patients, and the application of statistical predictive formulas to individual patients is often unfair or dangerous. The motivation to decide to withhold or withdraw support from individual very-low-birth-weight infants may stem from their propensity for prolonged hospitalization, generating large hospital bills and leading to unnecessary suffering before they ultimately die. There is also much stress and frustration among nursery staff members. Predictive models would be better used for the demonstration of objective cause for at least relative optimism in some patients.

The conclusion of Lipper and co-workers that we should anticipate the need for expansion of resources for special education because of increasing numbers of children with special needs is probably wise, not because the rate of injury among long-term survivors is increasing but simply because the absolute number of children with such needs is increasing. Perhaps the best way to conclude is that, despite impressive recent advances in neonatology, outcomes for extremely premature, very-low-birth-weight infants, (500–750 g) remain uneven. There are no simple algorithms for care as yet, but the humane limitation of treatment for extremely premature low-birth-weight infants is probably an important option to consider under some circumstances (4).—D.K. Stevenson, M.D.

References

1. Stevenson DK, Peterson KR: Update on the outcome of neonates with birth weights less than 801 grams. In Press.
2. Stevenson DK, et al: *J Perinatol* 8:82,
3. Fischer AF, et al: *Pediatrics* 77:615, 1986.
4. Young EWD, Stevenson DK: *Am J Dis Child* 144:549, 1990.

Very Low Birth Weight Children: Behavior Problems and School Difficulty in a National Sample

McCormick MC, Gortmaker SL, Sobol AM (Harvard School of Public Health; Harvard Med School)
J Pediatr 117:687–693, 1990

17–7

The early childhood course of infants of very-low-birth-weight (VLBW) infants remains uncertain; most samples have been small. A review was made of data from the 1981 National Health Interview Survey–Child Health Supplement, which collected information on 11,699 children aged 4–17 years. The Behavioral Problem Index (BPI) was used, and questions were asked about adjustment at school.

School difficulty was identified in one third of the study group, compared with one fifth of heavier LBW infants and 14% of normal-weight infants. The VLBW children were more likely to have high scores on the hyperactive subscale of the BPI. Hyperactive behavior correlated with school difficulty, the need to repeat a grade, and placement in special education. Independent risk factors for school difficulty included maleness, black race, more siblings, a low family income, and the absence of either parent.

This study certainly justifies concern over the long-term behavioral and academic status of VLBW children, although a majority of such children are free of problems. Intensive educational intervention before age 3 years seems to produce cognitive gains and a better behavioral outcome, but it is not clear whether these results translate into improved school performance.

▶ This commentary is contributed by Maureen Hack, M.B., Ch.B., Professor of Pediatrics, Director of the Follow-Up Program, Rainbow Babies and Childrens Hospital, Case Western Reserve University School of Medicine:

▶ This analysis of the National Health Interview Survey, Child Health Supplement, adds to the growing evidence of the school age difficulties of children born with very low weight. The histories of children aged 4–17 years were collected in 1981, thus these children were born during the years 1964–1977. The dramatic improvement in survival of VLBW infants since this time has resulted in a greater number of survivors of lower birth weight who have experienced many more neonatal problems and are more likely to have residual chronic illness. In the absence of a decrease in the VLBW rate, improvement in the quality of inner city schools, and state and federal funding to enforce public law 99–457, which mandates early intervention for children at risk, I predict that a similar survey in 2007 will demonstrate even poorer outcomes. The time to act is now.—M. Hack, M.B., Ch.B.

Increased Survival Rate in Very Low Birth Weight Infants (1500 Grams or Less): No Association With Increased Incidence of Handicaps
Grögaard JB, Lindstrom DP, Parker RA, Culley B, Stahlman MT (Vanderbilt Univ)
J Pediatr 117:139–146, 1990   17–8

Survival rates in very-low-birth-weight infants (VLBW) (≤1,500 g) have increased substantially. There is concern that this increased salvage may translate to an increased prevalence of neurodevelopmental handicaps. To address this concern, the incidence of major handicaps was studied in 1,919 VLBW infants born between 1976 and 1985. Of these, 632 were followed for up to 7 years of age; definitive assessment of all handicaps was available in 462 patients evaluated at age 18 months or older. The outcome of infants grouped by 250-g birth weight intervals was compared for 2 periods, 1976–1980 and 1981–1985.

The survival rate increased in all birth weight groups in 1981–1985. The overall incidence of major handicap was 18% (83 of 462). Severe retinopathy of prematurity occurred in 5.5% of the population, neurosensory hearing loss in 5.4%, cerebral palsy (CP) in 7.6%, and mental retardation (IQ ≤70) in 6.5%. More than 1 handicap was present in 6.7%, the most common combination being CP and mental retardation.

The overall incidence of major handicap decreased significantly from 27.2% in 1976–1980 to 12.1% in 1981–1985, particularly in the 500–750 g and 751–1,000 g birth weight groups. The decrease in handicaps was significant for mental retardation, retinopathy of prematurity, and neurosensory hearing loss, but not for CP. The incidence of multiple

Synthetic Estimates of Handicap Rates

Handicap	Period 1 (1976–1980)		Period 2 (1981–1985)	
	Estimated (%)	Observed (%)	Estimated (%)	Observed (%)
Retinopathy of prematurity	5.4	8.4	4.2	3.7
Cerebral palsy	7.3	8.4	7.3	7.1
Hearing loss	7.9	10.6	3.3	2.1
Mental retardation	7.1	10.69	5.1	3.9
Any handicap	18.7	27.2	14.7	12.1
Multiple handicaps	7.3	11.7	5.2	3.5

(Courtesy of Grögaard JB, Lindstrom DP, Parker RA, et al: *J Pediatr* 117:139–146, 1990.)

handicaps also fell significantly in the second 5-year period, particularly in the 2 lowest birth weight groups. Because patients lost to follow-up represented 55% of the eligible population, synthetic estimates of handicap rates were prepared, using inpatient morbidity factors, to determine whether the reduction in differences between the population followed and the group lost to follow-up between the 2 periods could explain the observed decrease in handicap rates. The synthetic estimates showed a lower incidence of all handicaps except for CP in the second period (table). An increased survival rate in VLBW infants need not be associated with a parallel increase in major handicaps.

▶ This paper has lent itself to vigorous discussion. The discussion, however, of necessity interchangebly takes into consideration facts, speculation, imagination, and perhaps some wishful thinking. The facts indisputably prove that the mortality rates for low-birth-weight babies have declined progressively since 1975. Moreover, among those infants who were followed, a reduced rate of handicaps was observed. Unfortunately, less than half of the original cohort were actually closely followed. What has happened to the rest of the subjects is purely speculative. Imaginative modeling is used to compute the probabilities of various outcomes for the infants whose actual status has not been verified. To concur with the title, i.e., increased survival, no association with an increased incidence of handicaps, we have to believe the calculations. I would like to accept this premise but will await confirmation from additional research involving regional rather than local data and with all of the subjects accounted for at follow-up.

Nothing is so firmly believed as what is least known.—M.E. de Montaigne.

A.A. Fanaroff, M.B.B.Ch.

Birthweight Ratio and Outcome in Preterm Infants

Morley R, Brooke OG, Cole TJ, Powell R, Lucas A (MRC Dunn Nutrition Unit; Univ of Cambridge, England; The Ryegate Ctr, Sheffield, England)

Arch Dis Child 65:30–34, 1990   17–9

The outlook of preterm infants relative to their size for gestation at birth is not clear, possibly because of the customary approach of defining outcomes in terms of small- or appropriate-for-gestation categorization. Brooke et al. defined a continuous variable to define size for gestation, termed the "birth weight ratio," which is calculated as the infant's birth

Birth Weight Ratio and Neurodevelopmental Outcome at 18 Months

| | *Birthweight ratio groups* | | | | |
	<0·8	*0·8 to <0·9*	*0·9 to <1·0*	*1·0 to <1·1*	*≥1·1*
No followed up	56	54	76	77	66
No (%) with neurological impairment	5 (9)	4 (7)	12 (16)	8 (10)	9 (14)
No (%) with neurodevelopmental impairment*	5 (9)	8 (15)	16 (21)	14 (18)	12 (18)
Mean (SD) Bayley mental development index	100 (17)	98 (20)	99 (17)	99 (21)	103 (20)
Mean (SD) Bayley motor development index	91 (19)	88 (16)	90 (19)	86 (20)	88 (17)
Mean (SD) language subscore as quotient	96 (18)	93 (18)	92 (20)	96 (19)	101 (19) †

*Neurodevelopmental impairment was diagnosed as neurologic impairment or mental index <70.
†P < .01, for language subscore in infants with birth weight ratios 1.1 or above compared with all infants with a ratio of <1.1.
(Courtesy of Morley R, Brooke OG, Cole TJ, et al: *Arch Dis Child* 65:30–34, 1990.)

weight divided by the reference median weight for the infant's gestation. Birth weight ratio was calculated in 429 infants born before 31 weeks' gestation, and the relationship between birth weight ratio and outcome in the neonatal period and at 18 months' post term was investigated.

The birth weight ratio corresponding to the 3rd, 10th, 90th, and 97th birth centiles was remarkably constant at gestations from 25 to 30 weeks. An increasing birth weight ratio was significantly associated with a progressive and significant decrease in the need for mechanical ventilation and postneonatal mortality. Similarly, an increasing birth weight ratio was significantly associated with a progressive increase in mean weight, length, and head circumference at 18 months post term. Overall, there was no association between birth weight ratio and neurodevelopmental outcome at 18 months post term. However, children with the largest weights for gestation (birth weight ratio ≥ 1.1) had significantly higher language scores than all other children (table).

With increasing birth weight for gestation, preterm infants have a progressively better prognosis in terms of the need for respiratory support or death in the early months, as well as progressively improved long-term growth performance. Dichotomous categorization into small- or appropriate-for-gestation groups is inadequate as a prognostic index in preterm infants.

▶ The response to this publication will depend on whether you are a splitter or a lumper. The splitters probably will endorse the concept of the birth weight ratio, whereas the lumpers will say that using the ratio little is gained by subclassification. Working from first principles we accept that there is a better prognosis with advancing gestational age and increased birth weight. We are now examining whether a higher percentile at the same gestation is advantageous, and the data as presented support this assumption. My impression is that it may be useful to reclassify infants, but this series is too small to allow major conclusions. If thousands of infants could be plotted in this manner and if their outcome data were available, the issue could be resolved beyond reasonable doubt.—A.A. Fanaroff, M.B.B.Ch.

Prediction of Subsequent Motor and Mental Retardation in Newborn Infants Exposed to Alcohol in Utero by Computerized EEG Analysis

Ioffe S, Chernick V (Univ of Manitoba, Winnipeg)
Neuropediatrics 21:11–17, 1990   17–10

Fetal exposure to alcohol causes dysmorphology in the newborn. The degree of abnormality in the electroencephalogram (EEG) at birth may predict the degree of subsequent motor and mental handicap in children exposed to alcohol in utero, even in the absence of the classic fetal alcohol syndrome. The results of a follow-up study of control and alcohol-exposed infants who had EEG studies at birth were examined.

Thirty-eight infants of mothers with varying quantities of alcohol ingestion during pregnancy were enrolled in the prospective, blinded study.

Electroencephalograms were obtained at 40 weeks postconceptional age. Bayley Development Tests were given between 1.5 and 10 months of age. There was an inverse relationship between the total power of the EEG during rapid eye movement (REM) sleep and subsequent motor development. The total power of the EEG during quiet sleep was inversely related to subsequent mental development. In infants exposed to alcohol, EEG abnormalities were present even in the absence of fetal alcohol syndrome. Similar results were obtained from 16 older children born to abstainers or alcoholic mothers.

There is a striking inverse correlation between the EEG power during REM sleep at birth and subsequent motor development and the EEG power during quiet sleep and subsequent mental development. Infants exposed to alcohol in utero, even in the absence of fetal alcohol syndrome, had increased power of the EEG during REM and quite sleep at birth, that correlated with poor motor and mental outcomes. The measure of the power of the EEG during REM and quiet sleep at birth can therefore be used as a predictor of subsequent outcomes of infants exposed to alcohol in utero.

▶ Max Wiznitzer, M.D., Assistant Professor of Pediatrics, Division of Pediatric Neurology, Department of Pediatrics, Rainbow Babies and Children's Hospital, Cleveland, offers these words of wisdom regarding EEG interpretations:

▶ This is a thought-provoking study because of the reported EEG changes. It is not obvious intuitively why increased power is related to either motor or mental dysfunction, unless the power spectrum is associated with increased slow activity on the conventional EEG. The ability to predict outcome during the neonatal period would be quite useful in future planning for these children. Why a difference should arise between active (REM) and quiet sleep is not immediately obvious. The authors' explanation about variation in drinking patterns leading to effects on different stages of sleep presumes that excessive alcohol use will occur only during either the early or later parts of the pregnancy. This may not necessarily occur in most situations. Also, the scores on the Bayley developmental assessment reflect performance in the first year of life. What is needed is a longer prospective study of a larger cohort that will also identify children with attentional disorders and learning problems. Only then can the significance of any neonatal EEG changes be addressed.— M. Wiznitzer, M.D.

Effect of Medical and Social Risk Factors on Outcome of Prematurity and Very Low Birth Weight
Leonard CH, Clyman RI, Piecuch RE, Juster JP, Ballard RA, Behle MB (Mount Zion Hosp and Med Ctr, San Francisco)
J Pediatr 116:620–626, 1990   17–11

In addition to a high medical risk, very-low-birth-weight infants may have increased vulnerability to environmental stresses. It was hypothe-

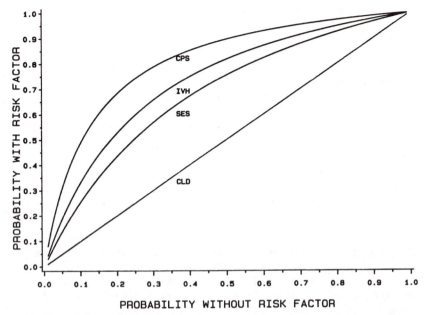

PROBABILITY WITHOUT RISK FACTOR

Fig 17–1.—Influence of CLD, SES, ICH, and parenting risk factor *(CPS)* on probability of abnormal cognitive outcome. *CLD* indicates risk associated with supplemental oxygen requirement for 50 days or longer compared with requirement for less than 30 days; *SES,* the risk associated with low SES; *IVH,* the risk associated with grade III or IV ICH compared with no ICH; *CPS,* the risk associated with CPS referral; *x-axis,* probability of abnormal outcome in absence of particular risk factor; *y-axis,* probability of abnormal outcome in presence of risk factor; *IVH,* intraventricular hemorrhage. (Courtesy of Leonard CH, Clyman RI, Piecuch RE, et al: *J Pediatr* 116:620–626, 1990.)

sized that some aspects of parenting may affect the cognitive outcome of these infants. In a prospective study, 129 of 326 infants with birth weights of 1,250 g or less were followed for more than 4½ years (mean, 60 months) to determine the independent effects of 2 medical risk factors, intracranial hemorrhage (ICH) and severe chronic lung disease (CLD), and a parenting risk factor, either abuse or neglect, on neurodevelopmental outcome.

Severe CLD in infants without ICH and a parenting risk factor was not related to the neurologic or cognitive outcome. In contrast, increasing grades of ICH correlated positively with an increasing rate of neurologic and cognitive deficits. Parenting risk in children with no ICH was not associated with abnormal neurologic outcome but was strongly associated with abnormal cognitive outcome. Low socioeconomic status (SES) did not explain the cognitive deficits in children with a parenting risk. Linear logistic regression analysis showed that the parenting risk factor was associated with the highest risk of later abnormality (Fig 17–1).

These findings indicate that infants with medical risk factors may have additional social risk factors. These infants may have heightened sensitivity to a suboptimal family environment. Both medical and social risk factors should be considered in the assessment of long-term sequelae of neonatal complications.

▶ In the past, the cognitive development of the small immature infant appeared to be closely correlated to the SES of the family (1). What is most disconcerting is that the parenting risk factor had an even greater effect on cognitive development than SES or intraventricular hemorrhage. A significant parenting risk factor was defined as a referral by a physician, nurse, or affiliated health professional to protective services for neglect or mild abuse. In the future, a more detailed study of the parents should be made before the infant is discharged from the hospital.—M.H. Klaus, M.D.

Reference

1. Drillien CM: *Pediatrics* 39:238, 1967.

Early Diet in Preterm Babies and Developmental Status at 18 Months
Lucas A, Morley R, Cole TJ, Gore SM, Lucas PJ, Crowley P, Pearse R, Boon AJ, Powell R (Med Research Council Dunn Nutritional Unit, Cambridge; MRC Biostatistics Unit, Cambridge; Norfolk and Norwich Hosp, Norwich; Jessop Hosp, Sheffield, England)
Lancet 335:1477–1481, 1990   17–12

Whether nutrition in early life has a long-term impact on neurodevelopmental outcome remains controversial. Two parallel studies on the long-term effects of early nutrition were conducted in 5 centers, with developmental data available at 18 months post term. A total of 424 preterm infants weighing less than 1,850 g at birth were studied. Infants of mothers who chose not to breast-feed were randomly assigned to receive a standard "term" formula or a nutrient-enriched "preterm" formula as the sole diet (trial A). In the second study, infants whose mothers chose to breast-feed were randomly allocated to term or preterm formula as a supplement to the mother's own milk (trial B); the median intake of mother's milk did not differ between infants given term and preterm formula.

A total of 377 survivors were available for 18-month post-term evaluation (median age, 82.6 weeks). Weight gain and head growth were significantly faster in infants fed preterm formula than in those fed standard formula in both trials. Infants fed preterm formula had significantly higher Bayley scores on mental and psychomotor development indices (Fig 17–2) and social quotients, as compared with infants fed term formula. These advantages were particularly striking in small-for-gestational age infants and males. In trial A, infants fed preterm formula had a 15-point advantage in motor development index compared with infants fed term formula; for infants born small for gestation, this advantage was 23 points. Infants fed preterm formula had a lower frequency of moderate developmental impairment (29%) than infants fed term formula (58%). There was also a small benefit in social maturity quotient in infants fed

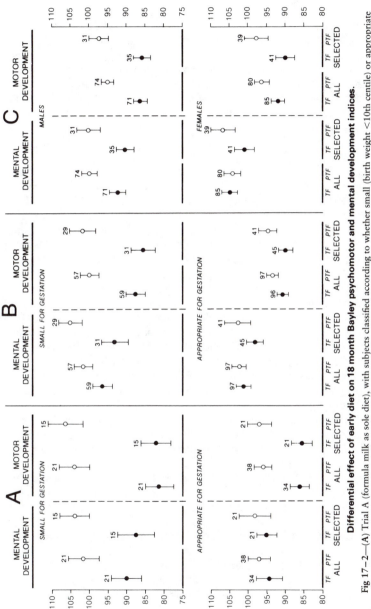

Fig 17–2—(A) Trial A (formula milk as sole diet), with subjects classified according to whether small (birth weight <10th centile) or appropriate size for gestation. (B) Trials A and B combined (formula milk as sole diet or supplement), with subjects classified as in (A). (C) Trials A and B combined, with subjects classified by sex. Bars represent mean (SE) neurodevelopmental scores; nos. above bars represent numbers of subjects. Selected infants refer to those who received the highest intakes of trial diet. (Courtesy of Lucas A, Morley R, Cole TJ, et al: *Lancet* 335:1477–1481; 1990.)

preterm formula. A short period of dietary manipulation in preterm infants has a significant impact on developmental status at 18 months; therefore, the first weeks of life may be critical for nutrition.

▶ Richard Umansky, M.D., Director of the Division of Child Development, Children's Hospital Oakland, Oakland, California, offers his thoughts:

▶ It is still relatively rare for clinical studies to examine the validity of established practices. This important study provides evidence of the developmental value to premature infants of a relatively short exposure early in infancy to the type of nutritionally enriched preterm formula (PTF) in general use in many parts of the world. The results were most pronounced in small-for-dates and male infants, whose Bayley mental and motor scores improved. They were less clear-cut in infants who received breast milk.

Several points require emphasis: First, as the authors note, the study was not designed to determine which constituents of the PTF were crucial in conferring the developmental advantage.

Second, one wonders whether the improved development associated with PTF was mediated through better physical growth; PTF resulted in better weight gain and head circumference growth during its use, but there was no correlation between such early indicators of improved growth and later development at 18 months. Also, this study did not examine the relationship between development at 18 months and physical growth status at that time.

Third, although the improvement conferred by PTF use on 18-month Bayley motor scores was greater than on Bayley mental scores, it may be less meaningful. At this age, the Bayley Motor Scale is based on comparatively few items, primarily measures of equilibrium and strength, and is not a general assessment of gross motor abilities. On the other hand, at 18 months, the Bayley Mental Scale is based on several times the number of items and assess a wide variety of cognitive and early language skills as well as incorporating a substantial fine motor component.

Fourth, the developmental advantage seen in the PTF group at 18 months may not be sustained. As noted by the authors, developmental testing early in life is of limited predictive value. At 18 months many attributes of mature intelligence are not readily measurable or have yet to emerge, e.g., abstract reasoning, use of symbols, reflective judgment. This may be true especially in premature infants because their "catch-up" process is not yet complete at this age.

Finally, the authors interpret the Vineland results as an indication that early diet may have a small but significant effect on how the premature infant subsequently adapts to its environment. The Vineland instrument is a questionnaire administered to caretakers. Supplemental information from the Infant Behavioral Record (derived during Bayley testing) would have been of interest. This record incorporates the results of direct infant observations of interpersonal responsiveness, emotional tone, attention to objects and goals, and activity level.

The authors should be congratulated for pursuing this valuable effort. One looks forward with anticipation to information to come from further follow-up of these youngsters in the preschool and school age years.—R. Umansky, M.D.

Birthweight Specific Trends in Cerebral Palsy

Pharoah POD, Cooke T, Cooke RWI, Rosenbloom L (Univ of Liverpool, England)

Arch Dis Child 65:602–606, 1990   17–13

Despite the overall improvement in provisions for neonatal care that has resulted in improved survival rates, the prevalence of cerebral palsy in low-birth-weight infants is increasing, with 25% to 40% of all cases of cerebral palsy occurring in 6% to 7% of low-birth weight infants. Data were analyzed from a register of 1,056 infants with cerebral palsy born to mothers resident in the Mersey region from 1967 to 1984. One hundred of the 331 with hemiplegia (30%), 152 of the 236 with diplegia (64%), and 115 of the 369 with quadriplegia (31%) weighed 2,500 g or less at birth.

There was no significant increase in the prevalence of cerebral palsy among infants with birth weights of greater than 2,500 g. In contrast, infants of low birth weight (1,501–2,500 g) had a two- to three-fold increase in the prevalence of cerebral palsy of all main clinical types up to 1977–1979, followed by a plateau or moderate decline thereafter. For very-low-birth-weight infants (1,500 g or lower) the increase started later with a five- to six-fold increase in the prevalence rate.

The rise in prevalence rates in both low-birth-weight groups was contributed to by all 3 main clinical types of cerebral palsy. The increased prevalence of cerebral palsy in low-birth-weight patients was accompanied by an increasing number who survived but did not have cerebral palsy.

There is an increasing prevalence of cerebral palsy among low-birth-weight infants. These changes could be the result of improved survival of prenatally impaired infants because of improved medical care, or a reflection of failure to maintain optimal conditions at or around the time of birth.

▶ Data from Liverpool can now be added to reports from Sweden, Ireland, and Norway that were described in the 1990 YEAR BOOK OF NEONATAL AND PERINATAL MEDICINE. These reports noted a marked increase in cerebral palsy in infants weighing less than 1,500 g at birth. A similar trend is observed in this report. There is a real cost to increasing the survival rates for small infants. A major question is whether this increase is secondary to intra- or extrauterine events.—M.H. Klaus, M.D.

The Long-Term Effects of Exposure to Low Doses of Lead in Childhood: An 11-Year Follow-Up Report

Needleman HL, Schell A, Bellinger D, Leviton A, Allred EN (Univ of Pittsburgh; Boston Univ; Children's Hosp, Boston; Harvard Med School)

N Engl J Med 322:83–88, 1990   17–14

Young children with increased levels of lead in dentin but no symptoms of plumbism have been found to have psychometric deficits and impaired school performance. One hundred thirty-two of the 270 initial subjects in 1 study were available for reassessment as young adults. Those who were followed up had had relatively lower levels of lead in dentin and higher IQ scores at initial assessment.

Impaired neurobehavioral function remained related to the lead content of teeth shed at ages 6–7 years. Subjects with levels of lead in dentin of greater than 20 ppm were at a much higher risk of dropping out of high school and of having reading disability. Higher levels of lead in childhood were associated with a lower class standing in high school, more absenteeism, and lower vocabulary and grammatical reasoning scores. In addition, higher levels of lead correlated with poorer hand-eye coordination and longer reaction times. When 10 children with clinical plumbism were included with the other subjects, a dose-response relationship was evident for both dropping out of school and having a reading disability.

Lead exposure, even in children who remain asymptomatic, can have lasting effects on success in school and in life. Because as many as 16% of children in the United States have increased blood levels of lead, the implications for preventing school failure are of great interest.

▶ It is interesting how the "safe" blood lead level keeps dropping every 5–10 years. The unique features of this study are the very long follow-up (11 years) and the upsetting findings. As we attempt to clean our environment, heavy metal poisoning continues to be a major problem for young infants and children.—M.H. Klaus, M.D.

Clinical Management Considerations in Long-Term Survivors With Trisomy 18
Van Dyke DC, Allen M (Univ of Iowa)
Pediatrics 85:753–759, 1990   17–15

Trisomy 18 is the second most common trisomy, with an incidence of approximately 1 in 8,000 births. As many as 90% or more of children with trisomy 18 die within the first year of life. To provide more information on the unique aspects of management of those children who survive, a review of the records of 6 patients with trisomy 18 who survived past the age of 1 year and of the trisomy 18 files of the Support Organization for Trisomy 18 and 13 was undertaken.

Of the 321 children with trisomy 18 recorded in the files, 124 survived beyond age 1 year, and some survived to ages 22, 23, and 35 years. Girls survive more frequently than boys. In addition to the medical problems that are unique to the syndrome, these patients present complex medical problems common to all persons with chromosomal abnormalities. Congenital heart disease, including septal defects with ventricular septal defects, is common, and children who survive longer have a second protective lesion (e.g., pulmonic stenosis). Cardiac management is primarily medical. Hemivertebrae is a common finding in these children, with scoliosis becoming apparent by age 3–6 months. Positioning, using an insert while seated, is the most acceptable form of modifying the scoliosis. Infection is an ongoing concern, with pneumonia being the cause of death in 3 of 6 case patients studied. Feeding problems are a major management issue, and most need nasogastric/gastrostomy supplementation, although some patients may go on to oral feeding. Growth in all parameters is always markedly less than the fifth percentile despite a high caloric intake.

Management does not include the child alone but also the family unit. Because the presence of a disabled child in any family has been linked to major family stressors, the family unit needs equally challenging care and support. These families experience a complex grieving process that combines both the reactive grief predominant in chronic illness and the preparatory grief associated with impending death. By knowing the unique but complex medical problems in long-term survivors with trisomy 18, as well as offering supportive care to the family, the physician can provide a service of significant benefit.

▶ Many physicians believe that they can be of little help to parents when the infant's condition is uniformly fatal. Birth of a trisomy 18 infant is a major attack on the integrated "self" of both parents and requires that they make a difficult set of complex adjustments. When a physician or caretaker spends time helping parents adjust and care for their sick infant, he is saying without words, "Even though you have had a malformed baby that I cannot repair, I care deeply about you and your family." This sensitive report should be read by all caregivers working in the perinatal period who manage those infants who are not perfect. As emphasized by the authors, ". . . the benefits to be gained from informed, empathic care are significant" and should never be underestimated.—M.H. Klaus, M.D.

18 Epidemiology

Enhancing the Outcomes of Low-Birth-Weight, Premature Infants: A Multisite, Randomized Trial
The Infant Health and Development Program, Stanford, Calif
JAMA 263:3035–3042, 1990   18–1

The Infant Health and Development Program is the first multisite, randomized clinical trial that evaluates the efficacy of combining early child development and family support services with pediatric follow-up in reducing developmental, behavioral, and other health problems among low-birth-weight (2,500 g or less) premature (37 weeks or younger) infants. A total of 985 infants, stratified by site and weight, were randomly assigned to receive an educational curriculum focused on child development, family support, and pediatric follow-up, or pediatric follow-up only.

At corrected age 36 months, the intervention group had significantly higher mean IQ scores than the follow-up group (mean difference in the heavier group was 13.2 and in the lighter group, 6.6). The intervention group had significantly fewer maternally reported behavior problems; a small but statistically significant increase in maternally reported minor morbidity was noted only in the light group. There was no difference in serious health problems.

These data demonstrate the effectiveness and safety of comprehensive and intensive early intervention in reducing the number of low-birth-weight premature infants at risk for later developmental disability. The long-term significance of these findings will be addressed in the continued follow-up of this cohort.

▶ This is a wonderful example of a multisite randomized trial. From the initial competition for the participating centers, through the study design, patient enrollment, follow-up, and data management, this trial can only be labeled first class. The goal of enhancing the outcomes of low-birth-weight premature infants is magnanimous and timely. The fairy tale would be complete if the hypothesis were proven and intervention enhanced the outcome of low-birth-weight infants. There is documentation of improved outcome and intellect in the group receiving the intervention. Unfortunately, in the lower birth weight categories, and these were by no means extremely low-birth-weight infants, the difference is only 6.6 points on the Stanford Binet. How will this translate with regard to school performance?

Nonetheless, there is a difference, and only continued observation of this cohort will demonstrate the full impact of the intervention. In the mean time, resources need to be marshalled to provide stimulating programs for many more at-risk graduates from the intensive care unit, notably those from lower socioeconomic strata.

"Success will require all our creativity, commitment and energy."—*Peter Lewis*

A.A. Fanaroff, M.B.B.Ch.

The Relation of Obstetrical Volume and Nursery Level to Perinatal Mortality

Mayfield JA, Rosenblatt RA, Baldwin L-M, Chu J, Logerfo JP (Univ of Washington)

Am J Public Health 80:819–823, 1990
18–2

Many experts are of the opinion that the dropping rates of neonatal and perinatal death seen in the United States in the past several decades are the result of more effective technological interventions combined with regionalization, a process that optimizes access to that technology. Volume is highly correlated with high technology, because a high volume of patients is needed to justify the expense of such technology.

Hospital delivery volume, nursery technology level, and perinatal outcome were studied in 226,164 white singleton births in the state of Washington from 1980 to 1983. Level III facilities, or neonatal intensive care units, were defined by the state licensing commission. Published criteria were used to define level II, or intermediate, and level I, or normal newborn, facilities. Infants weighing less than 2,000 g born in level III facilities had half the risk of perinatal death compared with those born in level I or II facilities. There was no significant improvement among level or volume groupings for infants of normal birth weight. According to a log linear regression model of hospital perinatal death rates, obstetric volume added minimal explanatory power to level of nursery care when birth weight and maternal risk were controlled (table). However, if all infants were delivered at a level III facility, the model predicts a higher number of deaths, mainly from a large number of normal birth weight infants dying at a slightly higher rate.

Observed Deaths and Deaths Predicted From the Model If All Births Occurred in 1 Type of Facility

Birthweight	Observed	Level I Volume 1000–2000	Level III Volume >2000
1000–1499 gm	234	425	213
1500–1999 gm	201	316	130
2000–2499 gm	221	204	264
2500–2999 gm	234	232	306
3000–3499 gm	251	301	281
3500–3999 gm	139	143	179
4000–4500 gm	47	35	81
>4500 gm	45	45	62
Total	1372	1701	1517

(Courtesy of Mayfield JA, Rosenblatt RA, Baldwin L-M, et al: *Am J Public Health* 80:819–823, 1990.)

The effect of hospital technology on perinatal mortality seems to be greater than that of volume. However, this benefits mostly low-birth-weight, high-risk infants. Further closing of smaller hospitals may even pose a risk for the normal-birth-weight infant. Assessment of practices and policies that encourage transferring obstetric patients must consider the outcomes for all segments of the population as a basis for effective policy decisions and efficient resource allocation.

▶ The results of the analysis of these 226,164 births were not fully anticipated. The increase in neonatal deaths of infants with a birth weight >2,500 g in level III units (table) was obviously unexpected. A similar observation was made in New York City (1), and Rosenblatt et al. (2) in New Zealand also noted increased infant mortality among full-term infants delivered in high-volume level III units. We should explore this observation in much greater depth before we push for closing smaller obstetric units. Is it possible that the environment in these large, high-volume obstetric units with their complex technology may have an adverse effect on normal laboring women, resulting in iatrogenic fetal distress, or is this the result of referral of the high-risk infant to these hospitals? We must explore these findings, especially because they don't meet our expectations.—M.H. Klaus, M.D.

References

1. Paneth N, et al: *Am J Dis Child* 141:60, 1987.
2. Rosenblatt RA, et al: *Lancet* 2:429, 1985.

European Community Collaborative Study of Outcome of Pregnancy Between 22 and 28 Weeks' Gestation
Working Group on the Very Low Birthweight Infant (McIlwaine GM, Glasgow Royal Maternity Hosp, Scotland)
Lancet 336:782–784, 1990

18–3

Comparing international perinatal mortality rates is difficult because legal criteria for registering livebirths and stillbirths differ among countries. Two disparate areas are the definition of livebirth and the variation in policy on the elective delivery of a very preterm fetus at risk of intrauterine death. Survival rates in several European countries were compared for very-low-birth-weight (VLBW) infants (less than 1,500 g).

In 7 populations (Denmark, Ireland, England, Greece, The Netherlands, Italy, and Scotland), there were pronounced differences in survival rates of VLBW infants of less than 1,000 g (Tables 1 and 2). The crude survival rate per 1,000 livebirths among infants born at 22–28 weeks' gestation was not different among 4 populations. More infants were born in the United Kingdom, and survival rates were higher in Scotland and England when the gestational age at birth was controlled for. Future international comparisons of outcome of pregnancy ending after 22 weeks

TABLE 1.—Survival Rates to Discharge Home per 1,000 Liveborn Infants 1983–1984

Country	Total Number livebirths 500–1499g.	500g. – 749g.	750g. – 999g.	1000g. – 1249g.	1250g. – 1499g.	TOTAL SURVIVAL RATE <1500g. (95% C.I.)
Denmark (Odense)	30	0	600	1000	1000	866 (745–988)
Ireland (Cork)	80	125	333	773	781	613 (506–719)
England (Oxford Region)	277	435	544	909	886	765 (715–815)
Greece (Athens)	459	154	317	478	706	521 (475–566)
Netherlands	1092	303	520	735	874	723 (697–750)
Italy (Naples, Trieste & Sardinia)	303	143	241	584	726	554 (499–610)
Scotland (Grampian)	70	0	526	563	1000	671 (561–781)
ALL REGIONS	2311					662 (643–682)

(Courtesy of Working Group on the Very Low Birthweight Infant: *Lancet* 336:782–784, 1990.)

would be facilitated if very preterm births were registered uniformly in all countries.

▶ The large differences in survival data are probably determined in part by regional variations in defining a livebirth, varying economic and social differences, and how infants are cared for in each country. To be able to make comparisons between countries, it may be necessary to take an Australian proposition and record the deaths of all infants of more than 20 weeks' gestation. It is useful to observe that the European Economic Community is not just interested in wheat and eggs but also does have a research consortium.—M.H. Klaus, M.D.

Predicting Death From Initial Disease Severity in Very Low Birthweight Infants: A Method for Comparing the Performance of Neonatal Units
Tarnow-Mordi W, Ogston S, Wilkinson AR, Reid E, Gregory J, Saeed M, Wilkie R (Univ of Dundee, Scotland; John Radcliffe Maternity Hosp, Oxford, England)
Br Med J 300:1611–1614, 1990   18–4

TABLE 2.—Proportion of Total Births Below 1,500 g by Birth-Weight Group

Area	No. total births 500-1499g.	Percentage of all births <1500g. who weighed				% of all births which weighed <1500g.
		500g. - 749g.	750g. - 999g.	1000g. - 1249g.	1250g. - 1499g.	
Denmark (Odense)	30	6.7	23.3	36.7	33.3	1.13
Ireland (Cork)	101	14.9	19.8	31.7	33.7	n/a
England (Oxford Region)	327	8.5	18.9	28.4	44.0	1.01
Netherlands*	1092	6.0	20.2	32.9	40.8	0.68
Italy (Naples, Trieste & Sardinia)	335	7.5	18.5	30.7	43.2	1.10
Scotland (Grampian)	99	18.2	26.5	23.2	32.0	1.38

Abbreviation: NA, not available.
*% of livebirths.
(Courtesy of Working Group on the Very Low Birthweight Infant: *Lancet* 336:782–784, 1990.)

In comparing the performance of various neonatal intensive care units, any comparison based on crude mortality or without correcting for major risk factors, particularly initial disease severity, may not be reliable. To determine which clinical variables and physiologic measures of disease severity best predict death in very-low-birth-weight (VLBW) infants (<1,500 g), a retrospective study was made of 262 VLBW infants who received mechanical ventilation in 2 different neonatal intensive care units. Various multiple logistic regression models of risk of death were used to compare the performance of these 2 neonatal units.

Among the 130 VLBW infants treated in hospital A, the mean levels of oxygenation in the first 12 hours of life, whether measured as inspired oxygen requirement, arterial/alveolar oxygen ratio, or alveolar-arterial oxygen difference, were more strongly associated with death than the 4 traditional risk factors, (e.g., low birth weight, short gestation, diagnosis of respiratory distress syndrome, and male sex). Low mean pH and low birth weight were both strongly associated with death.

Multiple logistic regression models were derived in infants from hospital A using the 4 traditional risk factors, all measures of oxygenation, and pH. The performance of these models in predicting death was tested in the 132 VLBW infants in hospital B. The sensitivity of the model using the 4 traditional risk factors in predicting death was only 31%. Adding the mean arterial/alveolar oxygen ratio and mean pH increased the sensitivity to 75%; replacing the mean arterial/alveolar oxygen ratio with the mean inspired oxygen requirement increased sensitivity further to 81%.

Comparisons of mortality between the hospitals was performed before and after correcting for major risk factors using appropriate regression models. The odds of death in hospital A vs. hospital B was .67 based on crude mortality rates alone and 1.21 after adjusting for the traditional risk factors. However, after correcting for traditional risk factors, mean inspired oxygen requirement, and mean pH, the odds of death in hospital A increased significantly to 3.27, even after adjusting for the time difference between each hospital cohort.

Crude comparisons of hospital mortality can be highly misleading, even after taking into account traditional risk factors. An accurate measure of initial disease severity would allow more reliable comparisons of perinatal outcome between neonatal units.

▶ This report and others like it have been developed to identify those physiologic measures and clinical variables that best predict death in VLBW infants. As in many other studies, the mean level of oxygenation, whether measured as the inspired oxygen requirement or the alveolar-arterial oxygen difference, was most predictive of the future. The authors strongly suggest that it should not be used to help in the decision of when to withdraw therapy. It is here that I disagree. In the past 8 years, more aggressive therapy of very small infants (500–700 g) has only increased the time before they die (survival time before death has increased from 4 hours to 36 days) and during the same time the quality of survival has not improved. A tool such as this can be used to help the parents and caretakers in deciding how their infant should be managed.—M.H. Klaus, M.D.

The Relationship of Unwed Status to Infant Mortality

Hein HA, Burmeister LF, Papke KR (Univ of Iowa)
Obstet Gynecol 76:763–768, 1990   18–5

To study potential factors associated with low birth weight and infant mortality, the incidence of infant deaths in offspring of unmarried women was compared with their married counterparts during 10 years in Iowa. Infant mortality was significantly higher in unwed mothers (Fig 18–1). The unwed population generally comprised poorly educated, younger women who frequently did not seek prenatal care. Because accessibility to obstetric and newborn care is good in all parts of Iowa, personal factors among unwed mothers may be more significant than lack of access to care in determining pregnancy outcome.

Although health care is accessible throughout the state of Iowa, unwed women had significantly fewer prenatal visits than married women. Unwed women also had a higher incidence of postneonatal death in term and near-term infants, those most likely to survive. Because unwanted

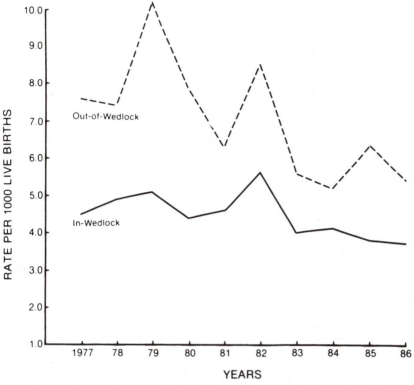

YEARS

Fig 18–1.—Infant mortality rate, 1977–1986, for birth weight 2,501–4,000 g. $\chi^2 = 43.79$; $P < .001$. (Courtesy of Hein HA, Burmeister LF, Papke KR: *Obstet Gynecol* 76:763–768, 1990.)

pregnancy has been associated with poor pregnancy outcome, increased education both in schools and for young adults is advocated to prevent unwanted pregnancy.

▶ Diana Petitti, M.D., Associate Professor, Department of Family and Community Medicine, University of California at San Francisco School of Medicine, offers her commentary.

▶ The study by Hein and colleagues contributes to the extensive literature on marital status as a correlate of pregnancy outcome, mainly because it was carried out in a setting in which direct financial barriers to access to prenatal care have been absent for a long time. The relationship of unmarried marital status with poor outcome persists in this setting, and the authors reasonably conclude that "financial access to the medical care system is not the major reason why unwed mothers have poor pregnancy outcomes." The authors note that unmarried women made fewer prenatal visits than married women. This finding, in the Iowa context, shows that removal of financial barriers to prenatal care is a necessary but not a sufficient condition for equality of care.

The study highlights the contribution of postneonatal mortality to the higher infant mortality rate in infants born to unmarried mothers. It is likely that this is true not only in Iowa. Traditional prenatal care will not have an impact on post-neonatal mortality. For women who are unmarried, parenting classes and ongoing provision of social services after the birth of the child must supplement the traditional approaches if this mortality rate is going to be lowered.

The authors suggest that intendedness is the central cause of poor pregnancy outcome among unmarried mothers. The subtle implication that the death of an unmarried woman's baby is because it was unwanted must be recognized. In the absence of real information on intendedness for women in this study, the contention that intendedness is a major cause of poor pregnancy outcome among unmarried women should be regarded as highly speculative.—D. Petitti, M.D.

Lack of Difference in Neonatal Mortality Between Blacks and Whites Served by the Same Medical Care System
Kugler JP, Connell FA, Henley CE (Madigan Army Med Ctr, Tacoma, Wash; Univ of Washington)
J Fam Pract 30:281–289, 1990   18–6

Neonatal mortality rates are twice as high in blacks as in whites, possibly because of the higher percentage of low birth weight (LBW) (<2,500 g) and premature births in blacks and a higher mortality rate in normal-weight black neonates. Because prenatal care can influence the risk of prematurity and LBW, a study was undertaken to assess the influence of health care systems on racial differences in LBW and neonatal mortality. A historical cohort analysis was conducted using birth and linked birth and death certificates of infants delivered in Pierce County, Washington, between 1982 and 1985. The 29,848 neonates were grouped based on race (black or white) and place of delivery (military or civilian facility).

Regardless of the health care system, LBW rates were about twofold higher among blacks. The neonatal mortality rate was twice as high in black infants born in cilivian facilities (12.23%) compared to white infants (5.4%). However, the neonatal mortality rate in black infants born in a military hospital (7.16%) was comparable to that of white infants (6.13%). The same risk trends were apparent even after controlling for marital status, age-parity risk, and income.

Analysis of birth-weight-specific neonatal mortality showed that the greatest difference in neonatal mortality was among normal-birth-weight infants. There was a marked excess in neonatal mortality among black infants with birth weights of more than 2,500 g born in civilian care, whereas the rate among black infants born in military care compared favorably with that of white infants. In these normal-weight infants, the effect of military care appeared to be most significant among infants of low-income women.

Military medical care appears to have a protective effect against neonatal mortality in black infants. The low-income, normal-weight black group may be the most sensitive to this protective effect. These findings suggest that infant mortality prevention should not focus only on LBW prevention, but also on comprehensive care for all pregnancies among the poor, particularly the black poor.

▶ Examining the data closely, black women in the military service had the same incidence of prematurity and LBW mortality as those in civilian life. The lower infant mortality rate among children born to black women in the military was surprisingly similar to that of normal-birth-weight infants. Nearly 50% of the excess neonatal deaths in civilian life were among infants with a normal birth weight. The major component of the difference in mortality rate between the civilian and military cohorts was in the number of deaths attributable to infectious causes. The authors suggest that the military is protective because it covers many areas of care, including general pediatrics, nutritional support, and close follow-up of at-risk families. Unfortunately, in the report we have only hints as to why infant mortality rates were reduced among black women cared for by the military.—M.H. Klaus, M.D.

Categories of Preventable Unexpected Infant Deaths

Taylor EM, Emery JL (Univ of Sheffield, England)
Arch Dis Child 65:535–539, 1990

18–7

Confidential inquiries into postperinatal deaths may be relevant to the implementation of preventive measures and health care planning in a community. In Sheffield, England, such inquiries have been carried out since 1973. During the years 1980–1988, 115 registered unexpected infant deaths (ages 1 week to 1 year) were classified in terms of possible preventability; the presence or absence of adverse family and social background factors was also noted in each case.

The overall rate of unexpected death in infancy from 1980 to 1988 was 2/1,000 live births. The mean age at death was 16 weeks. Of the 115 infants, 7 were considered to have had poor prognosis (group A), 45 had potentially treatable disease (group B), 32 had minor illnesses (group C), and 19 had no evidence of disease (group D). Four deaths were probably accidental (group E), and 8 were thought to have been the result of filicide (group F). Less than 20% of deaths corresponded to the classic definition of sudden infant death syndrome.

Infants who died during the course of potentially treatable disease had more adverse family and social factors. Typically, these families resided in the most underprivileged part of the community where health care had a low priority and ill health was the norm. The parents were less likely to own their own homes, own a car or have a telephone, and the mothers were young, tended to smoke, and had late antenatal care. These infants characteristically scored high in the "at risk for cot death" system. Infants who died of minor illnesses had similar backgrounds, but their families experienced greater levels of stress and the deaths appeared to be multifactorial. Maternal depression and a lack of maternal child bonding were common. Infants who died without terminal disease were younger and more likely to be boys. Demographically, their families were the only group not to differ from the controls and the general population. Deaths in group E and F occurred when there was acute social deprivation, crisis, or social incompetence. The findings of definite demographic differences among the groups confirm the heterogeneity of deaths registered as "unexpected death in infancy."

▶ This report continues a long-term (20-year) exploration of this difficult problem. The extensive interview with each family (2 hours) and thorough case discussion were unusually productive. The authors' view of cot death differs from that of most authors in the United States. In their evaluation of the family, a crisis refers to a serious event, e.g., a recent burglary of the home, a death in the family, or serious car accident. Likewise, in assessing adverse family background and social factors, only serious issues were included.

The divisions into 6 categories of cot death—(1) infants with a poor prognosis, (2) treatable disease, (3) minor disease, (4) no disease, (5) probable accident, (6) probable filicide—is a major step forward. Once this was done they found that most of the families categorized with treatable disease or minor disease had a much higher incidence of social morbidity, such as poor housing and domestic and financial problems compared to those with no disease or an accident. Initially, many deaths appeared to be unexplained, but with thorough exploration of the family a more reasonable diagnosis was usually discovered. Significantly, all of the probable filicides occurred in association with acute social deprivation, a severe crisis, or social incompetance, e.g., a mother who went to sleep on the sofa while under the influence of alcohol, drugs, or extreme fatigue. The full story of these deaths came out only during the confidental inquiry. Using this thorough approach markedly reduced the number of infants with truly unexplained deaths from 91% to 17%. Thus to reduce the death rate, the major focus changes from recommending apnea monitors to altering stress in high-risk families.—M.H. Klaus, M.D.

Interaction Between Bedding and Sleeping Position in the Sudden Infant Death Syndrome: A Population Based Case-Control Study
Fleming PJ, Gilbert R, Azaz Y, Berry PJ, Rudd PT, Stewart A, Hall E (Inst of Child Health, Bristol; Bath Unit for Research into Paediatrics, Bath; Bristol Maternity Hosp, Bristol; Royal United Hosp, Bath)
Br Med J 301:85–89, 1990   18–8

Several studies suggest a possible role of thermal stress, i.e., excessive bedding, in the etiology of sudden infant death syndrome (SIDS). Sleeping in the prone position has also been implicated. A case-control study was conducted to define the possible interaction between quantity of bedding and sleeping position with SIDS. Information on bedding, sleeping position, heating, and recent signs of illness were compared between 72 infants who had died suddenly or unexpectedly and 144 control infants matched for age and date with each index case. Parents of control infants were interviewed within 72 hours of the index infant's death. The mean age of the index infants was 94.4 days and of the control infants, 97 days.

Sixty-seven infants died of SIDS; the other 5 died of other causes. Infants who died of SIDS were significantly more likely to have been sleeping prone, to have been more heavily wrapped, and to have had heating all night, when compared with control infants. These differences were more pronounced in older infants (>70 days old). The risk of SIDS among older infants was 15.1-fold greater when nursed prone, compared with nursing supine on either side, and 25.2-fold greater when total thermal resistance of clothing and bedding exceeded 10 tog units, compared with less than 6 tog units. These data indicate that excess bedding and prone position are independently associated with an increased risk of SIDS, particularly among infants older than 70 days.

▶ This report strongly supports previous speculations that overheating and the prone position are singly and together strongly associated with an increased risk of SIDS. Until we have further studies refuting this report, it is probably time to recommend a change in our advice to parents and caregivers. Although most child care books recommend not overheating a febrile infant, a strong campaign will be required to reduce the amount of bedding. If the prone position and overheating are related to SIDS, what is the mechanism of the death? Should the United States Surgeon General order a change in practice? We await further data.— M.H. Klaus, M.D.

Cancer Risk Among Children of Atomic Bomb Survivors: A Review of RERF Epidemiologic Studies
Yoshimoto Y (Radiation Effects Research Found, Hiroshima)
JAMA 264:596–600, 1990   18–9

To the present, microcephaly among in-utero-exposed children of atomic bomb (A-bomb) survivors is the only teratogenic effect of ionizing radiation exposure observed in human beings. Recently, an increased prevalence of mental retardation related to A-bomb radiation exposure during weeks 8 through 15 of gestation was confirmed. Because somatic and germinal mutations are considered to promote cancer through many mechanisms, possible radiation-induced, somatic mutations in A-bomb survivors could increase their cancer risk compared. The Radiation Effects Research Foundation (RERF) investigated the possible genetic effects of biochemical mutations, cytogenetic abnormalities, untoward pregnancy outcomes, and survival of children born to A-bomb survivors, but no significant genetic effects were found.

Epidemiologic studies of cancer risk in children of atomic bomb survivors were carried out by the RERF. The children included 2 groups: (1) the in-utero-exposed children, (e.g., those born to mothers who were pregnant at the time of the bombing of Hiroshima and Nagasaki), and (2) the F_1 population that was conceived after the bombing and born to parents of whom 1 or both were atomic bomb survivors.

Even though from 1950 to 1984 only 18 cancer cases were confirmed among the in utero sample, the cancer risk appeared to increase significantly as maternal uterine dose increased. In the F_1 population, from May 1946 through December 1982, 43 cancer patients younger than 20 years were seen. In this group, cancer risk did not seem to increase significantly as parental gonadal dose increased. Follow-up of this population will continue to determine whether the patterns of adult-onset cancer have changed.

▶ Contributing her insights is Susan K. Cummins, M.D., Ph.D., Public Health Medical Officer, California Department of Health Services, Environmental, Epidemiology, and Toxicology Branch:

▶ This study estimates cancer risk in children exposed to atomic radiation from the bombing of Hiroshima and Nagaski. The author reports the cumulative cancer risk in 2 exposed groups: children exposed in utero and children conceived after the bombings to parent(s) who were exposed (the F_1 population). Although the in-utero-exposed group was small, 920 persons, a statistically significant excess cancer risk was identified in this group. Those with in utero exposure were 3.77 times more likely to have cancer than the unexposed comparison group. This group has not yet reached old age when cancer is most likely to occur, and their risk for cancer may continue to increase. The cancer risk in the F_1 population was the same as in the unexposed population.

This study supports the increasing body of evidence indicating an increased risk for cancer from in utero radiation exposure, but the results are limited by the small number of exposed subjects. Because only 13 cases of cancer occurred among the 920 in-utero-exposed subjects, no cancer site-specific analyses could be performed. As this cohort ages and more cancer develops, future analyses will be able to explore site-specific radiation effects.

Surprisingly, although the F_1 population was much larger (31,150 persons) no excess risk was identified in this group. As the author suggests, this may be because any excess cancer risk occurring in the F_1 population is extremely low and may not be identified with a cohort of this size. However, the data also suggest an alternative explanation. In contrast to the subgroups with lower levels of exposure, the cancer rate in the F_1 subgroup with very high parental exposure was 1.4 times that of the unexposed group. In the F_1 population, excess cancer may not result until a threshold of radiation exposure was reached by F_1 parent(s).

This is a remarkable study. Establishing a cohort in the chaos following wartime atomic explosions and tracking this cohort throughout their lifetime is difficult at best. The efforts of this investigator and others to identify the long-term health effects of radiation exposure during the Hiroshima and Nagasaki bombings have contributed to our understanding of the consequences of atomic radiation.—S.K. Cummins, M.D., Ph.D.

Supplemental Reading List

1. Abel Smith AE, Knight-Jones EB: The abilities of very low-birthweight children and their classroom controls. *Dev Med Child Neurol* 32:590–601, 1990.
2. Amato M, Howald H, Schneider H: Neurosonographic assessment of twin pairs in the perinatal period. *Eur Neurol* 30:9, 1990.
3. Baker SS, Baker RD, Cambell C: Short-term malnutrition in neonatal rabbits: Effect on function and synthesis of free radical metabolizing enzymes in the gastrointestinal tract. *J Pediatr Gastroenterol Nutr* 11:247–253, 1990.
4. Ben-Amitai D, Livshits G, Levi I, et al: The relative contribution of birth weight and gestational age on physical traits of newborn infants. *Early Hum Dev* 22:131–144, 1990.
5. Benacerraf BR, Saltzman DH, Estroff JA, et al: Abnormal karyotype of fetuses with omphalocele: Prediction based on omphalocele contents. *Obstet Gynecol* 75:317, 1990.
6. Bhatia P, Johnson KJ, Bell EF: Variability of abdominal circumference of premature infants. *J Pediatr Surg* 25:543–544, 1990.
7. Bignall S, Bailey PC, Bass CA, et al: The cardiovascular and oncotic effects of albumin infusion in premature infants. *Early Hum Dev* 20:191–201, 1989.
8. Bu'Lock R, Woolridge MW, Baum JD: Development of co-ordination of sucking, swallowing and breathing: Ultrasound study of term and preterm infants. *Dev Med Child Neurol* 32:669–678, 1990.
9. Burrows RF, Kelton JG: Low fetal risks in pregnancies associated with idiopathic thrombocytopenic purpura. *Am J Obstet Gynecol* 163:1147, 1990.
10. Calzolari E, Manservigi D, Garani GP, et al: Limb reduction defects in Emilia Romagna, Italy: Epidemiological and genetic study in 173 109 consecutive births. *J Med Genet* 27:353–357, 1990.
11. Chevaloer JY, Durandy Y, Batisse A, et al: Preliminary report: Extracorporeal lung support for neonatal acute respiratory failure. *Lancet* 335:1364, 1990.
12. Christenson RD: Hematopoiesis in the Fetus and Neonate, *Pediatr Res* 26:531, 1989.
13. Cohen HL, Haller JO, Pollack A: Ultrasound of the septum pellucidum: Recognition of evolving fenestrations in the hydrocephalic infant. *J Ultrasound Med* 9:377–383, 1990.
14. Crombleholme TM, Adzick NS, Longaker MT, et al: Reduced-size lung transplantation in neonatal swine: Technique and short-term physiological response. *Ann Thorac Surg* 49:55–60, 1990.
15. Crombleholme TM, Adzick NS, Hardy K, et al: Pulmonary lobar transplantation in neonatal swine: A model for treatment of congenital diaphramatic hernia. *J Pediatr Surg* 25:11–18, 1990.
16. Cussen L, Scurry J, Mitopoulos G et al: Mean organ weights of an Australian population of fetuses and infants. *J Paediar Child Health* 26:101, 1990.
17. Delight E, Goodall J: Love and Loss: Conversations With Parents of Babies With Spina Bifida Managed Without Surgery, 1971–1981, London, McKeith Press, 1990.
18. De Curtis M, Kempson C, Ventura V, et al: The relationship between fecal fat and water in very-low-birth-weight infants. *J Pediatr Gastroenterol Nutr* 11:63–65, 1990.
19. Eg-Andersen G, Pryds O, Zetterstrom R (eds): *Perspectives of Neonatology, Acta Pediatr Scand* (suppl 360), 1989.
20. Galdes-Sebaldt M, Sheller JR, Grogaard J, et al: Prematurity is associated with abnormal airway function in childhood. *Pediatr Pulmonol* 7:259–264, 1989.
21. Harger JH, Hsing AW, Tuomala RD, et al: Risk factors for premature rupture of fetal membranes: A multicenter case-control study. *Am J Obstet Gynecol* 163:130–137, 1990
22. Harrison MR, Adzick AS, Jennings RW, et al: Antenatal intervention for congenital cystic adenomatoid malformation. *Lancet* 336:985, 1990.
23. Heij HA, Ekkelkamp S: Diagnosis of congenital cystic adenomatoid malformation of the lung in newborn infants and children. *Thorax* 34:122–125, 1990.

24. Johnson AM, Palomaki GE, Haddow JE: Maternal serum fetoprotein levels in pregnancies among black and white women with fetal open spina bifida: A United States Collaborative Study, *Am J Obstet Gynecol* 162:328, 1990.

25. Kirkup W, Welch G: Normal but dead: Perinatal mortality in non-malformed babies of birthweight 2-5 kg and over in the Northern Region in 1983. *Br J Obstet Gynaecol* 97:381–392, 1990.

26. Lesko SM, Epstein MF, Mitchell AA: Recent patterns of drug use in newborn intensive care. *J Pediatr* 116:985–990, 1990.

27. McCleod RE Jr: Introduction. *J Pediatr* 117:51–544, 1990.

28. Merlob P, Aitkin I: Time trends (1980–1987) of ten selected informative morphogenetic variants in a newborn population. *Clin Genet* 38:33–37, 1990.

29. Michaelson KF, Skafte L, Badsberg JH, et al: Variation in macronutrients in human bank milk: Influencing factors and implications for human milk banking. *J Pediatr Gastroenterol Nutr* 11:229–239, 1990.

30. Moutet A, Fromont P, Farcet JP, et al: Pregnancy in women with immune thrombocytopenic purpura. *Arch Intern Med.* 150:2141, 1990.

31. Nicolini U, Tannirandorn Y, Gonzalez P, et al: Continuing controversy in alloimmune thrombocytopenia: Fetal hyperimmunoglobulinemia fails to prevent thrombocytopenia. *Am J Obstet Gynecol* 1163:1144, 1990.

32. Palomaki GE, Knight GJ, Holman MS, et al: Maternal serum α-fetoprotein screening for fetal Down syndrome in the United States: Results of a survey. *Am J Obstet Gynecol* 162:317, 1990.

33. Rigal E, Roze JC, Villers D, et al: Prospective evaluation of the protected specimen brush for the diagnosis of pulmonary infections in ventilated newborns. *Pediatr Pulmonol* 8:268, 1990.

34. Rooks JP, Weatherby NL, Ernst EKM, et al: Outcomes of care in birth centers. The national birth center study. *N Engl J Med* 321:1804–1811, 1989.

35. Roy RM, Betheras FR: The Melbourne Chart. A logical guide to neonatal resuscitation. *Anaesth Intens Care* 18:348, 1990.

36. Stahlman MT; Ethical issues in the nursery: Priorities versus limits. *J Pediatr* 115:410, 1989.

37. Thomas DFM: Fetal uropathy. *Br J Urol* 66:225–231, 1990.

38. Vannucci RC: Experimental biology of cerebral hypoxia-ischemia: Relation to perinatal brain damage. *Pediatr Res* 27:317–326, 1990.

39. Vettenranta K, Raivio KO: Xanthine oxidase during human fetal development. *Pediatr Res* 27:286–288, 1990.

40. Wolf B, Heard GS: Screening for biotinidase deficiency in newborns: Worldwide experience. *Pediatrics* 85:512–517, 1990.

41. Yngve D, Gross R: Late diagnosis of hip dislocation in infants. *J Pediatr Orthopaed* 10:777–779, 1990.

Subject Index

R

S

Author Index

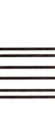

BUSINESS REPLY MAIL

FIRST CLASS   PERMIT No. 135   ST. LOUIS, MO.

POSTAGE WILL BE PAID BY ADDRESSEE

PAT NEWMAN
Mosby-Year Book, Inc.
11830 Westline Industrial Drive
P.O. Box 46908
St. Louis, Missouri 63146-9988

FREE Examination Privileges

Yes! I'd like to review a new Year Book. Please send me a FREE 30-day examination copy of the book(s) checked below:

[ ] Year Book of **Anesthesia**® (22137)	$57.95
[ ] Year Book of **Cardiology**® (22114)	$57.95
[ ] Year Book of **Critical Care Medicine**® (22091)	$54.95
[ ] Year Book of **Dermatology**® (22108)	$57.95
[ ] Year Book of **Diagnostic Radiology**® (22132)	$57.95
[ ] Year Book of **Digestive Diseases**® (22081)	$57.95
[ ] Year Book of **Drug Therapy**® (22139)	$57.95
[ ] Year Book of **Emergency Medicine**® (22085)	$57.95
[ ] Year Book of **Endocrinology**® (22107)	$57.95
[ ] Year Book of **Family Practice**® (20801)	$54.95
[ ] Year Book of **Geriatrics and Gerontology** (22121)	$54.95
[ ] Year Book of **Hand Surgery**® (22096)	$57.95
[ ] Year Book of **Hematology**® (20418)	$54.95
[ ] Year Book of **Health Care Management**® (21145)	$54.95
[ ] Year Book of **Infectious Diseases**® (20420)	$54.95
[ ] Year Book of **Infertility** (20414)	$54.95
[ ] Year Book of **Medicine**® (22087)	$57.95
[ ] Year Book of **Neonatal-Perinatal Medicine** (22117)	$54.95
[ ] Year Book of **Neurology and Neurosurgery**® (22120)	$57.95
[ ] Year Book of **Nuclear Medicine**® (22140)	$57.95
[ ] Year Book of **Obstetrics and Gynecology**® (22118)	$57.95
[ ] Year Book of **Occupational and Environmental Medicine** (22092)	$57.95
[ ] Year Book of **Oncology** (20415)	$54.95
[ ] Year Book of **Ophthalmology**® (22135)	$57.95
[ ] Year Book of **Orthopedics**® (20417)	$54.95
[ ] Year Book of **Otolaryngology – Head and Neck Surgery**® (22086)	$57.95
[ ] Year Book of **Pathology and Clinical Pathology**® (22104)	$57.95
[ ] Year Book of **Pediatrics**® (22088)	$54.95
[ ] Year Book of **Plastic and Reconstructive Surgery**® (22112)	$57.95
[ ] Year Book of **Psychiatry and Applied Mental Health**® (22110)	$57.95
[ ] Year Book of **Pulmonary Disease**® (22109)	$54.95
[ ] Year Book of **Speech Language and Hearing** (21144)	$59.95
[ ] Year Book of **Sports Medicine**® (20419)	$54.95
[ ] Year Book of **Surgery**® (22084)	$57.95
[ ] Year Book of **Ultrasound** (21170)	$75.00
[ ] Year Book of **Urology**® (20416)	$54.95
[ ] Year Book of **Vascular Surgery**® (22105)	$57.95

NAME/ACCT. NO.

ADDRESS

CITY/STATE/ZIP

Mosby-Year Book, Inc. • 11830 Westline Industrial Drive • St. Louis, MO 63146